INSTANT POT COOKBOOK FOR BEGINNERS

~1001~

Quick and Delicious Instant Pot Recipes for the Smart People on a Budget with 1000-Day Meal Plan

JASON WILLIAM

TABLE OF CONTENTS

- **DESCRIPTION** 1
- **INTRODUCTION** 2
- **BREAKFAST** 4
  - Mixed Mushroom Pate 4
  - Black Bean & Egg Casserole 4
  - Chicken Liver Breakfast 4
  - Spice Oatmeal 4
  - Barbeque Tofu 5
  - Instant Pot Cauliflower Soup 5
  - Beef Bourguignon Recipe 5
  - Cinnamon Bars 6
  - Beef Chuck Shoulder Roast Stew 6
  - Turkey Soup 6
  - Keto Vanilla Chia Seeds 7
  - Mushroom Chicken with Eggs 7
  - Beef Kale Patties 7
  - Pork with Mushrooms 8
  - Chicken with Spinach 8
  - Coconut Cherry Pancakes 8
  - Eggs with Mushrooms 9
  - Beef Chili 9
  - Pork Tenderloin Stew 9
  - Lamb Stew 10
  - Deviled Eggs 10
  - Beef Black Pepper Stew 11
  - Beef Stew with Eggplants 11
  - Cinnamon Pancakes 11
  - Chicken Veal Stew 12
  - Eggs with Scallions 12
  - Raspberry Mug Cake 12
  - Almond Porridge 13
  - Bacon Brussels Sprouts 13
  - Mushroom and Eggs Casserole 13
  - Banana Oatmeal 14
  - Easy and Cheesy Grits 14
  - Instant Nutritious Porridge 14
  - Pecan Sweet Potatoes 14
  - Breakfast Quiche 15
  - Mix Beans Rice 15
  - Coco Rice Pudding 15
  - Orange Marmalade Oatmeal 15
  - Eggs with Herbs de Provence 15
  - Cornmeal Porridge 16
  - Broccoli Egg Casserole 16
  - Apricot Cranberry Steel Cut Oats 16
  - Strawberry Compote 16
  - Breakfast Pudding 17
  - Rice Pudding 17
  - Mix Peppers Hash 17
  - Diced Turmeric Eggs 17
  - Veggie Quiche 18
  - Apple and Almond Porridge 18
  - Tomato Poached Eggs 18
  - Smoked Salmon Eggs 19
  - Carrot and Pecan Muffins 19
  - Beef Egg Muffins 19
  - Egg Bake with Carrots 20
  - Veggie and Beef Casserole 20
  - Sausage & Asparagus Dill 20
  - Simple Hardboiled Eggs 21
  - Breakfast Eggs Cheese 21
  - Kale Egg Breakfast Casserole 21
  - Easy Breakfast Casserole 22
  - Tomato Dill Frittata 22
  - Korean Steamed Eggs 22
  - Egg & Ham Casserole 23
  - Spicy Gluten-Free Pancakes 23
  - Cauliflower Pudding 23
  - Sausage and Cauliflower Mash . **Error! Bookmark not defined.**
  - Spinach and Mushroom Frittata**Error! Bookmark not defined.**
  - Egg and Asparagus Frittata **Error! Bookmark not defined.**
  - Vanilla Apple Cinnamon Breakfast Quinoa. **Error! Bookmark not defined.**
  - Apple Cinnamon Oatmeal Cups**Error! Bookmark not defined.**
  - Lentil Bolognese . **Error! Bookmark not defined.**
  - 20 Minute Jacket Potato ..... **Error! Bookmark not defined.**
  - Kielbasa with Sauerkraut and Potatoes .... **Error! Bookmark not defined.**
  - Macaroni and Cheese .... **Error! Bookmark not defined.**
  - Cheesy Chili Mac **Error! Bookmark not defined.**
  - Baked Blueberry Oatmeal 23
  - Poblano Cheese Frittata 24
  - Regular Oatmeal 24
  - Buckwheat Porridge 24
  - Crustless Tomato Spinach Quiche 25
  - Cheesy Instant Pot Goulash 25
  - Breakfast Burrito Casserole**Error! Bookmark not defined.**
- **MAINS** 26
  - Rice With Chicken And Veggies 26
  - Tomato Cream 26
  - Carrot Soup 26
  - Simple Chili 26
  - Lentils Soup 27
  - Easy Chicken Cacciatore 27
  - Sweet Paprika Pork Chops 27
  - Simple Pork Roast 28
  - Broccoli Cream 28
  - Coconut Chicken Mix 28
  - Fish Soup 28

Table Of Contents

- Italian Shrimp Mix 29
- Lemon Shrimp 29
- Cabbage And Beef Stew 29
- Shrimp And Tomatoes Mix 29
- Mackerel And Orange Sauce 30
- Fish Curry 30
- Salmon, Peas And Parsley Dressing 30
- Chili Salmon 30
- Tomato Shrimp 31
- Shrimp, Tomatoes And Potatoes 31
- Sausage And Beans Mix 31
- Duck And Veggies 31
- Duck, Carrots And Cucumbers 32
- Chinese Chicken 32
- Mexican Pork and Okra Salad 32
- Pork and Kale Meatballs 32
- Pork and Baby Spinach ...... **Error! Bookmark not defined.**
- Cinnamon Turkey Curry .... **Error! Bookmark not defined.**
- Basil Shrimp and Eggplants**Error! Bookmark not defined.**
- Mushroom and Chicken Soup ..**Error! Bookmark not defined.**
- Cod and Tomato Passata ... **Error! Bookmark not defined.**
- Chicken and Mustard Sauce**Error! Bookmark not defined.**
- Chicken and Avocado Mix **Error! Bookmark not defined.**
- Tomato and Pork Soup 33
- Cayenne Pork and Artichokes Stew 33
- Green Beans Soup 33
- Broccoli and Zucchini Soup 33
- Beef Soup 34
- Curry Tomato Cream 34
- Spinach Soup 34
- Cabbage Soup 34
- Cheesy Coconut Cream 34
- Eggplant Soup 35
- Sides 35
- Tomatoes and Cauliflower Mix 35
- Green Beans and Herbs 35
- Cauliflower Rice and Olives 36
- Rosemary Cauliflower 36
- Lemon Artichokes 36
- Celery and Broccoli Mix 36
- Zucchini Mix 36
- Dill Fennel Mix 37
- Mushrooms and Endives Mix 37
- Walnuts Green Beans and Avocado 37
- Thyme Brussels Sprouts 37
- Chives Broccoli Mash 37
- Creamy Endives 38
- Spinach and Kale Mix 38
- Thyme Tomatoes 38
- Lemon Brussels Sprouts and Tomatoes 38
- Creamy Fennel 39
- Saffron Bell Peppers 39
- Cabbage and Peppers 39
- Green Beans and Kale .... **Error! Bookmark not defined.**

SEAFOOD **40**
- Spicy Oyster Stew 40
- Tasty Monkfish Stew 40
- Carp Steaks with Aioli 40
- Lobster with Lime Cream 41
- Fast Ahi Tuna Salad 41
- Beer-Braised Alaskan Cod 41
- Favorite Fish Chili 42
- Stuffed Peppers with Haddock and Cheese 42
- Simple Swai with Wine Sauce 42
- Classic Garam Masala Fish 43
- Winter Tuna Salad 43
- Asian-Style Snapper Soup 43
- Trout Frittata with Cheese 44
- Prawn Salad in Mushroom "Buns" 44
- Creamy and Lemony Tuna Fillets 44
- Rainbow Trout with Buttery Veggies 45
- Easy Creole Sea Scallops 45
- Zucchini Stuffed with Tuna and Parmesan 45
- Norwegian Salmon Steaks with Garlic Yogurt ... 46
- Hot Chanterelles and Scampi Boil 46
- Refreshing Seafood Bowl 46
- Traditional Tiger Prawns with Butter Sauce 47
- Simple Party Seafood Dip 47
- Red Curry Perch Fillets 47
- Milky Mackerel Soup 48

BLUEFISH IN SPECIAL SAUCE **48**
- Grouper with Cremini Mushrooms and Sausage 48
- Easy King Crab with Mushrooms 48
- Seafood Jambalaya 49
- Shrimp Creole 49
- Salmon Casserole 50
- Tuna Chowder 50
- Salmon Soup 50
- Salmon Curry 51
- Salmon F4illets 51
- Spicy Salmon Meal**Error! Bookmark not defined.**
- Cheese Salmon .... **Error! Bookmark not defined.**
- Tangy Mahi-Mahi**Error! Bookmark not defined.**
- Mahi-Mahi with Tomatoes. **Error! Bookmark not defined.**
- Cod Platter .... **Error! Bookmark not defined.**
- Ready-to-Eat Dinner Mussels ...**Error! Bookmark not defined.**
- Butter-Dipped Lobsters 52
- Fish Curry Delight 52

~ III ~

Table Of Contents

Shrimp and Beans Mix........**Error! Bookmark not defined.**
Shrimp Curry.. 52
Seafood Gumbo 53
Saffron Chili Cod.. 53
Salmon and Endives... 53
Chili Tuna... 53
Mackerel and Shrimp Mix.. 54
Mackerel and Basil Sauce 54
Oregano Tuna... 54
Creamy Shrimp and Radish Mix 54
Marjoram Tuna... 55
Bacon Trout Mix 55
Tuna and Fennel Mix.. 55
Tilapia Salad... 55
Salmon and Dill Sauce 56
Tilapia and Olives Salsa 56
Catfish and Avocado Mix 56
Tilapia and Capers Mix 56
Glazed Salmon 57
Spicy Tilapia and Kale 57
Lime Glazed Salmon.. 57
POULTRY 58
Lemongrass Turkey.. 58
Cilantro Stuffed Chicken Breast 58
Turkey Bites and Mustard Sauce 58
Orange and Oregano Chicken....................................... 58
Cinnamon and Turmeric Chicken 59
Sweet Basil and Paprika Chicken 59
Thai Chili Chicken.. 59
Cumin and Cardamom Turkey...................................... 60
Turkey and Eggplant Mix... 60
Salsa Chicken Burrito Bowls.. 60
Mediterranean Chicken Orzo 60
Honey Garlic Chicken 61
Kun Pao Chicken.. 61
Buttery Lemon Chicken 61
Taco Ranch Chicken Chili 62
Korean Chicken Meatballs 62
Ground Turkey Lentil Chili 62
Honey Sesame Chicken.. 63
Green Chili Chicken Enchilada Soup 63
Root Beer Chicken Wings 64
Garlic Sesame Chicken... 64
BBQ Chicken with Potatoes... 64
Apple Balsamic Chicken 65
Butter Chicken 65
Chicken Corn Chowder 65
Chicken Tikka Masala.. 66
White Chicken Chili 66
Chicken Cacciatore... 67
Spicy Chicken... 67
Chicken and Grape Tomatoes 67
Chicken Dumplings 68
Chicken Tacos.. 68
BBQ Chicken Wings 68
Classic Turkey Cheese Gnocchi................................... 69
Turkey Stuffed Tacos 69
Rich taste Kung Pao Turkey... 69
Chicken Garlic .... **Error! Bookmark not defined.**
Chicken Recipe with Coca cola **Error! Bookmark not defined.**
Turkey and Smoked Paprika**Error! Bookmark not defined.**
Quick Dumplings**Error! Bookmark not defined.**
Easy Turkey Chili**Error! Bookmark not defined.**
Barbeque Honey Chicken ..**Error! Bookmark not defined.**
Crispy Chicken.... **Error! Bookmark not defined.**
Cheering Chicken Wings .... **Error! Bookmark not defined.**
Turkey with Garlic Herb Sauce.................................... 70
Braised Duck and Potatoes Recipe............................... 70
Taco Bowls 70
Stuffed Chicken Breast 71
Scampi Chicken 71
Potatoes with BBQ Chicken... 71
Chicken Curry with Honey 72
Delicious Chicken Sandwiches 72
Chicken Noodle Pho Recipe 72
Special Turkey Meatballs 73
Crack Chicken Recipe 73
Green Chilli Adobo Chicken 73
Chicken Curry with Honey 74
Chicken Bowl with Smoked Paprika 74
Chicken Dumplings.. 75
Sesame Chicken Teriyaki... 75
Chicken with Lettuce Wrap 75
Chicken with Black Beans.. 76
Steamed Garlic Chicken Breasts 76
Chicken with Cashew Butter 77
Lime Chicken with chillies 77
Instant Tso's Chicken .... **Error! Bookmark not defined.**
MEAT 78
Easy Caribbean Beef.. 78
Marjoram Leg of Lamb 78
Tomato Brisket 78
Dijon Meatloaf 79
Pork Chops with Brussel Sprouts 79
Shredded Chipotle Pork 79
Flavorful Braised Chuck 80
Balsamic Beef Roast 80
Lamb with Tomatoes and Zucchini 80
Basil Beef with Yams 80
Coconut Oil Pork Chops 81
Cinnamon and Orange Pork Shoulder.......................... 81
Beef Ribs with Button Mushrooms.............................. 82

Table Of Contents

Chili Braised Lamb Chops 82
Pork with Rutabaga and Apples 82
Instant Pot Italian Beef 82
Instant Pot Beef and Sweet Potato Stew 83
Healthy Instant Pot Ground Beef Jalapeno Stew 83
Tasty Pork Loin with Goat-Cheese Sauce 84
Traditional Pork Chili 84
Winter Pork and Bacon Soup 84
Burrito Bowl with Pork 85
Pork Shank with Cauliflower 85
Asian-Style Sirloin Pork Roast 86
Pork Sausages Peperonata Style 86
Mexican Style Pork Steaks 86
Cheesy Meatloaf with Bacon 87
B.B.B - Baby Back Ribs 87
Sticky Pork Spare Ribs 87
Yummy Stuffed Meatballs 88
Traditional Pork Roast 88
Pork Soup with Tortilla 88
Pork Shoulder with Herb Dijon Sauce 89
Traditional Pork Taco Bowl 89
Hearty Country-Style Pork Loin Ribs 89
Indian-Style Pork Vindaloo 90
Thai Pork Salad 90
Smoky Pork Ribs 90
Easy Pork Taco Frittata 91
Ruby Port-Braised Pork 91
Buffalo Pork Chowder 91
Greek-Style Pork Cutlets 92
Mediterranean Youvarlakia **Error! Bookmark not defined.**
Keto Lasagna .... **Error! Bookmark not defined.**
Traditional AlbóndigasSinaloenses .... **Error! Bookmark not defined.**
Italian Pork Tenderloin ...... **Error! Bookmark not defined.**
Beef and Cabbage Stew ...... **Error! Bookmark not defined.**
Pepperoni Pizza Bake .... **Error! Bookmark not defined.**
Winter Peasant Chowder ... **Error! Bookmark not defined.**
Italian Squash with Meat Sauce.**Error! Bookmark not defined.**
Traditional Kielbasa with Squash 92
Rich Beef, Bacon and Spinach Chili 93
Juicy Steak with Rainbow Noodles 93
Zettuccini with Pepperoni and Romano Sauce .. 93
Tasty Bottom Eye Roast in Hoisin Sauce 93
Winter Gulasch 94
Winter Beef Chowder 94
Italian-Style Beef Stew 95
Leberkäse with Sauerkraut 95
Holiday Bacon Meatloaf 95
Grandma's Cheeseburger Soup 96
Best Burgers with Kale and Cheese 96
Modern Beef Stroganoff 96
Hot Broccoli, Leek and Beef Chowder 97
Stew with Smoked Cheddar Cheese and Red Wine 97
Filet Mignon in Beer Sauce 97
French-Style Beef Shanks 98
Greek-Style Beef Curry 98
Beef Short Ribs with Cilantro Cream 98
Mexican Green Rice 99
New Orleans-Style Red Beans and Rice .... **Error! Bookmark not defined.**
13 Bean Soup ...... **Error! Bookmark not defined.**
Baked Beans .... **Error! Bookmark not defined.**
Red Beans and Rice .... **Error! Bookmark not defined.**
Rice Pudding .... **Error! Bookmark not defined.**
Mexican Rice and Beans ..... **Error! Bookmark not defined.**
Pinto Beans and Ham Hocks .... **Error! Bookmark not defined.**
Spanish Rice with Black Beans and Potatoes**Error! Bookmark not defined.**
Chicken & Rice ... **Error! Bookmark not defined.**
Pinto Beans .... **Error! Bookmark not defined.**
Cinnamon Brown Rice Pudding**Error! Bookmark not defined.**
Black Beans .... **Error! Bookmark not defined.**
Red Beans and Rice .... **Error! Bookmark not defined.**
Beans and Franks **Error! Bookmark not defined.**
Cilantro Lime Rice**Error! Bookmark not defined.**
Quinoa Black Bean Salad ... **Error! Bookmark not defined.**
Black Bean Soup. **Error! Bookmark not defined.**
VEGETABLES 100
Mashed Chili Carrots 100
Tasty Pepper Salad 100
Instant Pot Coconut Cabbage 100
Instant Pot Garlicky Mashed Potatoes 101
Instant Pot Ratatouille 101
Arugula, Orange &Kamut Salad 101
Sage-Infused Butternut Squash Zucchini Noodles 101
Cauliflower Tikka Masala 102
Barbecue Jackfruit 102
Cauliflower Risotto 103
Mexican-Inspired Posole 103
Mushroom Stir-Fry 104
Mashed Cauliflower with Spinach 104
Pesto Farfale 104
Spinach and Mushroom Risotto 104
Stuffed Eggplant 105

Table Of Contents

Veggie Patties 105
Leafy Risotto 105
Spaghetti "Bolognese" 106
Bean and Rice Bake 106
Broccoli & Tofu in a Tamari Sauce 106
Carrot and Sweet Potato Medley 107
Fruity Wild Rice Casserole with Almonds 107
Basil Risotto 107
Wheat Berries with Tomatoes 108
Black Bean Hash 108
Green Beans and Beets 108
Brussels Sprouts and Garlic 108
Bell Peppers and Rice 109
Garlic Peppers Mix 109
Bell Peppers and Pine Nuts 109
Bacon and Mustard Bell Peppers 109
Beets and Parmesan 109
Potatoes and Cheddar 109
Creamy Beets .... **Error! Bookmark not defined.**
Garlic Celeriac ..... **Error! Bookmark not defined.**
Creamy Zucchini **Error! Bookmark not defined.**
Spicy Zucchinis ... **Error! Bookmark not defined.**
Celery Sauté .... **Error! Bookmark not defined.**
Micro Greens Sauté .... **Error! Bookmark not defined.**
Dill Okra Mix ...... **Error! Bookmark not defined.**
Balsamic Cauliflower .... **Error! Bookmark not defined.**
Cauliflower and Collard Greens 110
Balsamic Collard Greens 110
Collard Greens and Apples Mix 110
Dill Endives and Chives 110
Nutmeg Endives 110
Wine-glazed Mushrooms 111
Steamed Artichoke 111
Green Beans with Tomatoes 111
Avocado Quinoa Salad 112
Pepper Salad 112
Asparagus Sticks 112
Instant Mashed Potato 113
Chickpea Hummus 113
Potato & Cauliflower Mash 113
Green Beans Salad 114
Tasty Corn Cobs 114
Vegetable Chickpea Salad ... **Error! Bookmark not defined.**
Boiled Bok Choy **Error! Bookmark not defined.**
Garlic with White Beets ...... **Error! Bookmark not defined.**
Italian Potato Salad .... **Error! Bookmark not defined.**
Cabbage with Bacon .... **Error! Bookmark not defined.**
Fresh Red Beets 114
Juicy Quinoa Olives 114
Cheese-filled Sweet Potatoes **Error! Bookmark not defined.**
Mayo Mushroom Salad .... **Error! Bookmark not defined.**

SOUPS AND STEWS 116
Tomato Soup 116
Potato and Corn Soup 116
Chicken and Kale Soup 116
Green Bean Soup 117
Pork and Cabbage Soup 117
Chicken and Mushroom Stew 117
Beef and Veggie Stew 118
Mixed Veggie Stew 118
Beef with Beans Chili 119
Three Beans Mix Chili 119
Full Meal Turkey Soup 120
Gourmet Mexican Beef Soup 120
Beef Soup 120
Bacon and Veggie Soup 121
Broccoli Soup 121
Spicy Parsnip Soup 121
Mexican-Style Chicken Soup 122
Traditional Bolognese Sauce 122
Ramen Spicy Soup with Collard Greens 122
Spicy Borscht Soup 123
Vichyssoise with Tofu 123
Hearty Winter Vegetable Soup 123
Leek and Potato Soup with Sour Cream 124
Two-Bean Zucchini Soup 124
Quick Chicken Rice Soup 124
Tomato & Rice Soup 124
Butternut Squash Curry 124
Creamy Quinoa and Mushroom Pilaf 125
Favorite Chicken Soup 125
Spicy Pork Soup 125
Garlic Pork Chop Soup ...... **Error! Bookmark not defined.**
Broccoli and Carrot Chowder .. **Error! Bookmark not defined.**

SNACKS AND APPETIZERS 126
Italian Mussels Appetizer 126
Spicy Italian Mussels 126
Seafood Platter 126
Spanish Clams Appetizer 126
Cheesy Clams 127
Artichokes Dip 127
Artichoke Appetizer 127
Wrapped Asparagus 127
Italian Sweet Potato And Lentils Dip 128
Apple Dip 128
Orange Cranberry Dip 128
Ginger And Onions Dip 128
Zucchini Dip 128

Table Of Contents

Garlic Mushroom Dip 129
Cauliflower Hummus 129
Turkey Meatballs 129
Chicken Meatballs 129
Pork Meatballs Appetizer 130
Chickpeas Spread 130
Apricot Dip 130
Whole Wheat Salad 130
Asian Sprouts Salad 131
Okra Salad 131
Leek Sticks 131
Balsamic Cabbage Appetizer Salad 131
Bell Pepper Dip 132
Chicken Appetizer Salad 132
Spinach Puffs 132
Basil Zucchini and Capers Dip 132
Lime Spinach and Leeks Dip 133
Chili Tomato and Zucchini Dip 133
Parmesan Mushroom Spread 133
Broccoli Dip 133
Ginger Cauliflower Spread 134
Radish Salsa 134
Mustard Greens Dip 134
Spinach and Artichokes Spread 134
Artichokes and Salmon Bowls 135
Salmon and Cod Cakes 135
Green Beans and Cod Salad 135
Shrimp and Leeks Platter 135
Balsamic Mussels Bowls 136
Tomato and Zucchini Salsa 136
Sweet Shrimp Bowls 136
Parsley Clams Platter 136
Zucchinis and Walnuts Salsa 136
Shrimp and Beef Bowls 137
Coconut Shrimp Platter 137
Marinated Shrimp 137
Eggplant and Spinach Dip 137
Balsamic Endives 138
Italian Asparagus 138
Fennel and Leeks Platter 138
Nutmeg Endives 138
Thyme Eggplants and 0Celery Spread .... **Error! Bookmark not defined.**
Shrimp and Okra Bowls ..... **Error! Bookmark not defined.**
Mushrooms Salsa **Error! Bookmark not defined.**
DESSERTS **139**
Coconut Cake 139
Yogurt Vanilla Lighter Cheesecake 139
Molten Lava Cake 139
Stuffed Peaches 140
Blueberry Jam 140
Vanilla Rice Pudding 140
Pressure Cooked Brownies 140

Almond Tapioca Pudding 141
Blondies with Peanut Butter 141
Gingery Applesauce 141
Peach Crumb 141
Pear Ricotta Cake 142
Lemon and Blackberry Compote 142
Poached Gingery Orange Pears 142
Caramel Flan 143
Strawberry Cream 143
Berry Compote 143
Creamy Coconut Peach Dessert 144
Banana and Almond Butter Bars 144
Fruity Sauce with Apples 144
Wine-Glazed Apples 144
Brown Fudge Cake 145
Chocolate Cheesecake 145
Maple-Glazed Flan 145
Almond Cheesecake 146
Crème Brûlée 146
Nutmeg Apple Crisp 146
Chocolate Crème Brûlée 147
Blueberry Cheesecake 147
Tapioca Pudding 147
Cherry Cheesecake 148
Lavender Crème Brûlée 148
Pumpkin Bundt Cake 148
Cinnamon Applesauce 149
Apple Bread Pudding 149
Orange Cheesecake 150
Banana Chocolate Chip Cake 150
Lemon Cheesecake 150
Rum Cheesecake 151
Vanilla Chocolate Brownies 151
Keto Coconut Bars 152
Keto Pecan Brownies 152
Choco Cinnamon Cake 153
Keto Mocha Brownies 153
Chocolate Cupcakes 153
Coconut Cohoco Brownies 154
Raspberry Muffins with Chocolate Topping 154
Matcha Cheesecake 155
Keto Mint Cake 155
Lemon Cake 156
Sweet Potato & Cinnamon Patties 156
Chocolate Chip Pudding 156
Choco Orange Muffins 157
Keto Gluten-Free Coconut Almond Cake ... 157
Choco Vanilla Pudding 157
Keto Orange Nut Cookies 158
Vanilla Cream with Raspberries **Error! Bookmark not defined.**
Chocolate Chips and Vanilla Cake .... **Error! Bookmark not defined.**
FAVORITES **159**

Table Of Contents

Family-Style Canapés 159
Yummy Egg Salad "Sandwich" 159
Beef Taco Wraps 159
Holiday Fish Sandwiches 159
Keto Muffins 160
Bacon Biscuits with Cheese 160
Special Chicken Liver Mousse 160
Chicken Legs with Spicy Mayo Sauce 161
Herbes de Provence Chicken Drumettes 161
Aromatic Chicken Chowder 161
Chicken Tacos 162
Traditional Chicken Stew 162
Chicken Teriyaki 163
Simple Chicken Carnitas 163
The Best Turkey Legs 163
Old-Fashioned Paprikash 164
Chicken Fillets with Cheese and Cream 164
Yummy Chicken Drumsticks 164
Special Beef Salad 165
Cozy Beef Soup 165
Mexican-Style Beef Chili 166
Hot and Spicy Beef Curry 166
Tender Beef Shoulder Roast**Error! Bookmark not defined.**
Special Beef Shawarma Bowls .. **Error! Bookmark not defined.**
Holiday Pork Chops with Squash Salad .... **Error! Bookmark not defined.**
1000-DAY MEAL 167
CONCLUSION 190

DESCRIPTION

An Instant pot is just a single appliance with multifunctional features. It can perform the task of the steamer, electric pressure cooker, warming pot and rice cooker. It speeds up the cooking process by using 70 percent less of energy. And now many manufacturers have ventured into the production of this appliance, which is smart, time-saving and is used by millions of people around the world. So if you are a type with a very tight work schedule, then this appliance is the right choice for you. The instant pot uses a pattern of cooking meals in a vessel that is sealed properly, holding the steam inside the pot below a pre-set pressure. As the water boiling point increases, so does the pressure increase as well. The built-up pressure allows the temperature to rise as well, thus making the cooking process quicker.

The instant pot cooking technique is best suitable to people who would rather prefer a time saving meal, as it's quicker and saves a lot of time, making the preparation of a low carb meal less cumbersome. But there are things you will need to know before you start using the instant pot, it is important to know the essentials like, how to release the steam and the function of the buttons.

Identifying a good instant pot has been one of the challenges many people have faced in the course of carrying out the low carb diet plan. There are several options available in the market where various manufacturers strive to give you the best quality but in turn makes the buying choices more complicated. It is advisable that you buy the instant pot according to their needs. The function, size, and version should be considered while purchasing the instant pot.

While Instant Pot is very easy to operate, problems may still arise especially if you don't handle it properly. Below you will find some practical safety tips for a comfortable cooking experience.

- You can't use Instant Pot for frying as high-temperature setting may cause the oil to start burning.
- Do not fill Instant Pot with a lot of ingredients as it will leave no space for the pressure to build up. Leave enough room for the air to move inside the pressure cooker.
- When using the quick pressure release, make sure that the valve is not facing in your direction. Beware of the hot steam; it might scald your face and body.

What do you gain from purchasing this book? You will have a detailed instruction guide of 600+ instant pot recipes with nutrition values. Here are the recipe categories covered in this guide.

- Breakfast
- Mains
- Sides
- Seafood
- Poultry
- Meat
- Vegetables
- Soups and Stews
- Snacks
- Desserts
- 1000-day meal plan

Make use of your Instant Pot!

INTRODUCTION

You must have heard it over and over that the Instant Pot is fast and very easy to use. It can be automated and makes cooking easy and will give you an awesome cooking experience. However, if you haven't tried it out, you may never find out the truth in these claims.

If you've got your own unit, that's a smart move. If you're still unable to use the appliance, this piece will assist you to do that effortlessly. Some amazing Instant Pot benefits

The list of benefits that you will use an Instant Pot will make up a huge list! Therefore, to keep things short and simple, below are some of the crucial ones that you should know about!

One Pot that does it all
The Instant Pot is designed to be extremely versatile and flexible to use. This single appliance has the capacity to be used as multiple cooking appliances, which not only saves your money but also your time as well! This is pretty much the "One Pot to Rule Them All"

Defrost-Be Gone

The Instant Pot is one of that rare appliances that actually allows you to directly cook frozen meals, saving a lot of time. The pressure method can easily defrost and tenderize frozen meat.

Easy cooking and cleaning
Let me start off with the most obvious one first! The Instant Pot will allow you to cook everything in just a single pot, which essentially means that you will be able to do all of your cooking without making a huge mess in the kitchen. The flawless sealing mechanism of the Instant Pot further helps to keep any kind of odor or debris locked inside the pot and the stainless-steel construction makes it very easy to clean.

Built to last
Since the Instant Pot is basically made Stainless Steel, this is an appliance that is made to last! And as an added bonus, the Stainless-Steel construction does not hamper with the flavors of the meal as well, so you can rest easy knowing that the flavors of your meal are preserved to perfection.

Chemical free Coating
Every single Instant Pot appliance is made following extremely high health standards. Therefore, no chemical coating is used in the interior part of the pot that helps the appliance to stay completely free from harmful chemicals that might otherwise hamper the flavor of your meal and negatively impact your health.

Delayed cooking mechanism
The delayed free cooking mechanism allows food to stay warm and moist as long as they are in the pot. This allows you to serve hot and delicious food, anytime you want, straight out of the pot!

Restaurant Quality Dish at Home
Yes, you read that right! Following the recipes found in this book and using the various functionalities of the Instant Pot, you will actually be able to create premium restaurant quality dishes right at home!

Saves space in Kitchen
The versatility of the Instant Pot and its capacity act as multiple appliances allow you to get rid of the steamer, Sauté pan, slow cooker, pressure cooker and a myriad of different appliances and use the Ninja Foodi for everything.

High-Pressure kills microbes
The excellent way in which the Instant Pot cook, ensure that the temperature inside is able to reach sufficiently high enough levels during pressure cooking to ensure that 99% of harmful microbes are killed during the process. In fact, the Instant Pot is even able to kill significantly more resistant microbes as well.

To keep things short and simple, the Instant Pot is at its core, one of the most advanced Electric Pressure cooker that

Introduction

comes packed with a wide variety of features that makes it one of the most versatile multi-cookers to date.

Here, you will learn the basics of the appliance and the step-by-step approach to cooking tasty meals with this unique cooking appliance.

1. Check the unit: First, unwrap your unit and make sure it meets all that you hoped for.
2. Consider the cleanliness: Check the unit and ensure that both the pot and lid are clean.

For the lid, ensure that the following parts are clean:

- Make sure the sealing ring is clean and properly installed.
- Float Valve is clean and easily goes up and down
- The steam release handle is clean and pointing to the ceiling position.

3. Decide what to cook: Do you have a list of recipes that you want to try out yourself? If yes, that's fine. Otherwise, we have lots of recipes in this book that you can start with.
4. Prepare your recipe ingredients. This, depending on the meal in question, can take minutes to hours to put together.
5. Placing the ingredients into the inner pot: For foods that require sautéing, frying, you need to first sauté the aromatics and meat in hot oil using the sauté function before proceeding with the rest ingredients.
6. However, for those that don't, all you have to do is place the ingredients into the pot and lock/seal the lid.
7. Install the lid and plug the unit: To lock/seal the lid, turn clockwise to the lock position. You can find more in this in the manual that came with your IP.
8. When everything is in place, you can now plug your Instant Pot to an outlet and wait to hear the beeping sound.
9. Select a cooking function as directed by the recipe: After putting the ingredients into the inner pot, lock and plug the unit into an outlet. Next, select a cooking program/function to either cook at high or low pressure, depending on the type of recipe and your preferred cook time.
10. To do this, you have lots of cooking functions which include the steam, soup, stew etc. at your disposal. Use the appropriate function to make the cooking easier for you, although many recipes/cookbooks simply recommend using the manual button in other to be more specific.
11. For more on the IP preset buttons and their functions, hop over to "Instant Pot Preset Button Functions Explained"
12. Releasing Pressure: After pressure cooking your meal for a preset number of minutes/hours, release the pressure from pot using either the natural or quick release method depending on the one directed by the recipe you're making. Serve the meal when you are through.

BREAKFAST

MIXED MUSHROOM PATE
Preparation Time: 25 minutes
Servings: 6
Ingredients:
- 1 lb. button mushrooms sliced
- 1 oz. dry porcini mushrooms
- 1 cup boiled water
- 1 bay leaf
- 1 tbsp. truffle oil
- 3 tbsp. grated parmesan cheese
- 1 tbsp. extra-virgin olive oil
- 1 shallot finely chopped
- 1/4 cup white wine
- 1 tbsp. butter
- Salt and pepper to the taste

Directions:
1. Put dry mushrooms in a bowl, add 1 cup boiling water over them and leave them aside for now.
2. Set your instant pot on sauté mode; add butter and the olive oil and heat them up.
3. Add the shallot; stir and cook for 2 minutes.
4. Add dry mushrooms and their liquid, fresh mushrooms, wine, salt, pepper, and bay leaf.
5. Stir; seal the instant pot lid and cook at High for 16 minutes.
6. Quick release the pressure, discard bay leaf and some of the liquid, transfer everything to your blender and pulse until you obtain a creamy spread
7. Add truffle oil and grated parmesan cheese; blend again, transfer to a bowl and serve.

BLACK BEAN & EGG CASSEROLE
Preparation Time: 30 minutes
Servings: 3
Ingredients:
- 1/2 can black beans; rinsed
- 4 large eggs; well-beaten
- 1/2 lb. mild ground sausage
- 1/4 large red onion; chopped.
- 1/2 red bell pepper; chopped.
- 1/4 cup green onions
- 1/4 cup flour
- 1/2 cup Cotija cheese
- 1/2 cup mozzarella cheese
- sour cream; cilantro to garnish

Directions:
1. Add sausage and onion to Instant Pot and select the *Sauté* function to cook for 3 minutes.
2. Combine flour with eggs and add this mixture to the sausages.
3. Add all the vegetables, cheeses and beans.
4. Secure the lid of instant pot and press *Manual* function key
5. Adjust the time to 20 minutes and cook at high pressure
6. When it beeps; release the pressure naturally and open the instant pot lid
7. Remove the inner pot; place a plate on top then flip the pot to transfer the casserole to the plate, Serve warm

CHICKEN LIVER BREAKFAST
Preparation Time: 20 minutes
Servings: 8
Ingredients:
- 3/4 lb. chicken liver
- 1 tsp. extra virgin olive oil
- 1 yellow onion, roughly chopped
- 1 tbsp. capers, drained and chopped.
- 1 tbsp. butter
- 1 bay leaf
- 1/4 cup red wine
- 2 anchovies
- Salt and black pepper to the taste

Directions:
1. Put the olive oil in your instant pot, add onion, salt, pepper, chicken liver, bay leaf and wine.
2. Stir; seal the instant pot lid and cook at High for 10 minutes.
3. Quick release the pressure, add anchovies, capers, and butter.
4. Stir, transfer to kitchen blender and pulse very well everything
5. Add salt and pepper to the taste, blend again; transfer to a bowl and serve with toasted bread slices

SPICE OATMEAL
Preparation Time: 18 minutes
Servings: 2
Ingredients:
- 1 cup old-fashioned rolled oats
- 1/4 cup grated extra-sharp cheddar
- 1 scallion; chopped.

- 2 cups water
- 1/4 tsp. paprika
- kosher salt and black pepper

Directions:
1. Add all the Ingredients to Instant Pot; except cheese.
2. Secure the lid of instant pot and press *Manual* function key
3. Adjust the time to 3 minutes and cook at high pressure
4. When it beeps; release the pressure naturally and open the instant pot lid. Stir in shredded cheese and serve

BARBEQUE TOFU

Preparation Time: 20 minutes
Servings: 6

Ingredients:
- 28 oz. firm tofu; cubed
- 12 oz. BBQ sauce
- 1 green bell pepper; chopped.
- 2 tbsp. extra virgin olive oil
- 4 garlic cloves; minced.
- 1 red bell pepper; chopped.
- 1 yellow onion; chopped.
- 1 celery stalk; chopped.
- Salt to the taste
- A pinch of curry powder

Directions:
1. Set your instant pot on Sauté mode; add the oil and heat it up
2. Add bell peppers, garlic, onion and celery and stir
3. Add salt and curry powder, stir and cook for 2 minutes
4. Add tofu, stir and cook 4 minutes more
5. Add BBQ sauce; then stir well and seal the instant pot lid and cook at High for 5 minutes
6. Quick release the pressure, open the instant pot lid, transfer to plates and serve

INSTANT POT CAULIFLOWER SOUP

Preparation Time 45 Minutes
Servings: 4

Ingredients:
- 32-ounce chicken stock
- 6 slices turkey bacon; cooked, diced.
- 1 head cauliflower; coarsely chopped.
- 1 green bell pepper; chopped
- 1 large yellow onion; diced.
- 2 cloves garlic; minced
- 1 tablespoon onion powder
- 1 tablespoon olive oil
- Salt; ground black pepper, to taste
- 2 cups cheddar cheese; shredded.
- 1 cup half and half
- 1 tablespoon Dijon mustard
- 4 dashes hot pepper sauce

Directions:
1. Turn on Instant Pot and press *Sauté* button.
2. Add olive oil, onion, and garlic. Cook for about 3 minutes to brown
3. Stir in cauliflower, green bell pepper, onion powder, salt, and pepper
4. Pour in chicken stock, then close and lock the lid.
5. Select *Soup* function and adjust the time to 35 minutes
6. Let the pressure release naturally for 10 minutes and then release any remaining pressure. Unlock and remove the lid
7. Stir in the remaining ingredients. Reselect *Sauté* function, and cook for about 5 minutes until bubbly. Serve hot

Nutrition Value: Calories: 404 ; Total Carbs: 3 g; Net Carbs: 1.4 g; Fat: 21 g; Protein: 47 g

BEEF BOURGUIGNON RECIPE

Preparation Time 55 Minutes
Servings: 5

Ingredients:
For bourguignon:
- 2-pounds beef sirloin; cut into-bite sized pieces
- 1 cup pearl onions; chopped
- 2 cups button mushrooms
- 3 cups beef broth
- 2 tablespoon arrowroot
- 4 bacon slices; chopped
- 1/4 cup balsamic vinegar
- 3 tablespoon butter
- 2 sage sprigs
- 2 thyme sprigs
- 1 teaspoon salt
- 1 teaspoon black pepper

Directions:
- Rinse the meat under cold running water and pat dry with a kitchen paper. Cut into bite-sized pieces and season with some salt and pepper, Set aside.
- Plug in the instant pot and press the *Sauté* button. Add butter to the inner pot and heat up. When melted, add mushrooms and onions. Cook for 10-12 minutes, stirring

constantly
- When done, transfer the mushrooms and onions to a large bowl. Cover with a lid and set aside.
- With the *Sauté* mode on, add bacon. Cook for 2-3 minutes or until crisp. Transfer the bacon to the bowl with mushrooms
- Now pour in the balsamic vinegar and broth. Stir in the arrowroot and add meat. Add the sage and thyme and seal the lid.
- Set the steam release handle to the *Sealing* position and press the *Manual* button. Set the timer for 30 minutes on high pressure
- When you hear the end signal, press the *Cancel* button and release the pressure naturally. Carefully open the lid and stir in the mushroom mixture. Serve it immediately.

Nutrition Value: Calories: 523; Total Fats: 25.5g; Net Carbs: 3.6g; Protein: 64.9g; Fiber: 0.8g

CINNAMON BARS

Preparation Time 25 Minutes
Servings: 2

Ingredients:
- 2 tablespoon coconut oil
- 1 cup unsweetened almond milk
- 1/3 cup pumpkin puree
- 2 tablespoon sesame seeds
- 1 tablespoon almonds; chopped
- 2 large eggs
- 1/3 cup hemp seeds
- 2 tablespoon swerve

Directions:
1. Line a small baking dish with some parchment paper, Set aside.
2. Place coconut oil and swerve in a microwave-safe bowl and microwave for 1 minute. Whisk together and transfer to a deep bowl along with the remaining ingredients.
3. Stir well and transfer to the prepared dish. Loosely cover with aluminum foil and set aside
4. Plug in the instant pot and pour in 1 cup of water in the inner pot. Position the trivet and place the baking dish on top
5. Seal the lid and set the steam release handle to the *Sealing* position. Press the *Manual* button and set the timer for 15 minutes on high pressure
6. When done, perform a quick pressure release by moving the pressure valve to the *Venting* position. Carefully open the lid and remove the dish
7. Chill for a while and cut into 4 bars. Serve it immediately.

Nutrition Value: Calories: 417; Total Fats: 36.7g; Net Carbs: 5g; Protein: 17g; Fiber: 3.9g

BEEF CHUCK SHOULDER ROAST STEW

Preparation Time 50 Minutes
Servings: 6

Ingredients:
For stew:
- 2 -pounds beef chuck shoulder roast; chopped
- 2 -pounds cauliflower; chopped into florets
- 2 tablespoon butter
- 5 cups beef broth
- 2 large onions; finely chopped.
- 3 tablespoon olive oil
- 1 cup cherry tomatoes
- 1 teaspoon smoked paprika
- 1/2 teaspoon garlic powder
- 1 teaspoon sea salt

Directions:
1. Plug in the instant pot and press the *Sauté* button. Grease the stainless steel insert with olive oil and heat up. Add onions and stir-fry until translucent
2. Season the meat with salt and add to the pot. Briefly brown, stirring constantly.
3. Now add tomatoes and pour in the beef broth. Stir well and seal the lid. Set the steam release handle and press the *Manual* button. Set the timer for 30 minutes on high pressure
4. When done; move the pressure valve to the *Venting* position to release the pressure.
5. Carefully, open the lid and add the remaining spices. Stir in the butter and add the chopped cauliflower. Seal the lid again and cook for another 4 minutes on the *Manual* mode
6. When done; release the pressure naturally and open the lid
7. Optionally, stir in one tablespoon of Greek yogurt and serve immediately

Nutrition Value: Calories: 470; Total Fats: 21.7g; Net Carbs: 9.4g; Protein: 53.8g; Fiber: 5.2g

TURKEY SOUP

Preparation Time 50 Minutes
Servings: 3

Ingredients:
For soup:
- 7-ounce turkey breast; chopped into bite-sized pieces

- 4 cups chicken broth
- 1 cup fresh celery leaves; chopped.
- 1/2 cup red bell peppers; finely chopped
- 1/4 teaspoon freshly ground white pepper
- 1 teaspoon salt

Directions:
1. Rinse the meat under cold running water and pat dry with some kitchen paper. Place on a clean work surface and cut into bite-sized pieces. Transfer to the pot along with red bell peppers.
2. Sprinkle with salt and freshly ground white pepper. Securely lock the lid.
3. Set the steam release handle to the *Sealing* position and press the *Manual* button
4. Set the timer for 35 minutes on high pressure
5. When done; release the pressure naturally and open the lid. Stir in the fresh celery and seal the lid again. Let it sit for 10 minutes. Serve it immediately.

Nutrition Value: Calories: 132; Total Fats: 3g; Net Carbs: 5.4g; Protein: 18.2g; Fiber: 1.1g

KETO VANILLA CHIA SEEDS

Preparation Time 15 Minutes
Servings: 2

Ingredients:
- 3 tablespoon chia seeds
- 2 tablespoon coconut oil
- 2 tablespoon Greek yogurt
- 2/3 cup unsweetened almond milk
- 1 teaspoon vanilla extract
- 1 teaspoon swerve
- 1/4 teaspoon salt

Directions:
1. Plug in the instant pot and press the *Sauté* button. Pour in the milk and add chia seeds. Cook for 5 minutes, stirring constantly.
2. Now add coconut oil and sprinkle with swerve, vanilla extract, and salt. Give it a good stir and pour in about 1/4 cup of water
3. Continue to cook for another 3-4 minutes
4. When done, press the *Cancel'* button and stir in Greek yogurt
5. Optionally, top with some fresh strawberries or seeds. Transfer to serving bowls and chill well before serving.

Nutrition Value: Calories: 227; Total Fats: 22.5g; Net Carbs: 2.4g; Protein: 6.1g; Fiber: 7.8g

MUSHROOM CHICKEN WITH EGGS

Preparation Time 40 Minutes
Servings: 2

Ingredients:
- 7-ounce boneless and skinless chicken breast; cut into bite-size pieces
- 1 cup button mushrooms; sliced
- 2 cups chicken stock
- 3 eggs
- 3 tablespoon olive oil
- 2 garlic cloves; crushed
- 2 tablespoon almond flour
- 1 teaspoon cayenne pepper
- 1 teaspoon salt
- 1/4 teaspoon black pepper

Directions:
1. Rinse the meat under cold running water and pat dry with a kitchen paper. Cut into bite-sized pieces and set aside
2. Plug in the instant pot and grease the inner pot with some oil. Add garlic and meat. Season with salt and cook for 3 minutes.
3. Now add mushrooms and continue to cook for 5 minutes.
4. Pour in the chicken stock and give it a good stir. Seal the lid and set the steam release handle to the *Sealing* position. Press the *Manual* button and set the timer for 9 minutes on high pressure
5. When done, perform a quick pressure release and open the lid. Press the *Sauté* button and cook until half of the liquid evaporates.
6. Now stir in the almond flour and sprinkle with cayenne pepper and black pepper. Cook for 5 minutes, stirring constantly
7. Finally, crack the eggs and cook until completely set. Serve it immediately.

Nutrition Value: Calories: 456g; Total Fats: 32.1g; Net Carbs: 3.2g; Protein: 39.4g; Fiber: 0.6g

BEEF KALE PATTIES

Preparation Time 25 Minutes
Servings: 4

Ingredients:
- 1-pound ground beef
- 1 tablespoon olive oil
- 1 large egg; beaten
- 1 cup fresh kale; finely chopped.
- 1 tablespoon almond flour
- 1/2 teaspoon dried rosemary; ground.
- 1/2 teaspoon black pepper; ground.
- 1/2 teaspoon dried oregano; ground.
- 1 teaspoon sea salt

Directions:
1. Rinse well the kale under cold running water using a large colander. Drain and finely chop, Set aside.
2. In a large mixing bowl, combine ground beef, kale, egg, and flour. Mix with your hands until well incorporated. Add flour and all spices. Mix again until smooth mixture. Shape about 8 patties, approximately 2-inch in diameter
3. Grease a fitting springform pan with some olive oil. Add the patties and set aside.
4. Plug in your instant pot and pour 1 cup of water in the stainless steel insert. Position a trivet on the bottom and place the pan on top. Securely lock the lid and adjust the steam release handle. Press the *Manual* button and set the timer for 15 minutes. Cook on *High* pressure
5. When done; perform a quick release of the pressure and open the pot. Remove the pan from the pot using oven mitts. Place on a wire rack and cool completely.
6. Optionally, brown the patties on *Saute* mode for 1 minute on both sides.

Nutrition Value: Calories: 279; Total Fats: 12.7g; Net Carbs: 1.9g; Protein: 36.9g; Fiber: 0.7g

PORK WITH MUSHROOMS
Preparation Time 20 Minutes
Servings: 2
Ingredients:
- 10-ounce pork; minced
- 1 tablespoon Dijon mustard
- 1 tablespoon olive oil
- 1 small zucchini; chopped
- 6-ounce button mushrooms; sliced
- 1 small onion; finely chopped
- 1/4 teaspoon dried basil; ground.
- 1/2 teaspoon black pepper; ground.
- 1/4 teaspoon garlic powder
- 1/2 teaspoon salt

Directions:
1. Plug in your instant pot and add the olive oil in the stainless steel insert. Press the *Saute* button and add onions. Stir-fry for 2-3 minutes and add minced pork. Sprinkle with garlic powder, salt, and pepper. Give it a good stir and cook for 3-4 minutes, or until browned.
2. Add zucchini and mushrooms. Pour 1 cup of water and close the lid. Adjust the steam release handle and press the *Manual* button. Set the timer for 6 minutes and cook on *High* pressure.
3. When you hear the cooker's end signal, perform a quick release of the pressure by turning the valve to the *Venting* position. Open the pot and press the *Saute* button
4. Stir in the Dijon mustard and sprinkle with dried thyme. Transfer to a serving plate

Nutrition Value: Calories: 312; Total Fats: 12.7g; Net Carbs: 6.4g; Protein: 41.3g; Fiber: 2.7g

CHICKEN WITH SPINACH
Preparation Time 50 Minutes
Servings: 3
Ingredients:
- 7 ounce boneless and skinless chicken breast; chopped into bite-sized pieces
- 1 garlic clove; crushed
- 1 cup fresh spinach; chopped
- 1 large leek; finely chopped
- 1 cup cottage cheese
- 3 tablespoon butter
- 1 cup avocado chunks
- 1 small onion, finely chopped
- 1/2 teaspoon dried rosemary
- 1 teaspoon salt

Directions:
1. Plug in the instant pot and press the *Sauté* button. Grease the inner pot with butter and heat up. Add chicken and sprinkle with salt. Cook for 12-15 minutes, stirring occasionally.
2. Now add avocado and continue to cook for 5 minutes. If necessary, add more olive oil
3. Finally, add onions, garlic, and chopped leeks. Give it a good stir and cook until completely soft
4. Add spinach and sprinkle with rosemary. Press the *Cancel* button and cover with the lid. Let it sit for 10 minutes
5. Remove from the pot and transfer to a deep bowl. Stir in the cottage cheese and serve immediately

Nutrition Value: Calories: 382g; Total Fats: 24.5g; Net Carbs: 5.8g; Protein: 31.2g; Fiber: 4g

COCONUT CHERRY PANCAKES
Preparation Time 20 Minutes
Servings: 3
Ingredients:
- 1 tablespoon coconut butter; melted
- 1/2 cup cream cheese; softened

- 1 teaspoon baking powder
- 2 tablespoon coconut milk
- 1 cup almond flour
- 3 large eggs; beaten
- 1/4 teaspoon nutmeg; ground.
- 1 teaspoon powdered stevia
- 1 teaspoon cherry extract

Directions:
1. In a large mixing bowl, combine coconut flour, baking powder, stevia, and nutmeg. Stir well using a kitchen spatula. Now; add eggs, cream cheese, coconut milk, nutmeg and cherry extract. With a whisking attachment on, beat until smooth and creamy
2. Plug in your instant pot and grease the stainless steel insert with coconut butter. Pour about 1/3 of the mixture and securely lock the lid. Adjust the steam release handle and press the *Manual* button. Set the timer for 5 minutes and cook on *High* pressure.
3. When you hear the cooker's end signal, perform a quick release of the pressure by moving the valve to the *Venting* position. Open the pot and repeat the process with the remaining batter.
4. Top with some plain yogurt and sprinkle with some shredded coconut. Serve it immediately.

Nutrition Value: Calories: 350; Total Fats: 31.3g; Net Carbs: 4.2g; Protein: 12.1g; Fiber: 3g

EGGS WITH MUSHROOMS

Preparation Time 25 Minutes
Servings: 1

Ingredients:
- 1/2 cup button mushrooms; sliced
- 2-ounce fresh arugula
- 1-egg
- 2 tablespoon olive oil
- 1/4 teaspoon chili flakes
- 1 tablespoon dried thyme

Directions:
1. Place mushrooms in a large sieve and rinse under cold running water. Pat dry with a kitchen towel making sure to wipe away any extra debris.
2. Using a sharp paring knife, slice each mushroom in half, lengthwise, but keep the stems on, Set aside
3. Plug in the instant pot and add butter to the stainless steel insert. Press the *Sauté* button and melt it.
4. Add mushrooms and cook for 4-5 minutes, or until the liquid evaporates
5. Now; add arugula and give it a good stir. Optionally, add one tablespoon of olive oil for some extra taste. Cook for one minute
6. Finally, crack the eggs and cook until set – for 2 minutes. Season with dried thyme and sprinkle with chili flakes
7. Turn off the pot and carefully transfer the mixture to a serving plate using a large kitchen spatula. Serve it immediately

Nutrition Value: Calories: 325; Total Fats: 32.8g; Net Carbs: 2.3g; Protein: 8.1g; Fiber: 1.3g

BEEF CHILI

Preparation Time 45 Minutes
Servings: 3

Ingredients:
For chili:
- 1-pound beef stew meat
- 2 garlic cloves; crushed
- 1 cup fire-roasted tomatoes; chopped
- 2 small red chilies; finely chopped.
- 2 tablespoon olive oil
- 2 tablespoon butter
- 1/2 green bell pepper; chopped
- 1/2 teaspoon freshly ground black pepper
- 1/4 teaspoon stevia powder
- 1 teaspoon salt

Directions:
1. Plug in the instant pot and grease the inner pot with olive oil. Press the *Sauté* button and heat up. Add onions, garlic, and chopped chili. Sauté for 3-4 minutes stirring constantly.
2. Now add the remaining ingredients and seal the lid. Set the steam release handle to the *Sealing* position and press the *Manual* button. Set the timer for 25 minutes on high pressure
3. When done; press the *Cancel'* button and release the pressure naturally. Let it sit, covered, for 10-15 minutes before serving
4. For a better taste, briefly brown the meat before cooking. Optionally, sprinkle with some finely chopped parsley before serving

Nutrition Value: Calories: 450; Total Fats: 26.6g; Net Carbs: 3.6g; Protein: 46.8g; Fiber: 1.1g

PORK TENDERLOIN STEW

Preparation Time 50 Minutes
Servings: 3

Ingredients:

For stew:
- 1-pound pork tenderloin; chopped.
- 1 small onion; chopped.
- 4 cup beef broth
- 1 cup tomatoes; chopped
- 1/4 cup apple cider vinegar
- 3 tablespoon oil
- 2 tablespoon butter
- 1/4 teaspoon black pepper; freshly ground.
- 1/4 teaspoon garlic powder
- 2 bay leaves
- 1/2 salt
- 1 teaspoon dried marjoram

Directions:
1. Grease the bottom of the inner pot with oil and press the *Sauté* button. Heat up the oil and add butter. Allow it to melt and then add onions. Cook for 3-4 minutes.
2. Now add chopped meat and season with salt, marjoram, black pepper, and garlic powder. Give it a good stir and continue to cook for 5-6 minutes stirring constantly
3. Pour in the broth and apple cider. Add bay leaves and tomatoes.
4. Seal the lid and set the steam release handle to the *Sealing* position. Press the *Manual* button and set the timer for 35 minutes on high pressure
5. When you hear the end signal, perform a quick pressure release by moving the pressure valve to the *Venting* position. Carefully open the lid and remove the bay leaves. Optionally, sprinkle with some Parmesan cheese and serve immediately.

Nutrition Value: Calories: 480; Total Fats: 28.6g; Net Carbs: 4.7g; Protein: 46.9g; Fiber: 1.2g

LAMB STEW
Preparation Time 45 Minutes
Servings: 3
Ingredients:
For stew:
- 1-pound lamb leg; chopped into bite-sized pieces
- 6 garlic cloves; crushed
- 4 cups vegetable stock
- 2 tablespoon butter; for serving
- 2 cups cabbage; shredded
- 1 thyme sprig
- 1 bay leaf
- 1 rosemary sprig
- 1 teaspoon sea salt

Directions:
1. Combine the ingredients in the pot and pour in the stock. Stir well and optionally season with some more salt or pepper.
2. Seal the lid and set the steam release handle to the *Sealing* position. Press the *Meat* button and set the timer for 35 minutes.
3. When you hear the end signal, press the *Cancel'* button and release the pressure naturally
4. Using oven mitts, move the pressure valve to the *Venting* position to release any remaining pressure
5. Carefully open the lid and stir in butter. Let it sit for 2-3 minutes and serve immediately.

Nutrition Value: Calories: 378; Total Fats: 19g; Net Carbs: 3.9g; Protein: 44.1g; Fiber: 2g

DEVILED EGGS
Preparation Time 30 Minutes
Servings: 4
Ingredients:
- 12 eggs
- 1/4 cup sour cream
- 2 tablespoon butter
- 1 tablespoon Dijon mustard
- 2 teaspoon lemon juice
- 2 tablespoon parsley; finely chopped.
- 1 teaspoon sea salt

Directions:
1. Plug in your Instant Pot and pour in 1 cup of water. Set the steaming insert and gently place egg in it. Securely close the lid and set the steam release handle to *Sealing* position. Press the *Manual* button and set the timer to 7 minutes.
2. Now prepare the deviled eggs stuffing. In a medium-sized bowl, combine sour cream, butter, cilantro, Dijon, and lime juice. Season with salt and mix well using a hand mixer. You want to get a nice and creamy mixture
3. When you hear the end signal, set the steam valve to *Venting* position to perform a quick pressure release. Open the lid and gently remove the eggs. Chill for a while.
4. Meanwhile, prepare the ice bath. Take a large bowl and pour in 4 cups of ice cold water. Optionally, add 2 cups of ice cubes to speed up the cooling process. Place eggs in it and cool them completely. This will stop the cooking process and prevent the eggs of being overcooked

5. Gently peel the eggs and slice them in half, lengthwise. Remove the yolks and place them in the cream mixture. Stir well to combine avoiding any large pieces
6. Place the cream mixture in a large piping pastry bag with a star tip. Pipe about 1 tablespoon of the mixture at the center of each egg and transfer to a serving plate.

Nutrition Value: Calories: 274; Total Fats: 22.1g; Net Carbs: 1.8g; Protein: 17.4g; Fiber: 0.2g

BEEF BLACK PEPPER STEW

Preparation Time 45 Minutes
Servings: 6
Ingredients:
For stew:
- 2 -pounds beef stew meat
- 3 large onions, chopped
- 1 cup cherry tomatoes
- 5 garlic cloves, crushed
- 3 tablespoon oil
- 4 cups beef broth
- 1 teaspoon peppercorn
- 1 teaspoon cayenne pepper
- 1 teaspoon salt
- 1/2 teaspoon black pepper, freshly ground.

Directions:
1. Grease the inner pot with oil and press the *Sauté* button. Add onions and garlic. Cook for 3-4 minutes, stirring constantly.
2. Now add the meat, salt, pepper, peppercorn, cayenne pepper, and tomatoes. Stir in the meat and pour in the broth. Give it a good stir and seal the lid.
3. Set the steam release handle and press the *Manual* mode. Cook for 20 minutes on high pressure
4. When done, release the pressure naturally and open the lid. Serve hot and enjoy!

Nutrition Value: Calories: 406; Total Fats: 17.3g; Net Carbs: 7.6g; Protein: 50.4g; Fiber: 2g

BEEF STEW WITH EGGPLANTS

Preparation Time 60 Minutes
Servings: 6
Ingredients:
For stew:
- 2 -pounds beef stew meat
- 1 cup eggplant; cut into chunks
- 6 bacon slices
- 4 cups beef broth
- 1 cup cherry tomatoes; chopped
- 1 large onion; finely chopped.
- 4 tablespoon butter
- 3 garlic cloves; crushed
- 1 bay leaf
- 1 teaspoon dried thyme
- 1/2 teaspoon salt

Directions:
1. Place eggplant in a large sieve and generously sprinkle with salt. Toss well and let it sit for 10-15 minutes.
2. Grease the bottom of your pot with butter. Add onions and garlic. Cook for 3-4 minutes or until translucent. Add cherry tomatoes and continue to cook until all the liquid has evaporated.
3. Now add the meat and briefly brown stirring constantly
4. Finally, pour in the beef broth and season with salt and thyme. Add bay leaves and give it a good stir
5. Seal the lid and set the steam release handle to the *Sealing* position. Press the *Meat* button
6. When you hear the end signal, perform a quick pressure release and open the lid. Serve and enjoy.

Nutrition Value: Calories: 498; Total Fats: 26.1g; Net Carbs: 4.3g; Protein: 57g; Fiber: 1.4g

CINNAMON PANCAKES

Preparation Time 20 Minutes
Servings: 3
Ingredients:
- 1 cup almond flour
- 1 tablespoon coconut butter; melted
- 2 tablespoon milk
- 2 large eggs
- 1/2 teaspoon baking powder
- 1/2 teaspoon vanilla extract
- 1 teaspoon cinnamon; ground.
- 1/2 teaspoon powdered stevia

Directions:
1. In a large mixing bowl, combine almond flour, baking powder, cinnamon, and stevia. Using a kitchen spatula, mix until combined.
2. Now; add eggs, vanilla extract, and milk. With a whisking attachment on, beat until smooth batter.
3. Plug in your instant pot and grease the stainless steel insert with coconut butter. Pour

about 1/3 of the mixture into the pot and securely lock the lid. Adjust the steam release handle and press the *Manual* button. Set the timer for 5 minutes and cook on *High* pressure.
4. When done; perform a quick release of the pressure and open the pot. Carefully remove the pancake to a serving plate. Repeat the process with the remaining batter.
5. Serve pancakes with some fresh raspberries

Nutrition Value: Calories: 312; Total Fats: 24.3g; Net Carbs: 5.7g; Protein: 12.9g; Fiber: 5.3g

CHICKEN VEAL STEW

Preparation Time 60 Minutes
Servings: 4

Ingredients:
For stew:
- 1-pound veal cuts; chopped into bite-sized pieces.
- 1-pound chicken boneless and skinless chicken breast; chopped into bite sized pieces.
- 3 tablespoon butter
- 2 tablespoon olive oil
- 5 cups beef broth
- 2 cups button mushrooms; sliced
- 1 cup cauliflower; chopped
- 1 cup cherry tomatoes; sliced
- 1 teaspoon salt
- 1 teaspoon smoked paprika
- 2 rosemary sprigs
- 1/2 black pepper; freshly ground.
- 1 tablespoon cayenne pepper

Directions:
1. Rinse well the meat and chop into bite-sized pieces. Generously sprinkle with salt and pepper. Place in two separate bowls and set aside.
2. Plug in the instant pot and grease the inner pot with olive oil. Press the *Sauté* button and add chopped veal. Cook for 4-5 minutes stirring constantly. Now add the chicken breast and continue to cook for another 3-4 minutes
3. Add mushrooms, cauliflower, and tomatoes. Sprinkle with cayenne pepper and smoked paprika. Continue to cook for 10 minutes
4. Finally, pour in the broth. Add rosemary sprigs and optionally season with some more salt and pepper to taste. Stir well and seal the lid
5. Set the steam release handle to the *Sealing* position and press the *Manual* button. Set the timer for 13 minutes on high pressure
6. When done, release the pressure naturally and carefully open the lid. Remove the rosemary sprigs and stir in the butter. Serve hot and enjoy.

Nutrition Value: Calories: 572; Total Fats: 29.5g; Net Carbs: 3.9g; Protein: 68.6g; Fiber: 1.5g

EGGS WITH SCALLIONS

Preparation Time 10 Minutes
Servings: 1

Ingredients:
- 1/4 cup scallions; finely chopped.
- 3 tablespoon butter
- 1/4 teaspoon garlic powder
- 2 eggs
- 1/4 teaspoon black pepper
- 1/2 teaspoon sea salt

Directions:
1. Plug in the instant pot and pour in 1 cup of water. Set the steam basket in the inner pot and set aside
2. In a small, heat-proof bowl, crack eggs and season generously with salt, pepper, and garlic powder.
3. Sprinkle with chopped scallions and place in the steam basket.
4. Seal the lid and set the steam release handle to the *Sealing* position. Press the *Manual* button and set the timer for 5 minutes
5. When you hear the end signal, perform a quick pressure release and open the lid
6. Using oven mitts remove the bowl and chill for a while before serving

Nutrition Value: Calories: 439; Total Fats: 43.4g; Net Carbs: 1.9g; Protein: 11.9g; Fiber: 0.7g

RASPBERRY MUG CAKE

Preparation Time 10 Minutes
Servings: 3

Ingredients:
- 4 large eggs
- 1/4 cup fresh raspberries
- 1/2 cup cream cheese
- 1/2 teaspoon baking powder
- 1/2 cup heavy whipping cream
- 1/2 cup almond flour
- 1/4 teaspoon vanilla extract
- 1/4 teaspoon powdered stevia

Directions:

1. In a large mixing bowl, combine eggs, cream cheese, almond flour, and baking powder. With a whisking attachment on, beat until well combined and smooth.
2. Pour the mixture into oven-safe mugs and set aside
3. Plug in your instant pot and pour 1 cup of water in the stainless steel insert. Position a trivet and place mugs on top.
4. Securely lock the lid and adjust the steam release handle. Press the *Manual* button and set the timer for 3 minutes. Cook on *High* pressure.
5. Meanwhile, combine heavy whipping cream with powdered stevia and vanilla extract. Beat until combined and set aside
6. When you hear the cooker's end signal, perform a quick release of the pressure by moving the valve to the *Venting* position. Open the pot and transfer the mugs to a wire rack using oven mitts.
7. Top each mug with raspberry cream and serve immediately.

Nutrition Value: Calories: 418; Total Fats: 36.5g; Net Carbs: 5.1g; Protein: 15.8g; Fiber: 2.7g

ALMOND PORRIDGE

Preparation Time 10 Minutes
Servings: 2

Ingredients:
- 1 cup unsweetened almond milk
- 2 tablespoon chia seeds
- 3 tablespoon coconut oil
- 1 teaspoon vanilla extract
- 1 teaspoon swerve
- 3 tablespoon hemp seeds
- 1/4 teaspoon salt
- Fresh raspberries; optional for topping

Directions:
1. Plug in the instant pot and grease the inner pot with coconut oil. Add hemp seeds and chia seeds
2. Pour in 1/2 cup of water and press the *Sauté* button. Cook for 5 minutes, stirring constantly
3. Now pour in the almond milk and sprinkle with salt, vanilla extract, and swerve.
4. Optionally, add a few drops of stevia extract. Stir well and cook for another 5 minutes.
5. When done, press the *Cancel'* button and transfer the porridge to a serving bowl. Optionally, top with a couple of fresh raspberries and serve.

Nutrition Value: Calories: 380; Total Fats: 37.4g; Net Carbs: 2.3g; Protein: 11g; Fiber: 6.2g

BACON BRUSSELS SPROUTS

Preparation Time 15 Minutes
Servings: 3

Ingredients:
- 1 cup Brussels sprouts; chopped.
- 3-ounce bacon; cut into bite-sized pieces
- 1 tablespoon balsamic vinegar
- 4 large eggs; beaten
- 1 tablespoon olive oil
- 1 tablespoon green onions; finely chopped
- 1/2 teaspoon smoked paprika; ground.
- 1 teaspoon garlic powder
- 1 teaspoon sea salt

Directions:
1. Plug in your instant pot and grease the stainless steel insert with olive oil. Press the *Saute* button and add Brussels sprouts. Sprinkle with garlic powder, paprika and salt. Stir well and cook for 5 minutes.
2. Now; add beaten eggs, onions, and balsamic vinegar. Give it a good stir and cook for 2-3 more minutes. Turn off the pot and stir in the bacon immediately. Let it stand for 10 minutes before serving

Nutrition Value: Calories: 307; Total Fats: 23.3g; Net Carbs: 3.3g; Protein: 20.1g; Fiber: 1.4g

MUSHROOM AND EGGS CASSEROLE

Preparation Time: 15 minutes
Servings: 3

Ingredients:
- 1/2 cup cremini mushrooms; cooked and sliced
- 3 eggs
- 1/4 cup heavy cream
- 1/2 small onion chopped.
- 1/2 cup cooked ham or bacon
- 1/2 cup cheddar cheese
- Sea salt and pepper; to taste

Directions:
1. Add 1 cup water to Instant Pot and place the trivet inside.
2. Add all the Ingredients to a bowl except cheese and whisk well
3. Take a heatproof container and pour the egg mixture into it
4. Place the container over the trivet.

5. Secure the lid of instant pot and press *Manual* function key
6. Adjust the time to 10 minutes and cook at high pressure.
7. When it beeps; release the pressure naturally and open the instant pot lid. Drizzle the shredded cheese on top and serve hot

BANANA OATMEAL

Preparation Time: 11 minutes
Servings: 4

Ingredients:
- 2 bananas sliced
- 2 cups old-fashioned oats
- 2¼ cups water
- 2¼ cups milk
- 1 tbsp. sugar
- 2 tbsp. molasses
- 4 tbsp. chopped toasted pecans

Directions:
1. Add oats, milk, water and sugar into Instant Pot.
2. Secure the lid of instant pot and press *Manual* function key
3. Adjust the time to 6 minutes and cook at high pressure.
4. When it beeps; release the pressure naturally and open the instant pot lid
5. Stir the prepared oatmeal. Serve with banana slices and pecans on top. Then drizzle molasses on it

EASY AND CHEESY GRITS

Preparation Time: 20 minutes
Servings: 4

Ingredients:
- 4 oz. cheddar cheese; grated
- 2 tsp. salt
- 3 tbsp. butter
- 1 ¾ cup half and half
- 2 tbsp. coconut oil
- 3 cups water
- 1 cup stone ground grits
- Butter for serving

Directions:
1. Set your instant pot on sauté mode; add grits, stir them for 3 minutes
2. Add oil, half, and half, water, salt, butter and cheese; then stir well. close the instant pot lid and cook on High for 10 minutes
3. Release the pressure naturally, leave cheesy grits aside for 15 minutes, transfer to breakfast bowls; add butter on top and serve.

INSTANT NUTRITIOUS PORRIDGE

Preparation Time: 8 minutes
Servings: 4

Ingredients:
- 1 cup cashews (raw, unsalted)
- 1/2 cup Pepitas; shelled
- 1 cup Pecan halves
- 4 tsp. coconut oil; melted
- 2 tbsp. maple syrup or honey
- 1 cup unsweetened dried coconut shreds
- 2 cups water

Directions:
1. Add all the Ingredients to a blender, except water, maple syrup and coconut oil. Blend well to form a smooth mixture
2. Add the prepared mixture along with water, coconut oil and maple syrup to Instant Pot
3. Secure the lid of instant pot and press *Porridge* option
4. Adjust the time to 3 minutes and let it cook
5. When it beeps; release the pressure naturally and open the instant pot lid.
6. Stir the prepared mixture and serve in a bowl. Garnish with fresh fruits and cashews on top

PECAN SWEET POTATOES

Preparation Time: 20 minutes
Servings: 8

Ingredients:
- 1 cup pecans chopped
- 1 tbsp. lemon peel
- 1/2 cup brown sugar
- 1 tbsp. cornstarch
- 1/4 cup butter
- 1/4 cup maple syrup
- 1/4 tsp. salt
- 1 cup water
- 3 sweet potatoes peeled and sliced
- Whole pecans for garnish

Directions:
1. Pour the water in your instant pot; add lemon peel, brown sugar and salt and stir
2. Add potatoes, seal the instant pot lid and cook at High for 15 minutes.
3. Release the pressure and transfer the potatoes to a serving plate
4. Select sauté mode on your instant pot; add the butter and melt it
5. Add pecans, maple syrup, cornstarch and stir very well
6. Pour this over the potatoes, garnish with whole pecans and serve

BREAKFAST QUICHE

Preparation Time: 40 minutes
Servings: 4

Ingredients:
- 1/2 cup ham, diced
- 1 cup sausage; already cooked and ground.
- 2 green onions; chopped.
- 1/2 cup milk
- 6 eggs, whisked
- 1 cup cheese; shredded.
- 4 bacon slices; cooked and crumbled
- 1 ½ cups water
- Salt and black pepper to taste

Directions:
1. Put the water in your instant pot and leave it aside for now.
2. In a bowl; mix eggs with salt, pepper, milk, sausage, ham, bacon, onions and cheese and stir everything well.
3. Pour this into a baking dish, cover with some tin foil, place the dish in the steamer basket of your instant pot, cover and cook at High for 30 minutes.
4. Release the pressure naturally for 10 minutes, then release remaining pressure by turning the valve to 'Venting', and carefully open the lid, take the quiche out and leave it aside for a few minutes to cool down.
5. Cut the quiche, arrange it on plates and serve

MIX BEANS RICE

Preparation Time: 27 minutes
Servings: 4

Ingredients:
- 1 cup whole mung beans
- 1 cup white basmati rice
- 1/2 tsp. turmeric powder
- 1/2 tsp. sea salt
- 2 inches ginger; grated or chopped.
- 3 tsp. shredded coconut
- bunch of cilantro; chopped.
- 6 cups water
- 1/2 cup cremini mushrooms; sliced

Directions:
1. Add all the Ingredients to Instant Pot
2. Secure the lid of instant pot and press *Manual* function key
3. Adjust the time to 15 minutes and cook at high pressure.
4. When it beeps; release the pressure naturally and open the instant pot lid.
5. Stir the prepared mixture and serve in a bowl. Garnish with mushroom slices on top

COCO RICE PUDDING

Preparation Time: 15 minutes
Servings: 2

Ingredients:
- 1/2 cup basmati rice; short grain
- 1 cup coconut milk
- Whipped cream and coconut flakes (garnish
- 3/4 cup water
- 1/2 cup coconut cream
- 2 tbsp. maple syrup
- Pinch of sea salt

Directions:
1. Add all the Ingredients to Instant Pot
2. Secure the lid of instant pot and press *Manual* function key
3. Adjust the time to 10 minutes and cook at high pressure.
4. After it beeps; release the pressure naturally and open the instant pot lid.
5. Stir the prepared pudding and serve in a bowl. Add whipped cream and coconut flakes on top.

ORANGE MARMALADE OATMEAL

Preparation Time: 11 minutes
Servings: 4

Ingredients:
- 2 tbsp. orange marmalade
- 2 cups old-fashioned oats
- 2¼ cups water
- 2¼ cups milk
- 1/2 tsp. salt
- 1/2 tsp. ground cinnamon
- 1/4 cup sugar
- 2 tbsp. plain low-fat Greek yogurt
- Orange and kiwi slices to garnish

Directions:
1. Add all the Ingredients to Instant Pot.
2. Secure the lid of instant pot and press *Manual* function key
3. Adjust the time to 6 minutes and cook at high pressure.
4. When it beeps; release the pressure naturally and open the instant pot lid
5. Stir the prepared oatmeal and serve in a bowl. Garnish with orange and kiwi slices on top

EGGS WITH HERBS DE PROVENCE

Preparation Time: 20 minutes
Servings: 3

Ingredients:

- 3 eggs
- 1/2 tsp. Herbs de Provence
- 1/2 small onion chopped.
- 1/2 cup cooked ham or bacon
- 1/4 cup heavy cream
- 1/2 cup chopped kale leaves
- 1/2 cup cheddar cheese
- Sea salt and pepper; to taste

Directions:
1. Add 1 cup of water to Instant Pot and place the trivet inside.
2. Add all the Ingredients to a bowl except cheese and whisk well
3. Take a heatproof container and pour the egg mixture into it. Place the container over the trivet.
4. Secure the lid of instant pot and press *Manual* function key
5. Adjust the time to 10 minutes and cook at high pressure.
6. When it beeps; release the pressure naturally and open the instant pot lid. Drizzle shredded cheese on top and serve hot

CORNMEAL PORRIDGE

Preparation Time: 16 minutes
Servings: 6

Ingredients:
- 1¼ cups yellow cornmeal; fine
- 6 cups water
- 1¼ cups milk
- 2½ sticks cinnamon
- 5 pimento berries
- 1¼ tsp. vanilla extract
- 3/4 tsp. nutmeg; ground
- 3/4 cup sweetened condensed milk

Directions:
1. Add 5 cups water and milk to Instant Pot.
2. Mix the cornmeal with 1 cup of water and add it to the pot
3. Stir in vanilla extract, pimento berries, nutmeg and cinnamon sticks.
4. Secure the lid of instant pot and press *Manual* function key
5. Adjust the time to 6 minutes and cook at high pressure.
6. When it beeps; release the pressure naturally and open the instant pot lid
7. Stir in sweetened condensed milk. Serve and enjoy.

BROCCOLI EGG CASSEROLE

Preparation Time: 30 minutes
Servings: 3

Ingredients:
- 1/2 lb. broccoli florets
- 3 eggs
- 1/4 cup heavy cream
- 1/2 cup cheddar cheese
- 1/2 small onion chopped.
- 1/2 cup cooked ham or bacon
- Sea salt and pepper; to taste

Directions:
1. Add 1 cup water to Instant Pot and place the trivet inside.
2. Add all the Ingredients to a bowl except cheese and whisk well
3. Take a heatproof container and pour the egg mixture into it
4. Place the container over the trivet
5. Secure the lid of instant pot and press *Manual* function key
6. Adjust the time to 20 minutes and cook at high pressure.
7. When it beeps; release the pressure naturally and open the instant pot lid. Drizzle shredded cheese on top and serve hot.

APRICOT CRANBERRY STEEL CUT OATS

Preparation Time: 15 minutes
Servings: 4

Ingredients:
- 2 tbsp. dried cranberries
- 2 cups steel-cut oats
- 3 cups water
- 4 tbsp. butter
- 2 cups freshly squeezed orange juice
- 2 tbsp. raisins
- 2 tbsp. chopped. dried apricots
- 2 tbsp. pure maple syrup
- 1/2 tsp. ground cinnamon
- 4 tbsp. chopped pecans
- 1/4 tsp. salt

Directions:
1. Add all the Ingredients to Instant Pot
2. Secure the lid of instant pot and press *Manual* function key
3. Adjust the time to 10 minutes and cook at high pressure.
4. After it beeps; release the pressure naturally and open the instant pot lid.
5. Stir the prepared oatmeal and serve in a bowl. Garnish with fresh strawberries on top.

STRAWBERRY COMPOTE

Preparation Time: 25 minutes

Servings: 4

Ingredients:

- 2 lb. fresh strawberries washed; trimmed and cut in half
- 1/4 cup sugar
- 2 oz. fresh orange juice
- 1/2 tsp. ground ginger
- 1 vanilla bean; chopped.

Directions:

1. Add all the Ingredients to Instant Pot.
2. Secure the lid of instant pot and press *Manual* function key
3. Adjust the time to 15 minutes and cook at high pressure.
4. When it beeps; release the pressure naturally and open the instant pot lid
5. Stir the prepared compote, let it thicken as it cools, Serve on toast and enjoy

BREAKFAST PUDDING

Preparation Time: 15 minutes
Servings: 4

Ingredients:

- 1/3 cup tapioca pearls
- 1 ¼ cup whole milk
- 1/2 cup sugar
- 1 ½ cups water
- Zest from 1/2 lemon

Directions:

1. Put 1 cup water in your instant pot.
2. Put tapioca pearls in a heat proof bowl add milk, 1/2 cup water, lemon zest and sugar
3. Stir everything, place the bowl in the steamer basket of the pot, close the instant pot lid and cook at High for 10 minutes.
4. Quick release the pressure; transfer pudding to cups and serve.

RICE PUDDING

Preparation Time: 15 minutes
Servings: 3

Ingredients:

- 1/2 cup basmati rice
- 1 cup milk
- 3/4 cup water
- 1/2 cup coconut cream
- 2 tbsp. maple syrup
- Pinch of sea salt
- 1 tsp. vanilla extract
- Strawberry jam (garnish)

Directions:

1. Add all the Ingredients to Instant Pot
2. Secure the lid of instant pot and press *Manual* function key
3. Adjust the time to 10 minutes and cook at high pressure.
4. When it beeps; release the pressure naturally and open the instant pot lid
5. Stir the prepared pudding and serve in a bowl. Add the strawberry jam on top.

MIX PEPPERS HASH

Preparation Time: 35 minutes
Servings: 3

Ingredients:

- 2 bacon slices; chopped.
- 1/2 green bell pepper; chopped.
- 6 eggs
- 1/2 yellow bell pepper; chopped.
- 1/2 cup cheddar cheese
- 1/2 red bell pepper; chopped.
- 1/4 tsp. black pepper
- 1/4 tsp. salt
- 1 tbsp. milk
- 6-inch springform pan

Directions:

1. Add bacon to Instant Pot and select the *Sauté* function to cook for 3 minutes.
2. Transfer the crispy cooked bacon to the greased *spring pan*
3. Add all the bell peppers on top of bacon
4. Crack all the eggs in a bowl and whisk them well with the milk
5. Pour the eggs mixture over the bell peppers in the spring pan.
6. Sprinkle salt and pepper on top and cover with aluminum foil
7. Pour some water into Instant Pot; set the trivet inside and then place the covered spring pan over the trivet.
8. Press the *Manual* key; adjust its settings to High pressure for 15 minutes.
9. When it is done; do a Natural release to release the steam
10. Remove the lid and the spring pan. Transfer the hash to a plate, Sprinkle cheddar cheese on top then serve

DICED TURMERIC EGGS

Preparation Time: 5 Mins
TotalTime: 15 Mins
Servings: 3

Ingredients:

- 6 Eggs
- ½ tsp Turmeric Powder
- ¼ tsp dried Parsley

- Pinch of Pepper
- 1 ½ cups Water

Direction
1. Pour the water into your Instant Pot and lower the trivet.
2. Grease a baking dish and crack the eggs into it, but make sure not to break the yolks.
3. Place the baking dish on the trivet and put the lid on.
4. Turn clockwise to seal and set the IP to MANUAL.
5. Cook on HIGH for 4 minutes.
6. Do a quick pressure release and remove the baking dish from the IP.
7. Transfer the egg 'pie' onto a cutting board.
8. Sprinkle the spices over and dice the eggs finely with a knife.
9. Serve and enjoy!

Nutrition Values:
Calories 130
Total Fats 8g
Carbs: 2g
Protein 10g
Dietary Fiber: 0g

VEGGIE QUICHE

Preparation Time: 8 Mins
Total Time: 25 Mins
Servings: 4
Ingredients:
- 8 Eggs
- ¼ cup Almond Milk
- 1 Green Onion, sliced
- ½ cup chopped Kale
- 1 Tomato, chopped
- ½ Red Bell Pepper, diced
- 1 Carrot, shredded
- ½ tsp dried Parsley
- Pinch of Pepper
- Pinch of Paprika
- 1 ½ cups Water

Direction
1. Pour the water into your IP.
2. In a large bowl, whisk together the eggs, almond milk, pepper, and paprika.
3. Add the veggies and stir to combine well.
4. Grease a round pie pan and pour the egg and veggie mixture into it.
5. Lower the trivet into the IP and place the pan on it.
6. Put the lid on and turn clockwise to seal.
7. Set your Instant Pot to MANUAL and cook on HIGH for 20 minutes. Do a natural pressure release.
8. Serve and enjoy!

Nutrition Values:
Calories 170
Total Fats 10g
Carbs: 6.1g
Protein 13.5g
Dietary Fiber: 1.4g

APPLE AND ALMOND PORRIDGE

Preparation Time: 2 Mins
Total Time: 5 Mins
Servings: 1
Ingredients:
- 1 tbsp Almond Butter
- 1 medium Gala Apple, grated
- 2 tbsp Flaxseed
- 3 tbsp ground Almonds
- ½ cup Almond Milk
- Pinch of Cinnamon

Direction
1. Place all of the ingredients in your Instant Pot.
2. Give it a good stir to combine.
3. Put the lid on and seal.
4. Set the Instant Pot to MANUAL and cook on HIGH for about 3 minutes.
5. Do a quick pressure release.
6. Stir once before serving and enjoy!

Nutrition Values:
Calories 443
Total Fats 18.5g
Carbs: 40g
Protein g
Dietary Fiber: 13.2g

TOMATO POACHED EGGS

Preparation Time: 8 Mins
TotalTime: 15 Mins
Servings: 1
Ingredients:
- 1 Tomato, chopped
- 4 Eggs
- ½ Onion, diced
- ¼ tsp Smoked Paprika
- Pinch of Turmeric
- Pinch of Pepper
- 1 ½ cups Water

Direction
1. Pour the water into the Instant Pot and lower the trivet.
2. Grease 4 ramekins and set aside.
3. In a bowl, beat the eggs with the paprika, pepper, and turmeric.

4. Add the diced onion and tomatoes and stir to combine.
5. Divide the eggs between the ramekins.
6. Place the ramekins on the trivet and put the lid on.
7. Set the Instant Pot to STEAM and cook for 5 minutes.
8. Do a quick pressure release.
9. Serve and enjoy!

Nutrition Values:
Calories 195
Total Fats 14g
Carbs: 6.5g
Protein 10g
Dietary Fiber: 1.5g

SMOKED SALMON EGGS

Preparation Time: 3 Mins
TotalTime: 10 Mins
Servings: 4

Ingredients:
- 4 Eggs
- 1 tbsp Olive Oil
- 4 slices of Smoked Salmon
- 1 tsp chopped Chives
- 1 cup of Water

Direction
1. Pour the water into your Instant Pot and lower the trivet.
2. Grease 4 ramekins with the olive oil.
3. Place a slice of salmon inside each of the ramekins.
4. Crack an egg on top.
5. Sprinkle with the chives and cover the ramekins with foil.
6. Place the ramekins on the trivet.
7. Put the lid on and seal.
8. Set your Instant Pot to MANUAL and cook on HIGH for 5 minutes.
9. Serve and enjoy!

Nutrition Values:
Calories 240
Total Fats 17g
Carbs: 2g
Protein 19g
Dietary Fiber: 0g

CARROT AND PECAN MUFFINS

Preparation Time: 25 Mins
Total Time: 40 Mins
Servings: 8

Ingredients:
- ½ cup chopped Pecans
- 1 tsp Baking Powder
- ¼ cup Coconut Oil
- ½ cup Almond or Coconut Milk
- 3 Eggs
- 1 cup Almond Flour
- 1/3 cup Pure Applesauce
- 1 tsp Apple Pie Spice
- 1 cup shredded Carrots

Direction
1. Pour the water into your Instant Pot and then lower the trivet.
2. In a mixing bowl, place all of the ingredients except the pecans and the carrots.
3. Beat with an electric mixer until fluffy and smooth.
4. Fold in the pecans and the carrots.
5. Divide the mixture between 8 silicone muffin cups and place the muffin cups on the trivet.
6. Set the Instant Pot to MANUAL and cook on HIGH for 15 minutes.
7. Do a quick pressure release.
8. Serve and enjoy!

Nutrition Values:
Calories 265
Total Fats 25g
Carbs: 6g
Protein 6g
Dietary Fiber: 2g

BEEF EGG MUFFINS

Preparation Time: 15 Mins
Total Time: 25 Mins
Servings: 2

Ingredients:
- 4 Eggs
- 1 Green Onions, sliced
- ¼ cup ground Beef
- ¼ cup diced Bell Peppers
- Pinch of Pepper
- ¼ tsp dried Parsley
- ½ tbsp Olive Oil
- 1 ½ cups Water

Direction
1. Set your Instant Pot to SAUTE and heat the olive oil in it.
2. Add the beef and cook until it becomes brown.
3. Transfer to a bowl.
4. Add the eggs to the bowl and beat along with the pepper.
5. Stir in the remaining ingredients and divide the mixture between 4 silicone muffin cups.
6. Pour the water into the IP and lower the trivet.

7. Place the muffin cups on the trivet and close the lid.
8. Cook on HIGH for 8 minutes.
9. Do a quick pressure release.
10. Serve and enjoy!

Nutrition Values:
Calories 236
Total Fats 16g
Carbs: 2.2g
Protein 20g
Dietary Fiber: 0.6g

EGG BAKE WITH CARROTS

Preparation Time: 10 Mins
Total Time: 20 Mins
Servings: 4

Ingredients:
- 8 Eggs
- 1 cup shredded Carrots
- 2 cups shredded Sweet Potatoes
- ¼ tsp Turmeric Powder
- ¼ tsp Thyme
- ¼ tsp Parsley
- 2 tsp Olive Oil
- ½ cup Almond Milk

Direction
1. Set the Instant Pot to SAUTE and heat the olive oil in it.
2. Add the potatoes and carrots and cook for about 2 minutes, stirring occasionally.
3. Meanwhile, beat the eggs and almond milk in a bowl.
4. Stir in the herbs and spices and pour the mixture over the veggies.
5. Close the lid and press CANCEL.
6. Set the IP to MANUAL and cook on HIGH for 7 minutes.
7. Do a quick pressure release.
8. Serve and enjoy!

Nutrition Values:
Calories 220
Total Fats 7g
Carbs: 17.2
Protein 6g
Dietary Fiber: 2g

VEGGIE AND BEEF CASSEROLE

Preparation Time: 15 Mins
Total Time: 40 Mins
Servings: 4

Ingredients:
- 1 tbsp Coconut Oil
- 6 Eggs, beaten
- 8 ounces ground Beef
- 1 tsp minced Garlic
- ¾ cup sliced Leek
- 1 Sweet Potato, shredded
- ¾ cup chopped Kale
- 1 ½ cups Water

Direction
1. Set your Instant Pot to SAUTE and add the coconut oil to it.
2. When melted, add the leeks and cook for 2 minutes.
3. Add the beef and cook until it becomes brown.
4. Stir in the garlic and kale and cook for 1 more minute.
5. Transfer the mixture to a bowl.
6. Add the eggs and potatoes to the bowl and stir well to combine everything.
7. Transfer the mixture to a greased baking dish.
8. Pour the water into your Instant Pot and lower the trivet.
9. Place the prepared dish on the trivet and close the lid.
10. Set the IP to MANUAL and cook on HIGH for 25 minutes.
11. Do a quick pressure release. Serve and enjoy!

Nutrition Values:
Calories 425
Total Fats 30g
Carbs: 13g
Protein 24g
Dietary Fiber: 1.6g

SAUSAGE & ASPARAGUS DILL

Preparation Time: 10 Mins
Total Time: 50 Mins
Servings: 5

Ingredients :
- Coconut oil, for greasing the dish
- 1 pound breakfast sausage
- ¼ cup coconut milk
- 8 free range eggs, beaten
- ½ cup coconut cream
- 1 tbsp. minced fresh dill
- 6-8 stalks asparagus, chopped
- 1 thinly sliced leek
- ¼ tsp. garlic powder
- Sea salt and pepper

Directions :
1. Grease a square baking dish and set aside.
2. Place the sausage in a pan set over medium heat; break them into small pieces.
3. Cook for a few minutes and add asparagus

and leeks; continue cooking for about 5 minutes more or until sausage is no longer pink.
4. Remove the pan from heat, discarding excess fat.
5. Whisk together eggs, garlic powder, dill, cream, salt and pepper in a bowl; pour the mixture into the prepared baking dish and add the sausage mixture; mix well.
6. Add water to the instant pot and insert a trivet; place the dish onto the trivet and lock lid.
7. Cook on high for 25 minutes and then let pressure come down on its own.
8. Remove the casserole and cut into equal slices.

Nutrition Values:
Calories 442
Total Fats 18.5g
Carbs: 59.8g
Protein 14.8g
Dietary Fiber: 10.5g

SIMPLE HARDBOILED EGGS

Preparation Time: 3 Mins
Total Time: 10 Mins
Servings: 6

Ingredients:
- 12 Eggs
- 1 cup of Water

Direction
1. Pour the water into the Instant Pot and place the eggs inside.
2. Put the lid on and then turn it clockwise to seal.
3. After the chiming sound, set the Instant Pot to MANUAL.
4. Cook on HIGH for 7 minutes.
5. Release the pressure quickly.
6. Prepare an ice bath and place the eggs inside.
7. Let cool until safe to handle.
8. Peel and serve as desired.
9. Enjoy!

Nutrition Values:
Calories 140
Total Fats 9g
Carbs: 1.8g
Protein 12g
Dietary Fiber: 0g

BREAKFAST EGGS CHEESE

Preparation Time: 10 Mins
Total Time: 40 Mins
Servings: 6

Ingredients:
- 1/2 cup coconut cream
- 6 eggs
- 1 cup cooked ham
- 1 red onion, chopped
- 1 cup vegan cheddar cheese
- 1 cup chopped kale leaves
- 1 tspHerbes de Provence
- 1/8 tsp. sea salt
- 1/8 tsp. pepper

Direction
1. In a bowl, whisk together coconut cream and eggs until well combined; stir in the remaining ingredients and pour the mixture into a heatproof bowl or dish, cover.
2. Add a cup of water in your instant pot and place a trivet over water.
3. Add the bowl and lock lid; cook on high for 20 minutes and then release pressure naturally.
4. Serve hot with a glass of fresh orange juice.

Nutrition Values:
Calories 285
Total Fats 18.3g
Carbs: 14.4g
Protein 16.6g
Dietary Fiber: 5g

KALE EGG BREAKFAST CASSEROLE

Preparation Time: 15 Mins
Total Time: 45 Mins
Servings: 6

Ingredients:
- 2 tablespoons coconut oil
- 1 ⅓ cups sliced leek
- 2 teaspoons minced garlic
- 1 cup chopped kale
- 8 eggs
- ⅔ cups sweet potato, peeled and grated
- 1 ½ cups breakfast sausage,

Direction
1. Set your instant pot to sauté mode and melt coconut oil;
2. Stir in garlic, leeks, and kale and sauté for about 5 minutes or until tender; transfer the veggies to a plate and clean the pot.
3. Whisk together eggs, beef sausage, sweet potato and the sautéed veggies in a large bowl until well blended; pour the mixture in a heatproof bowl or pan.
4. Add water to the instant pot and insert a trivet; place the bowl onto the trivet and lock lid.
5. Cook on manual for 25 minutes and then let pressure come down on its own.
6. Remove the casserole and cut into equal slices.

Nutrition Values:
Calories 280
Total Fats 19g
Carbs: 7g
Protein 25g
Dietary Fiber: 1g

EASY BREAKFAST CASSEROLE

Preparation Time: 25 Mins
Total Time: 50 Mins
Servings: 6

Ingredients:
- 1½ pound breakfast sausage
- 1 large yam or sweet potato, diced
- 2 tbsp. melted coconut oil
- 10 eggs, whisked
- ½ tsp. garlic powder
- 2 cups chopped spinach
- ½ yellow onion, diced
- ½ tsp. sea salt

Direction
1. Coat a 9x12 baking dish with cooking spray.
2. Toss the diced sweet potatoes in coconut oil and sprinkle with salt. Set aside.
3. Set a sauté pan over medium heat; add yellow onion and sauté for about 4 minutes or until fragrant.
4. Stir in breakfast sausage and cook for about 5 minutes or until the sausages are no longer pink.
5. Transfer the sausage mixture to the baking dish and add spinach and sweet potatoes.
6. Top with eggs and sprinkle with garlic powder and salt. Mix until well combined and pour the mixture in a heatproof bowl or pan.
7. Add water to the instant pot and insert a trivet; place the dish onto the trivet and lock lid.
8. Cook on high for 25 minutes and then let pressure come down on its own.
9. Remove the casserole and cut into equal slices.

Nutrition Values:
Calories 76
Total Fats 5.2g
Carbs: 0.9g
Protein 6.5g
Dietary Fiber: 0.2g

TOMATO DILL FRITTATA

Preparation Time: 10 Mins
Total Time: 30 Mins
Servings: 4

Ingredients:
- 8 free-range eggs, whisked
- 2 tbsp. chopped fresh chives
- 2 tbsp. chopped fresh dill
- 4 tomatoes, diced
- 1 tsp. red pepper flakes
- 2 garlic cloves, minced
- Coconut oil, for greasing the pan
- Sea salt
- Black pepper

Direction
1. Grease a cast iron skillet or saucepan and set aside.
2. In a large bowl, whisk together the eggs; beat in the remaining ingredients until well mixed.
3. Pour the egg mixture into the prepared pan and pour the mixture in a heatproof bowl or pan.
4. Add water to the instant pot and insert a trivet; place the pan onto the trivet and lock lid.
5. Cook on high for 20 minutes and then let pressure come down on its own.
6. Remove the casserole and cut into equal slices.
7. Garnish the frittata with extra chives and dill to serve.

Nutrition Values:
Calories 166
Total Fats 10.3g
Carbs: 7.2g
Protein 12.7g
Dietary Fiber: 1.9g

KOREAN STEAMED EGGS

Preparation Time: 5 Mins
Total Time: 10 Mins
Servings: 1

Ingredients:
- 1 large egg
- pinch of sesame seeds
- 1 tsp chopped scallions
- 1/3 cup cold water
- pinch of garlic powder
- pinch of salt
- pinch of pepper

Direction
1. In a small bowl, whisk together water and eggs until frothy; strain the mixture through a fine mesh into a heat proof bowl.
2. Whisk in the remaining ingredients until well combined; set aside.
3. Add a cup of water to an instant pot and place a steamer basket or trivet in the pot; place the bowl with the mixture over the basket and lock lid.

4. Cook on high for 5 minutes and then natural release pressure.
5. Serve hot with a glass of freshly squeezed orange juice.

Nutrition Values:
Calories 76
Total Fats 5.2g
Carbs: 0.9g
Protein 6.5g
Dietary Fiber: 0.2g

EGG & HAM CASSEROLE

Preparation Time: 10 Mins
Total Time: 35 Mins
Servings: 4

Ingredients:
- 1 cup almond milk
- 10 large eggs
- 2 cups shredded vegan cheddar cheese
- 1 cup chopped ham
- 1/2 onion, diced
- 4 medium red potatoes, chopped
- 1 teaspoon salt
- 1 teaspoon pepper

Direction
1. Grease an instant pot with nonstick cooking spray and add two cups of water; insert a steamer basket.
2. Whisk almond milk and eggs in a bowl until well blended; beat in cheese, onion, ham, potatoes, salt and pepper until well combined.
3. Transfer the egg mixture into a heatproof bowl and insert into the pot. Lock lid and press manual button; set for 25 minutes.
4. When done, let pressure come down on its own and then serve the quiche with your favorite toppings.

Nutrition Values:
Calories 528
Total Fats 30g
Carbs: 41.1g
Protein 26.9g
Dietary Fiber: 5.8g

SPICY GLUTEN-FREE PANCAKES

Preparation Time: 10 Mins
Total Time: 26 Mins
Servings: 4

Ingredients:
- 4 tablespoons coconut oil
- 1 cup coconut milk
- ½ cup tapioca flour
- ½ cup almond flour
- 1 teaspoon salt
- ½ teaspoon chili powder
- ¼ teaspoon turmeric powder
- ¼ teaspoon black pepper
- ½ inch ginger, grated
- 1 serrano pepper, minced
- 1 handful cilantro, chopped
- ½ red onion, chopped

Direction
1. In a bowl, combine coconut milk, tapioca flour, almond flour and spices until well blended; stir in ginger, Serrano pepper, cilantro, and red onion until well combined.
2. Grease the interior of the instant pot with coconut oil; pour in the batter and seal the pot with vent closed; set pressure to low and cook for 30 minutes.
3. Serve the crispy pancakes with freshly squeezed orange juice.

Nutrition Values:
Calories 447
Total Fats 34.6g
Carbs: 34g
Protein 4.6g
Dietary Fiber: 3.3g

CAULIFLOWER PUDDING

Preparation Time: 5 Mins
Cook Time: 20 Mins
Servings: 4

Ingredients:
- 1½ cups unsweetened coconut milk or unsweetened almond milk
- 1 cup water
- 1 cup cauliflower rice pulse florets in food processor until rice-like consistency
- 2 teaspoons organic ground cinnamon powder
- 1 teaspoon pure vanilla extract
- Pinch of salt

Direction
1. Add all ingredients to Instant Pot. Stir until combined.
2. Press "Manual" button. Cook on HIGH 20 minutes.
3. When done, naturally release pressure for 10 minutes, then quick release remaining pressure. Remove lid. Serve.

Nutrition Values:
Calories: 213; Fat: 21.6g, Carbohydrates: 6.3g, Protein: 2.7g, Dietary Fiber: 2.5g

BAKED BLUEBERRY OATMEAL

Preparation time: 5 minutes

Cooking time: 30 minutes
Total time: 35 minutes
Servings: 6

Ingredients:
- 2 ¼ cups of whole oats
- ½ cup of brown sugar
- 14 oz. of canned coconut milk, light or regular
- 3 cups of water
- 1 cup of blueberries frozen or fresh
- 1 tsp. of vanilla
- 1/8 tsp. of salt
- ¼ cup of gluten free flour blend

Directions:
1. Turn on your Pressure Cooker.
2. Add all the ingredients into the bottom of your Pressure Cooker.
3. Close and lock the lid in place and ensure that the valve is in sealing position.
4. Set to bake for about 30 minutes.
5. Unplug when the machine is cooking. Use a natural pressure release and carefully open the lid.
6. Serve warm and enjoy.

POBLANO CHEESE FRITTATA

Preparation time: 10 minutes
Cooking time: 30 minutes
Total time: 40 minutes
Servings: 4

Ingredients:
- 4 eggs
- 1 cup of half and half
- 10 oz. of diced canned green chilies
- ½-1 tsp. of salt
- ½ tsp. of ground cumin
- 1 cup of Mexican blend shredded cheese, divided
- ¼ cup of chopped cilantro

Directions:
1. In a medium bowl, beat the eggs and combine with half and half, diced green chilis, salt, cumin, and ½ cup of shredded cheese.
2. Pour the mixture into a 6-inch greased metal or silicone pan and cover with a piece of aluminum foil.
3. Pour 2 cups of water into the bottom of your Instant Pot and add the trivet in the pot. Place the covered pan on the trivet.
4. Select Manual function to cook on High Pressure for about 20 minutes.
5. When the time is up, use a natural pressure release for about 10 minutes, then quick release any remaining pressure.
6. Carefully open the lid and remove the pan from your Instant Pot. Scatter the remaining half cup of cheese on top of the quiche.
7. Place in a broiler and broil for about 5 minutes until cheese is bubbling and brown.
8. Serve and enjoy!

REGULAR OATMEAL

Preparation time: 6 minutes
Cooking time: 7 minutes
Total time: 13 minutes
Servings: 5

Ingredients:
- 1 cup of regular oats
- 3 cups of water or depending on your desired thickness of your Oatmeal.
- Optional Toppings: apples, blueberries, strawberries, bananas, pears, sliced dates, cinnamon, flax seed, flax seed, maple syrup or agave, all kinds of nuts, coconut flakes, or peanut butter etc.

Directions:
1. Add water and regular oats into the Instant Pot.
2. Close and lock the lid in place and ensure that the valve is in sealing position.
3. Press the manual setting to cook on high pressure for about 7 minutes.
4. When the time is up, use a natural pressure release for about 10 minutes.
5. Carefully open the lid once the pressure has been released.
6. Add the oatmeal into a bowl and add any optional toppings.
7. Serve and enjoy!

BUCKWHEAT PORRIDGE

Preparation time: 5 minutes
Cooking time: 25 minutes
Total time: 30 minutes
Servings: 4

Ingredients:
- 1 cup of raw buckwheat groats
- 3 cups of rice milk
- 1 banana, sliced
- ¼ cup of raisins
- 1 teaspoon of ground cinnamon
- ½ teaspoon of vanilla
- Chopped nuts, optional

Directions:
1. Gently rinse the buckwheat and add in your Instant Pot.
2. Add the rice milk, banana, raisins, cinnamon and vanilla into the bottom of your Instant

Pot.
3. Close and lock the lid in place and ensure that the valve is in sealing position.
4. Select Manual function to cook on High Pressure for about 6 minutes.
5. When the time is up, use a natural pressure release for about 20 minutes.
6. Carefully remove the lid and stir porridge with a long handled spoon.
7. Add more rice milk to individual bowls to achieve your desired consistency. Sprinkle with chopped nuts if desired.
8. Serve and enjoy!

CRUSTLESS TOMATO SPINACH QUICHE

Yield: 6
Preparation time: 10 minutes
Cooking time: 20 minutes
Total time: 30 minutes

Ingredients:
- 12 large eggs
- ½ cup of milk
- ½ tsp. of salt
- ¼ tsp. of fresh ground black pepper
- 3 cups fresh baby spinach, roughly chopped
- 1 cup of diced seeded tomato
- 3 large green onions, sliced
- 4 tomato slices, for topping
- ¼ cup of shredded Parmesan cheese

Directions:
1. Add a trivet into the bottom of your Instant Pot and pour 1 ½ cups of water.
2. In a medium bowl, whisk together the eggs, milk, salt and pepper. Add spinach, tomato, and green onions to a 1 ½ quart baking dish and give everything a good mix.
3. Add the egg mixture over the veggies and give everything a good stir to combine. Carefully add the sliced tomatoes on top and sprinkle with Parmesan cheese.
4. Place the dish on the trivet with a sling into the inner cooking pot of your Instant Pot. Close and lock the lid in place.
5. Press Manual function to cook on High Pressure for about 20 minutes. When the time is up, wait for about 10 minutes, then use a quick pressure release.
6. Carefully open the lid, remove the dish from your Instant Pot. Use a broiler to broil until lightly browned.
7. Serve and enjoy!

CHEESY INSTANT POT GOULASH

Preparation time: 15 minutes
Cooking time: 5 minutes
Total time: 20 minutes
Servings: 8

Ingredients:
- 1 pound of spicy sausage or ground beef
- 2 tablespoons of olive oil
- ½ large onion diced
- 1 bell pepper diced, optional
- 1 cup of beef broth
- 4 cup of uncooked pasta, 4 measuring cups full of uncooked pasta
- 24 ounces spaghetti sauce
- 14.5 ounces petite diced tomatoes
- 1 cup of heavy cream
- ¾ cup of parmesan cheese, grated
- ¾ cup of cheddar cheese, grated

Directions:
1. Press the Sauté function on your Instant Pot and add the olive oil.
2. Add the sausage or ground beef, onions and diced bell peppers. Sauté until the meat is no longer pink. Press the Cancel function.
3. Add in your beef broth, spaghetti sauce, diced tomatoes and the uncooked noodles and do not stir. Ensure that the noodles are submerged in the liquid.
4. Secure the lid in place and cook on High Pressure for 5 minutes. When the timer beeps, do a quick pressure release.
5. Carefully open the lid and stir in heavy cream and cheese. Stir until cheese is melted. The goulash will thicken as it cools.
6. Serve and enjoy!

MAINS

RICE WITH CHICKEN AND VEGGIES

Preparation time: 10 minutes
Cooking time: 20 minutes
Servings: 4

Ingredients:
- ½ cup coconut aminos
- 1/3 cup rice wine vinegar
- 2 teaspoons arrowroot powder
- 2 tablespoons olive oil
- 1 chicken breast, skinless, boneless and cubed
- ½ cup red bell pepper, chopped
- A pinch of black pepper
- 2 garlic cloves, minced
- ½ teaspoon ginger, grated
- ½ cup carrots, grated
- 1 cup white rice
- 2 cups water
- 1 cup broccoli florets
- ½ cup edamame beans

Directions:
1. In your instant pot, mix the aminos with the vinegar, arrowroot powder and oil and whisk well.
2. Add chicken, bell pepper, black pepper, cloves, ginger, carrots, rice, water, broccoli and edamame beans, cover and cook on High for 20 minutes.
3. Stir the whole mix once again, divide it into bowls and serve.
4. Enjoy!

Nutrition Value: calories 321, fat 12, fiber 6, carbs 22, protein 17

TOMATO CREAM

Preparation time: 10 minutes
Cooking time: 15 minutes
Servings: 4

Ingredients:
- 3 garlic cloves, minced
- 1 yellow onion, chopped
- 3 carrots, chopped
- 15 ounces tomato sauce, no-salt-added
- 1 tablespoon avocado oil
- 15 ounces roasted tomatoes, no-salt-added
- 1 cup low-sodium veggie stock
- 1 tablespoon tomato paste, no-salt-added
- 1 tablespoon basil, dried
- ¼ teaspoon oregano, dried
- 3 ounces coconut cream
- A pinch of black pepper

Directions:
1. In your instant pot, mix the garlic with the onion, carrots, tomato sauce, oil, tomatoes, stock, tomato paste, basil, oregano and black pepper, toss, cover and cook on High for 15 minutes.
2. Blend using an immersion blender, add the cream, toss, divide into bowls and serve.
3. Enjoy!

Nutrition Value: calories 271, fat 6, fiber 9, carbs 18, protein 7

CARROT SOUP

Preparation time: 10 minutes
Cooking time: 15 minutes
Servings: 4

Ingredients:
- 10 carrots, chopped
- 3 garlic cloves, minced
- 1 yellow onion, chopped
- 14 ounces coconut milk
- 1 and ½ cups veggie stock, low-sodium
- 1 tablespoon red curry paste
- 2 tablespoons cilantro, chopped

Directions:
1. In your instant pot, mix the carrots with the garlic, onion, milk, stock, curry paste and cilantro, toss, cover and cook on High for 15 minutes.
2. Blend using an immersion blender, ladle into bowls and serve.
3. Enjoy!

Nutrition Value: calories 251, fat 4, fiber 8, carbs 18, protein 6

SIMPLE CHILI

Preparation time: 10 minutes
Cooking time: 15 minutes
Servings: 4

Ingredients:
- 1 cup low-sodium chicken stock
- 2 tablespoons tomato paste
- 1 teaspoon cocoa powder
- 1 tablespoon avocado oil
- 1 yellow onion, chopped
- 2 garlic cloves, minced

- 1 pound chicken meat, ground
- 1 tablespoon chili powder
- 1 tablespoon cumin, ground
- 1 teaspoon oregano, dried
- 28 ounces canned kidney beans, no-salt-added, drained and rinsed
- 28 ounces canned tomatoes, no-salt-added
- 2 cups corn
- A pinch of black pepper

Directions:
1. In your instant pot, mix the stock with tomato paste, cocoa powder, oil, onion, garlic, chicken, chili powder, cumin, oregano, kidney beans, tomatoes, corn and black pepper, toss, cover and cook on High for 15 minutes.
2. Divide the chili into bowls and serve.
3. Enjoy!

Nutrition Value: calories 265, fat 6, fiber 9, carbs 19, protein 7

LENTILS SOUP

Preparation time: 10 minutes
Cooking time: 20 minutes
Servings: 4

Ingredients:
- 2 teaspoons olive oil
- ½ yellow onion, chopped
- 2 carrots, chopped
- 1 celery stalk, chopped
- 4 garlic cloves, minced
- 2 teaspoons cumin, ground
- 1 teaspoon turmeric powder
- 1 teaspoon thyme, dried
- 1 cup brown lentils, rinsed
- 4 cups veggie stock, low-sodium
- 7 ounces baby spinach

Directions:
1. Set your instant pot on sauté mode, add the oil, heat it up, add onions, celery and carrots, stir and cook for about 5 minutes.
2. Add garlic, cumin, turmeric, thyme, lentils and stock, cover and cook on High for 12 minutes.
3. Add spinach, cover, cook on High for 3 minutes more, ladle the soup into bowls and serve.
4. Enjoy!

Nutrition Value: calories 251, fat 4, fiber 8, carbs 16, protein 7

EASY CHICKEN CACCIATORE

Preparation time: 10 minutes
Cooking time: 20 minutes
Servings: 6

Ingredients:
- 8 chicken legs
- Black pepper to the taste
- 2 tablespoons avocado oil
- 1 yellow onion, chopped
- 3 carrots, chopped
- 1 red bell pepper, chopped
- ½ pound mushrooms, sliced
- 2 garlic cloves, minced
- 1 teaspoon oregano, dried
- ¼ teaspoon red pepper flakes
- 2 tablespoons basil, chopped
- 1 cup chicken stock, low-sodium
- 16 ounces canned tomatoes, no-salt-added and chopped
- 2 tablespoons parsley, chopped
- 1 teaspoon thyme, chopped
- ¼ cup balsamic vinegar

Directions:
1. In your instant pot, mix the chicken with black pepper, oil, onion, carrots, bell pepper, mushrooms, garlic, oregano, pepper flakes, basil, stock, tomatoes, vinegar and thyme, toss, cover and cook on High for 20 minutes.
2. Add parsley, toss, divide between plates and serve.
3. Enjoy!

Nutrition Value: calories 300, fat 7, fiber 9, carbs 19, protein 7

SWEET PAPRIKA PORK CHOPS

Preparation time: 10 minutes
Cooking time: 15 minutes
Servings: 4

Ingredients:
- 4 pork chops, boneless
- 1 tablespoon olive oil
- 1 cup chicken stock, low-sodium
- A pinch of black pepper
- 1 teaspoon sweet paprika

Directions:
1. Set your instant pot on sauté mode, add the oil, heat it up, add pork chops, brown for a few minutes on each side, add paprika, black pepper and stock, cover the pot, cook on High for 5 minutes, divide between plates and serve.
2. Enjoy!

Nutrition Value: calories 362, fat 4, fiber 8, carbs 19, protein 11

SIMPLE PORK ROAST

Preparation time: 10 minutes
Cooking time: 45 minutes
Servings: 12

Ingredients:
- ½ cup beef stock
- 1 tablespoon olive oil
- ¼ cup Jamaican spice mix, no-salt-added
- 4 pounds pork shoulder

Directions:
1. In a bowl, mix pork with oil and spice mix and rub well.
2. Set your instant pot on sauté mode, add pork, brown for a few minutes on each side, add stock, cover the pot and cook pork shoulder on High for 40 minutes.
3. Slice roast and serve
4. Enjoy!

Nutrition Value: calories 371, fat 6, fiber 7, carbs 17, protein 16

BROCCOLI CREAM

Preparation time: 10 minutes
Cooking time: 10 minutes
Servings: 4

Ingredients:
- 1 broccoli head, florets separated and roughly chopped
- 4 cups low-sodium chicken stock
- A pinch of black pepper
- ¼ teaspoon garlic powder
- 1 cup carrots, chopped
- 2 tablespoons olive oil
- 1 yellow onion, chopped
- 2 cups fat-free cheddar cheese, shredded
- 1 cup coconut cream

Directions:
1. Set your instant pot on sauté mode, add the oil, heat it up, add onion, stir and cook for 2-3 minutes.
2. Add carrots, broccoli, stock, garlic powder, salt and pepper, stir, cover, cook on High for 5 minutes, add cream, blend using an immersion blender, ladle into bowls, sprinkle cheese on top and serve.
3. Enjoy!

Nutrition Value: calories 300, fat 6, fiber 7, carbs 14, protein 9

COCONUT CHICKEN MIX

Preparation time: 10 minutes
Cooking time: 30 minutes
Servings: 4

Ingredients:
- 3 tomatoes, chopped
- 2 pounds chicken thighs, skinless, boneless and cubed
- 2 tablespoons olive oil
- 1 cup low sodium chicken stock
- 14 ounces coconut milk
- 2 garlic cloves, minced
- 1 cup white onion, chopped
- 3 red chilies, chopped
- Black pepper to the taste
- 1 tablespoon water
- 1 tablespoon ginger, grated
- 2 teaspoons coriander, ground
- 1 teaspoon cinnamon, ground
- 1 teaspoon turmeric powder
- 1 teaspoon fennel seeds, ground
- 1 tablespoon lime juice

Directions:
1. In your food processor, mix white onion with garlic, chilies, water, ginger, coriander, cinnamon, turmeric, fennel and black pepper and blend until you obtain a paste.
2. Set your instant pot on sauté mode, add the oil, heat it up, add the paste you made, stir and cook for 30 seconds.
3. Add chicken, tomatoes and stock, stir, cover the pot and cook on High for 15 minutes.
4. Add coconut milk, stir, cover the pot again and cook on High for 7 minutes more.
5. Add lime juice, stir, divide into bowls and serve.
6. Enjoy!

Nutrition Value: calories 381, fat 16, fiber 4, carbs 17, protein 17

FISH SOUP

Preparation time: 10 minutes
Cooking time: 20 minutes
Servings: 4

Ingredients:
- 1 yellow onion, chopped
- 12 cups low-sodium chicken stock
- 1 pound carrots, sliced
- 1 tablespoon olive oil
- Black pepper to the taste
- 2 tablespoons ginger, minced
- 1 cup water
- 1 pound white fish, skinless, boneless and cut into medium chunks

Directions:

1. Set your instant pot on sauté mode, add oil, heat it up, add onion, stir and cook for 4 minutes.
2. Add water, stock, ginger and carrots, stir, cover and cook on High for 8 minutes.
3. Blend soup using an immersion blender, add the fish and pepper, stir a bit, cover, cook on High for 6 minutes, ladle into bowls and serve hot.
4. Enjoy!

Nutrition Value: calories 261, fat 6, fiber 2, carbs 11, protein 9

ITALIAN SHRIMP MIX

Preparation time: 10 minutes
Cooking time: 20 minutes
Servings: 4

Ingredients:
- 8 ounces mushrooms, chopped
- 1 pound shrimp, peeled and deveined
- 1 yellow onion, chopped
- 1 asparagus bunch, cut into medium pieces
- Black pepper to the taste
- 2 tablespoons olive oil
- 2 teaspoons Italian seasoning
- 1 teaspoon red pepper flakes, crushed
- 1 cup fat-free cheddar cheese, grated
- 2 garlic cloves, minced
- 1 cup coconut cream
- 1 cup water

Directions:
1. Put the water in your instant pot, add steamer basket, add asparagus, cover, cook on High for 3 minutes, cool it down in a bowl filled with ice water, drain and leave aside.
2. Clean your instant pot, set it on sauté mode, add oil, heat it up, add mushrooms and onion, stir and cook for 3-4 minutes.
3. Add pepper flakes, Italian seasoning, pepper and asparagus, stir and cook for a few minutes more.
4. Add coconut cream, cheddar, garlic and shrimp, cover, cook on High for 4 minutes, divide between plates and serve.
5. Enjoy!

Nutrition Value: calories 275, fat 6, fiber 2, carbs 17, protein 8

LEMON SHRIMP

Preparation time: 10 minutes
Cooking time: 3 minutes
Servings: 4

Ingredients:
- 2 tablespoons olive oil
- 1 pound shrimp, peeled and deveined
- 2 tablespoons lemon juice
- Black pepper to the taste
- 2 tablespoons garlic, minced
- 1 tablespoon lemon zest, grated

Directions:
1. Set your instant pot on sauté mode, add the oil, heat it up, add garlic, shrimp, lemon juice, lemon zest and pepper, stir, cover, cook on High for 3 minutes, divide between plates and serve with a side salad
2. Enjoy!

Nutrition Value: calories 209, fat 1, fiber 3, carbs 16, protein 9

CABBAGE AND BEEF STEW

Preparation time: 10 minutes
Cooking time: 1 hour and 20 minutes
Servings: 6

Ingredients:
2 and ½ pounds beef brisket, fat removed
2 bay leaves
4 cups water
4 carrots, chopped
3 garlic cloves, chopped
1 cabbage head, roughly shredded
Black pepper to the taste

Directions:
1. Put the beef brisket in your instant pot, add water, pepper, garlic and bay leaves, cover and cook at High for 1 hour.
2. Add carrots and cabbage, stir, cover the pot again, cook on High for 6 minutes, divide into bowls and serve.
3. Enjoy!

Nutrition Value: calories 281, fat 8, fiber 3, carbs 21, protein 8

SHRIMP AND TOMATOES MIX

Preparation time: 10 minutes
Cooking time: 11 minutes
Servings: 4

Ingredients:
- 2 pounds shrimp, peeled and deveined
- 1 pound tomatoes, peeled and chopped
- 4 tablespoons olive oil
- 4 onions, chopped
- 1 teaspoon coriander, ground
- 1 teaspoon curry powder
- Juice of 1 lemon
- A pinch of black pepper

Directions:

1. Set the instant pot on sauté mode, add oil, heat it up, add onions, stir and cook for 5 minutes.
2. Add black pepper, coriander, curry, tomatoes, lemon juice and shrimp, stir, cover, cook on High for 6 minutes more, divide everything into bowls and serve.
3. Enjoy!

Nutrition Value: calories 201, fat 4, fiber 1, carbs 17, protein 15

MACKEREL AND ORANGE SAUCE

Preparation time: 10 minutes
Cooking time: 10 minutes
Servings: 4

Ingredients:
- 4 mackerel fillets, skinless and boneless
- 4 spring onions, chopped
- 1 teaspoons olive oil
- 1-inch ginger piece, grated
- Black pepper to the taste
- Juice and zest of 1 orange
- 1 cup low-sodium fish stock

Directions:
1. Season the fillets with black pepper and rub them with the olive oil.
2. Put stock, ginger, orange juice, orange zest and onions in your instant pot, add steamer basket, add fish fillets, cover and cook on High for 10 minutes.
3. Divide fish fillets between plates, drizzle the orange sauce all over and serve.
4. Enjoy!

Nutrition Value: calories 200, fat 4, fiber 9, carbs 19, protein 14

FISH CURRY

Preparation time: 10 minutes
Cooking time: 10 minutes
Servings: 6

Ingredients:
- 6 white fish fillets, skinless, boneless and cut into medium pieces
- 1 tomato, chopped
- 1 tablespoon olive oil
- 14 ounces coconut milk
- 2 onions, sliced
- 2 garlic cloves, minced
- 6 curry leaves
- 1 tablespoons coriander, ground
- 1 tablespoon ginger, finely grated
- ½ teaspoon turmeric powder
- Black pepper to the taste
- ½ teaspoon fenugreek, ground
- 2 tablespoons lemon juice

Directions:
- Set your instant pot on Sauté mode, add oil and curry leaves, fry for 1 minute, add ginger, onion, garlic, coriander, turmeric, fenugreek, coconut milk, tomatoes and fish, stir, cover and cook on Low for 10 minutes.
- Add black pepper to the taste, stir, divide into bowls, and serve with lemon juice drizzled on top.
- Enjoy!

Nutrition Value: calories 281, fat 6, fiber 9, carbs 14, protein 7

SALMON, PEAS AND PARSLEY DRESSING

Preparation time: 15 minutes
Cooking time: 15 minutes
Servings: 4

Ingredients:
- 16 ounces salmon fillets, boneless and skin-on
- 1 tablespoon parsley, chopped
- 10 ounces peas
- 9 ounces veggie stock, low-sodium
- 2 cups water
- ½ teaspoon oregano, dried
- ½ teaspoon sweet paprika
- 2 garlic cloves, minced
- A pinch of black pepper

Directions:
1. In your food processor mix garlic with parsley, oregano, paprika and stock and blend well.
2. Add the water to your instant pot, add steamer basket, add fish fillets inside, season them with black pepper, cover, cook on High for 10 minutes and divide between plates.
3. Add peas to the steamer basket, cover the pot again and cook at High for 5 minutes.
4. Divide the peas next to the fish fillets and serve with the parsley dressing you've made drizzled on top.
5. Enjoy!

Nutrition Value: calories 271, fat 6, fiber 9, carbs 19, protein 19

CHILI SALMON

Preparation time: 10 minutes
Cooking time: 7 minutes
Servings: 4

Ingredients:
- 4 salmon fillets, boneless and skin-on
- 2 tablespoons assorted chili pepper, chopped
- Juice of 1 lemon

- 1 lemon, sliced
- 1 cup water
- Black pepper to the taste

Directions:
1. Add the water to your instant pot, add steamer basket, add salmon fillets, season with black pepper, chili pepper and lemon juice, top with lemon slices, cover and cook on High for 7 minutes.
2. Divide salmon and lemon slices between plates and serve with a side salad.
3. Enjoy!

Nutrition Value: calories 281, fat 8, fiber 8, carbs 19, protein 7

TOMATO SHRIMP

Preparation time: 10 minutes
Cooking time: 10 minutes
Servings: 4

Ingredients:
- 1 and ½ pounds shrimp, peeled and deveined
- 2 tablespoons olive oil
- 1 cup yellow onion, chopped
- 2 tablespoons parsley, chopped
- 4 garlic cloves, minced
- 2 teaspoons hot paprika
- ½ cup fish stock, low-sodium
- 1 cup tomato sauce
- 1 teaspoon hot pepper, crushed
- ¼ teaspoon thyme, dried
- Black pepper to the taste

Directions:
1. Set your instant pot on Sauté mode, add the oil, heat it up, add shrimp, cook for 2 minutes and transfer to a platter.
2. Add onion, parsley, garlic, paprika, stock, tomato sauce, red pepper, thyme and pepper, stir, cover and cook on High for 4 minutes.
3. Add shrimp, cover again, cook on High for 2 minutes, divide between plates and serve.
4. Enjoy!

Nutrition Value: calories 251, fat 7, fiber 9, carbs 20, protein 7

SHRIMP, TOMATOES AND POTATOES

Preparation time: 10 minutes
Cooking time: 18 minutes
Servings: 4

Ingredients:
- 2 pounds shrimp, peeled and deveined
- 1 pound tomatoes, peeled and chopped
- 8 potatoes, cut into quarters
- 2 cups water
- 4 tablespoons olive oil
- 4 yellow onions, chopped
- 1 teaspoon coriander, ground
- 1 teaspoon curry powder
- Juice of 1 lemon

Directions:
1. Add the water to the pot, add steamer basket, add potatoes inside, cover, cook on High for 10 minutes, transfer them to a bowl and clean the pot.
2. Set the pot on Sauté mode, add oil, heat it up, add onions, stir and cook for 5 minutes.
3. Add coriander, curry, tomatoes, shrimp, lemon juice and return potatoes, stir, cover, cook on High for 3 minutes, divide into bowls and serve.
4. Enjoy!

Nutrition Value: calories 200, fat 4, fiber 8, carbs 18, protein 18

SAUSAGE AND BEANS MIX

Preparation time: 15 minutes
Cooking time: 30 minutes
Servings: 8

Ingredients:
- 1 pound smoked sausage, low-sodium and sliced
- 1 pound red beans, dried
- 1 bay leaf
- 2 tablespoons Cajun seasoning
- 1 celery stalk, chopped
- Black pepper to the taste
- ½ green bell pepper, chopped
- 1 teaspoon parsley, dried
- 5 cups water
- ¼ teaspoon cumin, ground
- 1 garlic clove, chopped
- 1 small yellow onion, chopped

Directions:
1. In your instant pot, mix beans with sausage, bay leaf, Cajun seasoning, celery, pepper, bell pepper, parsley, cumin, garlic, onion and water, stir, cover, cook on High for 30 minutes, divide mix into bowls and serve.
2. Enjoy!

Nutrition Value: calories 271, fat 6, fiber 8, carbs 29, protein 12

DUCK AND VEGGIES

Preparation time: 10 minutes
Cooking time: 20 minutes
Servings: 4

Ingredients:
- 1 duck, cut into medium pieces
- Black pepper to the taste
- 1 gold potato, cubed
- 1-inch ginger root, sliced
- 4 garlic cloves, minced
- 4 tablespoons coconut aminos
- 2 green onions, chopped
- 4 tablespoons low-sodium veggie stock
- ¼ cup water

Directions:
1. Set your instant pot on Sauté mode, add duck, stir and brown them for a few minutes.
2. Add garlic, ginger, green onions, aminos, black pepper, stock and water, stir, cover and cook on High for 18 minutes.
3. Add potatoes, stir, cover, cook on High for 5 minutes more, divide between plates and serve right away.
4. Enjoy!

Nutrition Value: calories 261, fat 8, fiber 8, carbs 18, protein 16

DUCK, CARROTS AND CUCUMBERS

Preparation time: 10 minutes
Cooking time: 40 minutes
Servings: 8

Ingredients:
- 1 duck, cut into medium pieces
- 1 cucumber, chopped
- 1 tablespoon low-sodium veggie stock
- 2 carrots, chopped
- 2 cups water
- Black pepper to the taste
- 1-inch ginger piece, grated

Directions:
1. Put duck pieces in your instant pot, add cucumber, carrots, stock, water, ginger and pepper, stir, cover, cook on Low for 40 minutes, divide between plates and serve.
2. Enjoy!

Nutrition Value: calories 206, fat 7, fiber 8, carbs 28, protein 16

CHINESE CHICKEN

Preparation time: 10 minutes
Cooking time: 15 minutes
Servings: 4

Ingredients:
- 5 pounds chicken thighs
- Black pepper to the taste
- ½ cup balsamic vinegar
- 1 teaspoon black peppercorns
- 4 garlic cloves, minced
- ½ cup coconut aminos

Directions:
1. In your instant pot, mix chicken with vinegar, aminos, pepper, garlic and peppercorns, stir, cover and cook on High for 15 minutes.
2. Divide chicken mix between plates and serve.
3. Enjoy!

Nutrition Value: calories 261, fat 7, fiber 8, carbs 18, protein 8

MEXICAN PORK AND OKRA SALAD

Preparation time: 10 minutes
Cooking time: 30 minutes
Servings: 4

Ingredients:
- 2 pounds pork sirloin, cubed
- A pinch of salt and black pepper
- 2 teaspoons garlic powder
- 1 tablespoon olive oil
- 1 and ½ cups okra
- 1 cup tomato passata
- 2 garlic cloves, minced
- 1 tablespoon smoked paprika

Directions:
1. Set the instant pot on Sauté mode, add the oil, heat it up, add the meat, garlic, salt and pepper and brown for 5 minutes.
2. Add the remaining ingredients, toss, put the lid on and cook on High for 25 minutes.
3. Release the pressure naturally for 10 minutes, divide everything between plates and serve for lunch.

Nutrition Value: calories 66, fat 3.9, fiber 2, carbs 2.7, protein 1.6

PORK AND KALE MEATBALLS

Preparation time: 10 minutes
Cooking time: 20 minutes
Servings: 6

Ingredients:
- 2 pounds pork stew meat, ground
- ¼ cup cheddar, grated
- 1 cup kale, chopped
- ¼ cup green onions, chopped
- 1 egg, whisked
- A pinch of salt and black pepper
- 1 tablespoon garlic, minced
- 1 tablespoon avocado oil
- 1 cup tomato passata
- ½ cup beef stock

Directions:
1. In a bowl, combine the meat with the cheese, kale, green onions, the egg, garlic, salt and pepper, stir well and shape medium meatballs out of this mix.
2. Set the instant pot on Sauté mode, add the oil, heat it up, add the meatballs and brown them for 2 minutes on each side.
3. Add the sauce and the stock, toss gently, put the lid on and cook on High for 15 minutes.
4. Release the pressure naturally for 10 minutes, divide everything between plates and serve for lunch.

Nutrition Value: calories 362, fat 16.1, fiber 1, carbs 4.4, protein 26.7

TOMATO AND PORK SOUP

Preparation time: 10 minutes
Cooking time: 25 minutes
Servings: 4

Ingredients:
- 1 and ½ pounds pork stew meat, cubed
- 8 cups chicken stock
- 15 ounces tomatoes, chopped
- A pinch of salt and black pepper
- 1 tablespoon chives, chopped

Directions:
1. In your instant pot, mix all the ingredients except the chives, put the lid on and cook on High for 25 minutes.
2. Release the pressure naturally for 10 minutes, divide the soup into bowls and serve.

Nutrition Value: calories 39, fat 4.3, fiber 1.2, carbs 3.4, protein 2.4

CAYENNE PORK AND ARTICHOKES STEW

Preparation time: 10 minutes
Cooking time: 25 minutes
Servings: 4

Ingredients:
- 1 spring onion, chopped
- 2 and ½ pounds pork stew meat, cubed
- 15 ounces canned tomatoes, chopped
- 2 red chilies, chopped
- 1 and ½ cups canned artichoke hearts, chopped
- 2 garlic cloves, minced
- 2 tablespoons avocado oil
- 1 tablespoon cayenne pepper
- A pinch of salt and black pepper
- 1 teaspoon basil, dried

Directions:
1. Set your instant pot on sauté mode, add the oil, heat it up add the onion and the meat and brown for 5 minutes.
2. Add the rest of the ingredients, put the lid on and cook on High for 20 minutes.
3. Release the pressure naturally for 10 minutes, divide the stew into bowls and serve.

Nutrition Value: calories 36, fat 6.4, fiber 2.1, carbs 3.5, protein 1.4

GREEN BEANS SOUP

Preparation time: 10 minutes
Cooking time: 15 minutes
Servings: 4

Ingredients:
- 2 tablespoons olive oil
- 1 shallot, chopped
- 1 teaspoon garlic, minced
- 1 red bell pepper, chopped
- 8 cups chicken stock
- 1 and ½ pounds green beans, trimmed and halved
- 1 cup tomatoes, chopped
- 1 tablespoon chili powder
- 1 cup coconut cream

Directions:
1. Set your instant pot on sauté mode, add the oil, heat it up, add the shallot and the garlic and sauté for 2 minutes.
2. Add the rest of the ingredients, put the lid on and cook on High for 13 minutes.
3. Release the pressure naturally for 10 minutes, divide the soup into bowls and serve.

Nutrition Value: calories 242, fat 22.9, fiber 2.8, carbs 8.9, protein 3.7

BROCCOLI AND ZUCCHINI SOUP

Preparation time: 10 minutes
Cooking time: 15 minutes
Servings: 4

Ingredients:
- 1 shallot, chopped
- 2 teaspoons avocado oil
- 1 pound broccoli florets
- 1 pound zucchinis, sliced
- 4 cups chicken stock
- 1 teaspoon basil, dried
- 1 tablespoon cilantro, chopped

Directions:
1. Set your instant pot on sauté mode, add the oil, heat it up, add the shallot and sauté for 2 minutes.
2. Add the broccoli and the rest of the ingredients, put the lid on and cook on High

for 12 minutes.
3. Release the pressure naturally for 10 minutes, ladle the soup into bowls and serve.

Nutrition Value: calories 70, fat 11.3, fiber 4.3, carbs 6.7, protein 5.3

BEEF SOUP

Preparation time: 10 minutes
Cooking time: 25 minutes
Servings: 4

Ingredients:
- 1 and ½ pound beef meat, cubed
- 2 tablespoons olive oil
- A pinch of salt and black pepper
- 1 cup scallions, chopped
- 1 tablespoon sweet paprika
- 6 cups veggie stock
- 1 tablespoon parsley, chopped

Directions:
1. Set your instant pot on sauté mode, add the oil, heat it up, add the meat and the scallions and brown for 5 minutes.
2. Add the rest of the ingredients, put the lid on and cook on High for 20 minutes.
3. Release the pressure naturally for 10 minutes, ladle the soup into bowls and serve.

Nutrition Value: calories 73, fat 7.3, fiber 1.3, carbs 2.9, protein 0.8

CURRY TOMATO CREAM

Preparation time: 10 minutes
Cooking time: 20 minutes
Servings: 4

Ingredients:
- 1 pound tomatoes, peeled and chopped
- A pinch of salt and black pepper
- 3 garlic cloves, minced
- 1 tablespoon cilantro, chopped
- 2 cups coconut cream
- 2 cups chicken stock
- 1 tablespoon red curry paste
- 2 tablespoons chives, chopped

Directions:
1. In your instant pot, combine the tomatoes with salt, pepper, garlic and the stock, put the lid on and cook on High for 20 minutes.
2. Release the pressure naturally for 10 minutes, transfer the soup to a blender, add the cream and curry paste, pulse well, divide into bowls and serve with the chives and cilantro sprinkled on top.

Nutrition Value: calories 320, fat 30.2, fiber 4.1, carbs 8.1, protein 4.2

SPINACH SOUP

Preparation time: 10 minutes
Cooking time: 20 minutes
Servings: 4

Ingredients:
- 2 teaspoons olive oil
- 1 scallion, chopped
- 1 celery stalk, chopped
- 4 cups baby spinach
- 4 garlic cloves, minced
- 2 teaspoons cumin, ground
- 6 cups veggie stock
- 1 teaspoon basil, dried

Directions:
1. Set your instant pot on sauté mode, add the oil, heat it up, add the scallion and garlic and sauté for 5 minutes.
2. Add the celery, cumin and the basil and sauté for 4 minutes more.
3. Add the spinach and the stock, put the lid on and cook on High for 10 minutes.
4. Release the pressure naturally for 10 minutes, ladle the soup into bowls and serve.

Nutrition Value: calories 37, fat 3.1, fiber 1, carbs 3, protein 1.4

CABBAGE SOUP

Preparation time: 6 minutes
Cooking time: 15 minutes
Servings: 4

Ingredients:
- 1 shallot, chopped
- 1 pound green cabbage, shredded
- 12 cups chicken stock
- 1 celery stalk, chopped
- 1 tablespoon olive oil
- A pinch of salt and black pepper
- 2 tablespoons dill, chopped

Directions:
1. Set your instant pot on sauté mode, add oil, heat it up, add the shallot and sauté for 2 minutes.
2. Add the rest of the ingredients, put the lid on and cook on High for 13 minutes.
3. Release the pressure fast for 6 minutes, ladle the soup into bowls and serve.

Nutrition Value: calories 92, fat 5.4, fiber 3.1, carbs 5.7, protein 3.9

CHEESY COCONUT CREAM

Preparation time: 5 minutes
Cooking time: 20 minutes
Servings: 4

Ingredients:
- 2 tablespoons olive oil
- ½ cup spring onions, chopped
- 6 cups chicken stock
- A pinch of salt and black pepper
- 2 tablespoons parsley, chopped
- 2 cups coconut cream
- 1 cup cheddar cheese, grated

Directions:
1. Set your instant pot on Sauté mode, add the oil, heat it up, add the spring onions and sauté for 2-3 minutes.
2. Add the rest of the ingredients, whisk, put the lid on and cook on High for 15 minutes.
3. Release the pressure naturally for 10 minutes, divide the soup into bowls and serve.

Nutrition Value: calories 313, fat 30.5, fiber 2, carbs 6.1, protein 7.4

EGGPLANT SOUP

Preparation time: 10 minutes
Cooking time: 15 minutes
Servings: 4

Ingredients:
- 1 tablespoon avocado oil
- 1 celery stalk, chopped
- 1 shallot chopped
- 3 eggplants, cubed
- 2 tomatoes, chopped
- 8 cups chicken stock
- A pinch of salt and black pepper
- 2 tablespoons rosemary, chopped

Directions:
1. Set your instant pot on Sauté mode, add the oil, heat it up, add the shallot and celery, stir and sauté for 3 minutes.
2. Add the eggplants and the rest of the ingredients, put the lid on and cook on High for 12 minutes.
3. Release the pressure naturally for 10 minutes, ladle the soup into bowls and serve.

Nutrition Value: calories 144, fat 5.7, fiber 0.2, carbs 5.3, protein 6.1

SIDES

Preparation time: 10 minutes
Cooking time: 12 minutes
Servings: 4

Ingredients:
- 4 garlic cloves, minced
- A pinch of salt and black pepper
- 2 pounds cherry tomatoes, halved
- 2 tablespoons olive oil
- 1 tablespoon dill, chopped
- ½ cups chicken stock
- ¼ cup basil, chopped

Directions:
1. Set your instant pot on sauté mode, add the oil, heat it up, add the garlic and sauté for 2 minutes.
2. Add the rest of the ingredients, put the lid on and cook on High for 10 minutes.
3. Release the pressure naturally for 10 minutes, divide the mix between plates and serve.

Nutrition Value: calories 109, fat 7.6, fiber 2.9, carbs 6.8, protein 2.5

TOMATOES AND CAULIFLOWER MIX

Preparation time: 10 minutes
Cooking time: 12 minutes
Servings: 4

Ingredients:
- ½ cup scallions, chopped
- 1 tablespoon avocado oil
- 1 pound cauliflower florets
- ½ cup chicken stock
- 2 cups cherry tomatoes, halved
- 1 tablespoon chives, chopped
- 2 tablespoons parsley, chopped

Directions:
1. Set your instant pot on Sauté mode, add the oil, heat it up, add the scallions and sauté for 2 minutes.
2. Add the rest of the ingredients, put the lid on and cook on High for 10 minutes.
3. Release the pressure naturally for 10 minutes, divide the mix between plates and serve as a side dish.

Nutrition Value: calories 55, fat 1.6, fiber 0.4, carbs 1.5, protein 3.5

GREEN BEANS AND HERBS

Preparation time: 10 minutes
Cooking time: 12 minutes
Servings: 4

Ingredients:
- 2 tablespoons avocado oil
- ½ teaspoon chili powder
- 1 pound green beans, trimmed and halved
- 1 and ½ cups chicken stock
- 1 tablespoon rosemary, chopped
- 1 tablespoon basil, chopped
- 1 tablespoon dill, chopped
- A pinch of salt and black pepper

- ½ cup almonds, chopped

Directions:
1. In your instant pot, combine the green beans with the chili and the rest of the ingredients. put the lid on and cook on High for 12 minutes.
2. Release the pressure naturally for 10 minutes, divide the mix between plates and serve as a side dish.

Nutrition Value: calories 119, fat 7.2, fiber 3.4, carbs 5.3, protein 4.9

CAULIFLOWER RICE AND OLIVES
Preparation time: 10 minutes
Cooking time: 15 minutes
Servings: 4

Ingredients:
- 1 cup cauliflower rice
- 1 and ½ cup chicken stock
- 1 cup black olives, pitted and sliced
- 1 tablespoon chives, chopped
- A pinch of salt and black pepper
- ½ cup cilantro, chopped

Directions:
1. In your instant pot, mix the cauliflower rice with the rest of the ingredients, put the lid on and cook on High for 15 minutes.
2. Release the pressure naturally for 10 minutes, divide the mix between plates and serve.

Nutrition Value: calories 40, fat 3.6, fiber 1.2, carbs 2.2, protein 0.3

ROSEMARY CAULIFLOWER
Preparation time: 10 minutes
Cooking time: 12 minutes
Servings: 4

Ingredients:
- 1 pound cauliflower florets
- 1 cup chicken stock
- 2 garlic cloves, minced
- A pinch of salt and black pepper
- 1 tablespoon rosemary, chopped
- 1 teaspoon hot chili sauce

Directions:
1. In your instant pot, combine the cauliflower with the stock and the rest of the ingredients, put the lid on and cook on High for 12 minutes.
2. Release the pressure naturally for 10 minutes, divide the mix between plates and serve.

Nutrition Value: calories 36, fat 2.4, fiber 1.5, carbs 2.3, protein 3.6

LEMON ARTICHOKES
Preparation time: 10 minutes
Cooking time: 12 minutes
Servings: 4

Ingredients:
- 4 artichokes, trimmed
- 1 tablespoon olive oil
- 1 tablespoon lemon juice
- 1 tablespoon chives, chopped
- 1 tablespoon sweet paprika
- 1 tablespoon parsley, chopped
- 2 cups water

Directions:
1. In a bowl, mix the artichokes with the oil and the other ingredients except the water and toss.
2. Put the water in your instant pot, add the steamer basket, put the artichokes inside, put the lid on and cook on High for 12 minutes.
3. Release the pressure naturally for 10 minutes, divide the artichokes between plates and serve.

Nutrition Value: calories 113, fat 4, fiber 2.4, carbs 3.5, protein 5.6

CELERY AND BROCCOLI MIX
Preparation time: 10 minutes
Cooking time: 12 minutes
Servings: 4

Ingredients:
- 2 garlic cloves, minced
- 1 tablespoon olive oil
- 1 and ½ cups broccoli florets
- 1 celery stalk, chopped
- ½ cups veggie stock
- A pinch of salt and black pepper
- 2 tablespoons lime juice

Directions:
1. Set your instant pot on sauté mode, add the oil, heat it up, add the garlic and celery and cook for 2 minutes.
2. Add the rest of the ingredients, put the lid on and cook on High for 10 minutes.
3. Release the pressure naturally for 10 minutes, divide the mix between plates and serve.

Nutrition Value: calories 33, fat 3.5, fiber 0.1, carbs 0.7, protein 0.1

ZUCCHINI MIX
Preparation time: 10 minutes
Cooking time: 20 minutes
Servings: 4

Ingredients:

- ½ cup veggie stock
- 3 zucchinis, sliced
- A pinch of salt and black pepper
- 1 tablespoon dill, chopped
- ½ teaspoon nutmeg, grated
- 2 tablespoons sweet paprika

Directions:
1. In your instant pot, mix the zucchinis with the rest of the ingredients, put the lid on and cook on Low for 20 minutes.
2. Release the pressure naturally for 10 minutes, divide the mix between plates and serve.

Nutrition Value: calories 40, fat 2.3, fiber 1.5, carbs 1.9, protein 2.5

DILL FENNEL MIX

Preparation time: 10 minutes
Cooking time: 10 minutes
Servings: 4

Ingredients:
- 2 fennel bulbs, sliced
- ¼ cup chicken stock
- A pinch of salt and black pepper
- 1 tablespoon dill, chopped
- 1 tablespoon parsley, chopped

Directions:
1. In your instant pot, mix the fennel with the stock and the rest of the ingredients, put the lid on and cook on High for 10 minutes.
2. Release the pressure naturally for 10 minutes, divide the mix between plates and serve.

Nutrition Value: calories 39, fat 3.2, fiber 1, carbs 2.9, protein 1.7

MUSHROOMS AND ENDIVES MIX

Preparation time: 10 minutes
Cooking time: 15 minutes
Servings: 4

Ingredients:
- 1 pound white mushrooms, sliced
- 2 spring onions, chopped
- 1 garlic clove, minced
- 2 endives, trimmed and halved
- 1 tablespoon balsamic vinegar
- 1 tablespoon chives, chopped
- 1 cup chicken stock

Directions:
1. In your instant pot, mix the mushrooms with the rest of the ingredients, put the lid on and cook on High for 15 minutes.
2. Release the pressure naturally for 10 minutes, divide the mix between plates and serve.

Nutrition Value: calories 31, fat 3.1, fiber 1.3, carbs 2.3, protein 3.9

WALNUTS GREEN BEANS AND AVOCADO

Preparation time: 10 minutes
Cooking time: 15 minutes
Servings: 6

Ingredients:
2 cups green beans, halved
- ½ cup chicken stock
- ½ cup walnuts, chopped
- 1 avocado, peeled, pitted and cubed
- ¼ teaspoon sweet paprika
- A pinch of salt and black pepper
- 2 teaspoons balsamic vinegar

Directions:
1. In your instant pot, mix the green beans with the stock and the rest of the ingredients, put the lid on and cook on High for 15 minutes.
2. Release the pressure naturally for 10 minutes, divide the mix between plates and serve.

Nutrition Value: calories 146, fat 12.8, fiber 2.5, carbs 6.7, protein 3.9

THYME BRUSSELS SPROUTS

Preparation time: 10 minutes
Cooking time: 12 minutes
Servings: 4

Ingredients:
- 2 and ½ pounds Brussels sprouts, halved
- 2 tablespoons olive oil
- A pinch of salt and black pepper
- 2 shallots, chopped
- ½ cups beef stock
- 1 tablespoon thyme, chopped

Directions:
1. Set your instant pot on Sauté mode, add the oil, heat it up, add the shallots and sauté for 2 minutes.
2. Add the rest of the ingredients, put the lid on and cook on High or 10 minutes.
3. Release the pressure naturally for 10 minutes, divide the mix between plates and serve as a side dish.

Nutrition Value: calories 64, fat 7.1, fiber 0.3, carbs 0.5, protein 0.4

CHIVES BROCCOLI MASH

Preparation time: 10 minutes
Cooking time: 12 minutes
Servings: 4

Ingredients:
- 1 broccoli, florets separated

- A pinch of salt and black pepper
- ½ teaspoon turmeric powder
- ½ cup chicken stock
- 1 tablespoon ghee, melted
- 1 tablespoon chives, chopped

Directions:
1. In your instant pot, mix the broccoli with the rest of the ingredients except the ghee and the chives, put the lid on and cook on High for 12 minutes.
2. Release the pressure naturally for 10 minutes, drain the broccoli, transfer it to a blender, add the ghee, pulse well, divide between plates, sprinkle the chives on top and serve.

Nutrition Value: calories 31, fat 3.3, fiber 0.1, carbs 0.3, protein 0.1

CREAMY ENDIVES

Preparation time: 10 minutes
Cooking time: 10 minutes
Servings: 4

Ingredients:
- 4 endives, trimmed and halved
- ½ cup chicken stock
- ¼ cup coconut cream
- 1 tablespoon dill, chopped
- 1 tablespoon smoked paprika

Directions:
1. In your instant pot, mix the endives with the rest of the ingredients, put the lid on and cook on High for 10 minutes.
2. Release the pressure naturally for 10 minutes, divide the mix between plates and serve as a side dish.

Nutrition Value: calories 43, fat 3.9, fiber 1.1, carbs 2.3, protein 0.9

SPINACH AND KALE MIX

Preparation time: 5 minutes
Cooking time: 10 minutes
Servings: 4

Ingredients:
- 1 and ½ pounds baby spinach
- ½ pound kale, torn
- 1 tablespoon ghee, melted
- A pinch of salt and black pepper
- 1 cup veggie stock
- 1 teaspoon nutmeg, ground
- 1 tablespoon chives, chopped

Directions:
1. In your instant pot, mix the spinach with the kale and the rest of the ingredients, toss, put the lid on and cook on High for 10 minutes.
2. Release the pressure fast for 5 minutes, divide the mix between plates and serve.

Nutrition Value: calories 59, fat 3.4, fiber 1, carbs 2.4, protein 1.8

THYME TOMATOES

Preparation time: 10 minutes
Cooking time: 10 minutes
Servings: 4

Ingredients:
- ½ cup veggie stock
- 1 pound cherry tomatoes, halved
- 1 tablespoon thyme, chopped
- A pinch of salt and black pepper
- 1 teaspoon chili powder
- 1 shallot, chopped
- 1 tablespoon olive oil

Directions:
1. Set the instant pot on Sauté mode, add the oil, heat it up, add the shallot and sauté for 2 minutes.
2. Add the tomatoes and the rest of the ingredients, put the lid on and cook on High for 8 minutes.
3. Release the pressure naturally for 10 minutes, divide the mix between plates and serve.

Nutrition Value: calories 54, fat 3.9, fiber 1.8, carbs 2.4, protein 1.1

LEMON BRUSSELS SPROUTS AND TOMATOES

Preparation time: 10 minutes
Cooking time: 15 minutes
Servings: 4

Ingredients:
- 1 pound Brussels sprouts, trimmed and halved
- ½ pound cherry tomatoes, halved
- 1 tablespoon lemon juice
- 1 tablespoon lemon zest, grated
- ¼ cup veggie stock
- 1 tablespoon rosemary, chopped
- A pinch of salt and black pepper

Directions:
1. In your instant pot, mix the Brussels sprouts with the tomatoes and the remaining ingredients, put the lid on and cook on High for 15 minutes.
2. Release the pressure naturally for 10 minutes, divide the mix between plates and serve as a side dish.

Nutrition Value: calories 64, fat 2.7, fiber 1.5, carbs 2, protein 4.5

CREAMY FENNEL

Preparation time: 5 minutes
Cooking time: 8 minutes
Servings: 4

Ingredients:
- 2 big fennel bulbs, sliced
- 2 tablespoons avocado oil
- 2 spring onions, chopped
- 2 shallots, minced
- 1 garlic clove, minced
- 1 and ½ cups coconut cream
- ¼ teaspoon nutmeg, ground
- A pinch of salt and black pepper

Directions:
1. Set your instant pot on Sauté mode, add the oil, heat it up, add spring onions, shallots and the garlic and sauté for 2 minutes.
2. Add the fennel and the rest of the ingredients, toss, put the lid on and cook on High for 6 minutes.
3. Release the pressure fast for 5 minutes, divide the mix between plates and serve as a side dish.

Nutrition Value: calories 58, fat 3.2, fiber 1, carbs 2.7, protein 0.3

SAFFRON BELL PEPPERS

Preparation time: 10 minutes
Cooking time: 10 minutes
Servings: 4

Ingredients:
- 2 yellow bell peppers, cut into strips
- 2 red bell peppers, thinly sliced
- 3 garlic cloves, minced
- 1 shallots, chopped
- A pinch of salt and black pepper
- 1 teaspoon saffron powder
- ¼ cup chicken stock
- 1 tablespoon cilantro, chopped

Directions:
1. In your instant pot, mix the peppers with the garlic and the rest of the ingredients, put the lid on and cook on High for 10 minutes.
2. Release the pressure naturally for 10 minutes, divide the mix between plates and serve.

Nutrition Value: calories 64, fat 2.4, fiber 1.7, carbs 1.9, protein 1.4

CABBAGE AND PEPPERS

Preparation time: 10 minutes
Cooking time: 15 minutes
Servings: 4

Ingredients:
- 2 red bell peppers, cut into strips
- 1 green cabbage head, shredded
- ½ cup chicken stock
- 1 tablespoon avocado oil
- 1 tablespoon sweet paprika
- A pinch of salt and black pepper
- 2 garlic cloves, minced
- 1 teaspoon lime zest, grated
- 1 teaspoon lime juice
- 1 tablespoon dill, chopped

Directions:
1. Set the instant pot on Sauté mode, add the oil, heat it up, add the garlic, lime zest and lime juice and sauté for 2 minutes.
2. Add the peppers and the rest of the ingredients, put the lid on and cook on High for 12 minutes.
3. Release the pressure naturally for 10 minutes, divide the mix between plates and serve.

Nutrition Value: calories 79, fat 2.6, fiber 0.4, carbs 1.4, protein 3.5

SEAFOOD

SPICY OYSTER STEW

Preparation Time: 15 minutes
Servings 4
Nutrition Values: 421 Calories; 25.6g Fat; 7g Total Carbs; 39.1g Protein; 2.3g Sugars

Ingredients
- 1 tablespoon ghee
- 1 medium-sized leek, chopped
- 2 cloves garlic, pressed
- 1 ½ cups double cream
- 1 ½ cups fish stock
- 2 tablespoons sherry
- 1 parsnip, trimmed and sliced
- 1 celery with leaves, diced
- 1 ½ pounds oysters, shucked
- Sea salt and ground black pepper, to taste
- 1 tablespoon paprika
- 1 or 2 dashes Tabasco
- 1/2 cup sour cream

Directions
1. Press the "Sauté" button to heat up your Instant Pot. Now, melt the ghee and cook the leek and garlic until aromatic.
2. Add coconut milk, fish stock, sherry, parsnip, celery, oysters, salt, pepper, paprika, and Tabasco.
3. Secure the lid. Choose "Manual" mode and Low pressure; cook for 6 minutes. Once cooking is complete, use a quick pressure release; carefully remove the lid.
4. Serve dolloped with chilled sour cream. Bon appétit!

TASTY MONKFISH STEW

Preparation Time: 40 minutes
Servings 6
Nutrition Values: 163 Calories; 7.6g Fat; 3.4g Total Carbs; 19.8g Protein; 1.6g Sugars

Ingredients
- Juice of 1 lemon
- 1 tablespoon fresh parsley
- 1 tablespoon fresh basil
- 1 teaspoon garlic, minced
- 1 tablespoon olive oil
- 1 ½ pounds monkfish
- 1 tablespoon butter
- 1 onion, sliced
- 1 bell pepper, chopped
- 1/4 teaspoon ground cumin
- 1/4 teaspoon turmeric powder
- 1/2 teaspoon cayenne pepper
- Sea salt and ground black pepper, to taste
- 2 cups fish stock
- 1/2 cup water
- 1/4 cup dry white wine
- 1 ripe tomato, crushed
- 2 bay leaves
- 1/2 teaspoon mixed peppercorns

Directions
1. In a ceramic dish, whisk the lemon juice, parsley, basil, garlic, and olive oil; add monkfish and let it marinate for 30 minutes.
2. Press the "Sauté" button to heat up your Instant Pot. Now, melt the butter and cook the onion and bell peppers until fragrant.
3. Add the remaining ingredients and gently stir to combine.
4. Secure the lid. Choose "Manual" mode and High pressure; cook for 6 minutes. Once cooking is complete, use a quick pressure release; carefully remove the lid.
5. Afterwards, discard bay leaves and ladle your stew into serving bowls. Serve hot.

CARP STEAKS WITH AIOLI

Preparation Time: 10 minutes
Servings 4
Nutrition Values: 315 Calories; 24.8g Fat; 0.6g Total Carbs; 21.1g Protein; 0.1g Sugars

Ingredients
1 pound carp steaks
- 2 tablespoons ghee
- 1 teaspoon granulated garlic
- 1 teaspoon onion powder
- 1/2 teaspoon dried dill
- Salt, to taste
- 1/4 teaspoon freshly ground black pepper
- 1/2 teaspoon cayenne pepper

For Aioli:
- 1 egg yolk
- 1 teaspoon garlic, minced
- 1 tablespoon fresh lemon juice
- 1/2 cup extra-virgin olive oil
- 1/3 teaspoon Dijon mustard

Directions
1. Start by adding 1 ½ cups water and a steamer

basket to the Instant Pot. Now, place the fish in the steamer basket.
2. Drizzle the fish with melted ghee; sprinkle granulated garlic, onion powder, dill, salt, black pepper, and cayenne pepper over the fish.
3. Secure the lid. Choose "Manual" mode and High pressure; cook for 4 minutes. Once cooking is complete, use a quick pressure release; carefully remove the lid.
4. Then, make your homemade aioli by mixing the egg yolk, garlic, and lemon juice. Add olive oil and mix with an immersion blender; add mustard and mix again.
5. Serve the prepared carp steaks with the homemade aioli on the side. Bon appétit!

LOBSTER WITH LIME CREAM

Preparation Time: 15 minutes
Servings 4
Nutrition Values: 322 Calories; 26.5g Fat; 1.8g Total Carbs; 19.3g Protein; 0.7g Sugars
Ingredients
- 1 pound lobster tails
- 1 tablespoon Creole seasoning blend
- Lime Cream Sauce:
- 1 stick butter
- 2 tablespoons shallots, finely chopped
- 1/4 teaspoon salt
- 1/4 teaspoon black pepper
- 1/4 teaspoon cayenne pepper
- 2 tablespoons lime juice
- 1/4 cup heavy cream

Directions
1. Prepare the Instant Pot by adding 1 ½ cups of water and a steamer basket to the bottom of the inner pot.
2. Place lobster tails in the steamer basket. Sprinkle with Creole seasoning blend.
3. Secure the lid. Choose "Manual" mode and Low pressure; cook for 3 minutes. Once cooking is complete, use a quick pressure release; carefully remove the lid.
4. Wipe down the Instant Pot with a damp cloth. Now, press the "Sauté" button and melt the butter.
5. Now, add the shallots, salt, black pepper, and cayenne pepper; cook for 1 minute and add lime juice and heavy cream. Cook until the sauce has reduced.
6. Spoon the sauce over the fish and serve right now. Bon appétit!

FAST AHI TUNA SALAD

Preparation Time: 10 minutes + chilling time
Servings 4
Nutrition Values: 252 Calories; 12.8g Fat; 5.8g Total Carbs; 27.8g Protein; 3g Sugars
Ingredients
1 cup water
- 2 sprigs parsley
- 2 sprigs thyme
- 2 sprigs rosemary
- 1 lemon, sliced
- 1 pound ahi tuna
- 1/3 teaspoon ground black pepper
- 1 cup cherry tomatoes, halved
- 1 head lettuce
- 1 red bell pepper julienned
- 1 carrot julienned
- Sea salt, to taste
- 2 tablespoons extra-virgin olive oil
- 1 teaspoon Dijon mustard

Directions
1. Pour 1 cup of water into the Instant Pot; add the parsley, thyme, rosemary, and lemon; place a metal trivet inside.
2. Lower the fish onto the trivet; sprinkle with ground black pepper.
3. Secure the lid. Choose "Manual" mode and High pressure; cook for 4 minutes. Once cooking is complete, use a quick pressure release; carefully remove the lid.
4. Place the other ingredients in a salad bowl; toss to combine. Add flaked tuna and toss again. Serve well-chilled.

BEER-BRAISED ALASKAN COD

Preparation Time: 10 minutes
Servings 4
Nutrition Values: 310 Calories; 23.5g Fat; 2.7g Total Carbs; 17.9g Protein; 0g Sugars
Ingredients
- 1 pound Alaskan cod fillets
- 1/2 cup butter
- 1 cup white ale beer
- 1 tablespoon fresh basil, chopped
- 1 teaspoon fresh tarragon, chopped
- 2 garlic cloves, minced
- 1 teaspoon whole black peppercorns
- 1/2 teaspoon coarse sea salt

Directions
1. Add all of the above ingredients to your Instant Pot.
2. Secure the lid. Choose "Manual" mode and Low pressure; cook for 3 minutes. Once

cooking is complete, use a quick pressure release; carefully remove the lid.
3. Serve right away. Bon appétit!

FAVORITE FISH CHILI

Preparation Time: 10 minutes
Servings 4

Nutrition Values: 213 Calories; 12.7g Fat; 5.9g Total Carbs; 17.1g Protein; 2.1g Sugars

Ingredients
- 2 tablespoons olive oil
- 1 red onion, coarsely chopped
- 1 teaspoon ginger-garlic paste
- 1 celery stalk, diced
- 1 carrot, sliced
- 1 bell pepper, deveined and thinly sliced
- 1 jalapeño pepper, deveined and minced
- 2 ripe Roma tomatoes, crushed
- 1/2 pound snapper, sliced
- 1/2 cup water
- 1/2 cup broth, preferably homemade
- 2 tablespoons fresh coriander, minced
- Sea salt and ground black pepper, to taste
- 1/2 teaspoon cayenne pepper
- 1 bay leaf
- 1/4 teaspoon dried dill
- 1/2 cup Cheddar cheese, grated

Directions
1. Press the "Sauté" button to heat up your Instant Pot. Now, heat the olive oil and cook the onion until translucent and tender.
2. Now, add the remaining ingredients, except for the grated Cheddar cheese.
3. Secure the lid. Choose "Manual" mode and High pressure; cook for 6 minutes. Once cooking is complete, use a quick pressure release; carefully remove the lid.
4. Ladle into individual bowl and serve garnished with grated Cheddar cheese. Bon appétit!

STUFFED PEPPERS WITH HADDOCK AND CHEESE

Preparation Time: 15 minutes
Servings 3

Nutrition Values: 352 Calories; 20.1g Fat; 6.6g Total Carbs; 35.3g Protein; 2.6g Sugars

Ingredients
- 3 bell peppers, stems and seeds removed, halved
- 3/4 pound haddock fillets. Flaked
- 1 cup Romano cheese, grated
- 4 tablespoons scallion, chopped
- 2 garlic cloves, minced
- 4 tablespoons fresh coriander, chopped
- 1 tablespoon ketchup
- Sea salt and ground black pepper, to taste
- 1 teaspoon cayenne pepper
- 1/2 cup tomato sauce
- 1 cup water
- 2 ounces Pepper-Jack cheese, shredded

Directions
1. In a mixing bowl, thoroughly combine the fish, Romano cheese, scallions, garlic, coriander, ketchup, salt, black pepper, and cayenne pepper; mix to combine well.
2. Now, divide this mixture among pepper halves. Add 1 cup of water and a metal rack to your Instant Pot.
3. Arrange the peppers on the rack. Top each pepper with tomato sauce.
4. Secure the lid. Choose "Manual" mode and High pressure; cook for 10 minutes. Once cooking is complete, use a natural pressure release; carefully remove the lid.
5. Lastly, top with Pepper-Jack cheese, cover and allow the cheese to melt. Serve warm and enjoy!

SIMPLE SWAI WITH WINE SAUCE

Preparation Time: 15 minutes
Servings 4

Nutrition Values: 109 Calories; 3.3g Fat; 1.2g Total Carbs; 17.6g Protein; 0.5g Sugars

Ingredients
- 1 tablespoon butter, melted
- 2 garlic cloves, minced
- 2 tablespoon green onions, chopped
- 1 teaspoon fresh ginger, grated
- 1 pound swai fish fillets
- 1/2 cup port wine
- 1/2 tablespoon lemon juice
- 1 teaspoon parsley flakes
- 1/2 teaspoon chili flakes
- Coarse sea salt and ground black pepper, to taste
- 1/2 teaspoon cayenne pepper
- 1/4 teaspoon ground bay leaf
- 1/2 teaspoon fennel seeds

Directions
1. Press the "Sauté" button to heat up your Instant Pot. Now, melt the butter and cook the garlic, green onions and ginger until softened and aromatic.
2. Add the remaining ingredients and gently stir

3. Secure the lid. Choose "Manual" mode and Low pressure; cook for 6 minutes. Once cooking is complete, use a quick pressure release; carefully remove the lid.
   4. Serve warm over cauli rice. Bon appétit!

CLASSIC GARAM MASALA FISH

Preparation Time: 15 minutes
Servings 4

Nutrition Values: 159 Calories; 7.4g Fat; 4.7g Total Carbs; 18.1g Protein; 2.2g Sugars

Ingredients

- 2 tablespoons sesame oil
- 1/2 teaspoon cumin seeds
- 1/2 cup leeks, chopped
- 1 teaspoon ginger-garlic paste
- 1 pound cod fillets, boneless and sliced
- 2 ripe tomatoes, chopped
- 1/2 teaspoon turmeric powder
- 1/2 teaspoon garam masala
- 1 ½ tablespoons fresh lemon juice
- 1 tablespoon fresh parsley leaves, chopped
- 1 tablespoon fresh dill leaves, chopped
- 1 tablespoon fresh curry leaves, chopped
- Coarse sea salt, to taste
- 1/4 teaspoon ground black pepper, or more to taste
- 1/2 teaspoon smoked cayenne pepper

Directions

1. Press the "Sauté" button to heat up the Instant Pot. Now, heat the sesame oil. Once hot, sauté the cumin seeds for 30 seconds.
2. Add the leeks and cook an additional 2 minutes or until translucent. After that, add the ginger-garlic paste and cook for 40 seconds more.
3. Add the other ingredients and stir to combine.
4. Secure the lid. Choose "Manual" mode and Low pressure; cook for 6 minutes. Once cooking is complete, use a quick pressure release; carefully remove the lid. Bon appétit!

WINTER TUNA SALAD

Preparation Time: 10 minutes
Servings 4

Nutrition Values: 163 Calories; 4.7g Fat; 5.4g Total Carbs; 23.5g Protein; 2.1g Sugars

Ingredients

- 1 pound tuna steaks
- 2 Roma tomatoes, sliced
- 1 red bell pepper, sliced
- 1 green bell pepper, sliced
- 1 head lettuce
- 2 tablespoons Kalamata olives, pitted and halved
- 1 red onion, chopped
- 2 tablespoons balsamic vinegar
- 2 tablespoons extra-virgin olive oil
- Sea salt, to taste
- 1/2 teaspoon chili flakes

Directions

1. Prepare your Instant Pot by adding 1 ½ cups of water and steamer basket to the inner pot.
2. Place the tuna steaks in your steamer basket. Place the tomato slices and bell peppers on top of the fish.
3. Secure the lid. Choose "Manual" mode and High pressure; cook for 4 minutes. Once cooking is complete, use a quick pressure release; carefully remove the lid. Flake the fish with a fork.
4. Divide lettuce leaves among serving plates to make a bad for your salad. Now, add olives and onions. Drizzle balsamic vinegar and olive oil over the salad.
5. Sprinkle salt and chili flakes over your salad. Top with the prepared fish, tomatoes, and bell peppers. Enjoy!

ASIAN-STYLE SNAPPER SOUP

Preparation Time: 10 minutes
Servings 4

Nutrition Values: 218 Calories; 6.9g Fat; 6.2g Total Carbs; 31.2g Protein; 2.4g Sugars

Ingredients

- 1 teaspoon toasted sesame seeds
- 1/2 cup scallions, chopped
- 2 cloves garlic, minced
- 1 pound snapper
- 1/2 teaspoon fine sea salt
- 1/3 teaspoon black peppercorns, freshly ground
- 1/2 teaspoon dried grated lemon peel
- 1/3 teaspoon dried marjoram
- 1/3 cup dry white wine
- 1 tablespoon dark soy sauce
- 1 ½ cups Chinese cabbage, shredded
- 2 tablespoons fresh coriander, chopped
- 1 carrot, diced
- 1 celery, diced
- 4 cups roasted vegetable broth
- 1 jalapeño pepper, minced

- 1 teaspoon Chinese five-spice powder

Directions
1. Press the "Sauté" button to heat up the Instant Pot. Now, heat the oil and sauté the scallions until tender and fragrant.
2. Add the remaining ingredients. Secure the lid. Choose "Manual" mode and High pressure; cook for 6 minutes. Once cooking is complete, use a quick pressure release; carefully remove the lid.
3. Ladle into individual serving bowls and serve garnished with fresh chives, if desired. Bon appétit!

TROUT FRITTATA WITH CHEESE

Preparation Time: 15 minutes
Servings 3
Nutrition Values: 408 Calories; 24.2g Fat; 3.6g Total Carbs; 42.3g Protein; 1.8g Sugars

Ingredients
- 1 ½ tablespoons olive oil
- 3 plum tomatoes, sliced
- 1 teaspoon dried basil
- 1/2 teaspoon dried oregano
- 3 trout fillets
- 1/2 teaspoon cayenne pepper, or more to taste
- 1/3 teaspoon black pepper
- Salt, to taste
- 1 bay leaf
- 1 cup Pepper-Jack cheese, shredded

Directions
1. Prepare your Instant Pot by adding 1 ½ cups of water and a metal rack to the bottom of the inner pot.
2. Now, grease a baking dish with olive oil. Place the slices of tomatoes on the bottom of the baking dish. Sprinkle the basil and oregano over them.
3. Now, add fish fillets; season with cayenne pepper, black pepper, and salt. Add bay leaf. Lower the baking dish onto the rack.
4. Secure the lid. Choose "Manual" mode and High pressure; cook for 10 minutes. Once cooking is complete, use a quick pressure release; carefully remove the lid.
5. Lastly, top with Pepper-Jack cheese, seal the lid and allow the cheese to melt. Serve warm. Bon appétit!

PRAWN SALAD IN MUSHROOM "BUNS"

Preparation Time: 20 minutes
Servings 4
Nutrition Values: 436 Calories; 29.2g Fat; 5.5g Total Carbs; 37.1g Protein; 2.1g Sugars

Ingredients
- 1 ½ pounds prawns, peeled and deveined
- Juice of one lemon, freshly squeezed
- 2/3 cup water
- 1/2 teaspoon sea salt
- 1/4 teaspoon chili flakes
- 1 red onion, chopped
- 1 celery stalk with leaves, chopped
- 1 bell pepper, chopped
- 1 ½ tablespoons balsamic vinegar
- 1 cup mayonnaise
- 1 teaspoon yellow mustard
- 2 heaping tablespoons fresh cilantro, chopped
- 8 large Portobello mushroom caps, stems removed
- 1 tablespoon olive oil

Directions
1. Toss the prawns, lemon juice, and water into your Instant Pot.
2. Secure the lid. Choose "Manual" mode and Low pressure; cook for 2 minutes. Once cooking is complete, use a quick pressure release; carefully remove the lid.
3. Allow your prawns to cool completely.
4. Then, toss the prawns with sea salt, chili flakes, onion, celery, bell pepper, vinegar, mayonnaise, and mustard. Gently stir to combine and set aside.
5. Now, drizzle 1 tablespoon of olive oil over Portobello mushroom caps and roast them for 10 to 13 minutes at 450 degrees F.
6. To assemble your sandwiches, divide the prepared shrimp salad among roasted Portobello mushroom caps. Garnish with fresh cilantro and serve right now.

CREAMY AND LEMONY TUNA FILLETS

Preparation Time: 10 minutes
Servings 4
Nutrition Values: 175 Calories; 6.9g Fat; 1.9g Total Carbs; 25.2g Protein; 0.3g Sugars

Ingredients
- 1 cup water
- 1/3 cup lemon juice
- 2 sprigs fresh rosemary
- 2 sprigs fresh thyme
- 2 sprigs fresh parsley
- 1 pound tuna fillets
- 4 cloves garlic, pressed
- Sea salt, to taste

- 1/4 teaspoon black pepper, or more to taste
- 2 tablespoons butter, melted
- 1 lemon, sliced

Directions
1. Prepare your Instant Pot by adding 1 cup of water, lemon juice, rosemary, thyme, and parsley to the bottom. Add a steamer basket too.
2. Now, place tuna fillets in the steamer basket. Place the garlic on the top of fish fillets; sprinkle with salt and black pepper.
3. Drizzle the melted butter over the fish fillets and top with the sliced lemon.
4. Secure the lid. Choose "Manual" mode and Low pressure; cook for 3 minutes. Once cooking is complete, use a quick pressure release; carefully remove the lid. Serve warm and enjoy!

RAINBOW TROUT WITH BUTTERY VEGGIES

Preparation Time: 20 minutes
Servings 4
Nutrition Values: 341 Calories; 17.7g Fat; 6.4g Total Carbs; 38.3g Protein; 1.2g Sugars
Ingredients
- 1 ½ pounds rainbow trout fillets
- 4 tablespoons butter
- Sea salt and ground black pepper, to taste
- 1 bunch of scallions
- 1 pound mixed greens, trimmed and torn into pieces
- 1/2 cup chicken broth
- 1 tablespoon apple cider vinegar
- 1 teaspoon cayenne pepper

Directions
1. Start by adding 1 cup water and a steamer basket to your Instant Pot.
2. Now, add the fish to the steamer basket. Drizzle 1 tablespoon of the melted butter over them and sprinkle with salt and black pepper.
3. Secure the lid. Choose "Manual" mode and Low pressure; cook for 12 minutes. Once cooking is complete, use a quick pressure release; carefully remove the lid.
4. Wipe down the Instant Pot with a damp cloth; then, warm the remaining 3 tablespoons of butter. Once hot, cook the scallions, greens, broth, vinegar and cayenne pepper until the greens start to wilt.
5. Serve the prepared trout fillets with the sautéed greens on the side. Bon appétit!

EASY CREOLE SEA SCALLOPS

Preparation Time: 10 minutes
Servings 4
Nutrition Values: 163 Calories; 4.7g Fat; 6.1g Total Carbs; 22.6g Protein; 0g Sugars
Ingredients
- 2 teaspoon butter, melted
- 1 ½ pounds sea scallops
- 2 garlic cloves, finely chopped
- 1 (1-inch piece fresh ginger root, grated
- 1/3 cup dry white wine
- 2/3 cup fish stock
- Coarse sea salt and ground black pepper, to taste
- 1 teaspoon Creole seasoning blend
- 2 tablespoons fresh parsley, chopped

Directions
1. Press the "Sauté" button to heat up the Instant Pot. Now, melt the butter. Once hot, cook the sea scallops until nice and browned on all sides.
2. Now, stir in the garlic and ginger; continue sautéing for 1 minute more or until fragrant. Dump the remaining ingredients, except for the fresh parsley, into your Instant Pot.
3. Secure the lid. Choose "Manual" mode and High pressure; cook for 1 minutes. Once cooking is complete, use a quick pressure release; carefully remove the lid.
4. Serve garnished with fresh parsley and enjoy!

ZUCCHINI STUFFED WITH TUNA AND PARMESAN

Preparation Time: 15 minutes
Servings 4
Nutrition Values: 203 Calories; 9.5g Fat; 6.1g Total Carbs; 22.5g Protein; 2.8g Sugars
Ingredients
- 1 tablespoon olive oil
- 1 yellow onion, finely chopped
- 1 garlic clove, smashed
- 3/4 pound tuna fillets, chopped
- 1/4 cup Parmesan cheese, grated
- 2 tablespoons fresh cilantro, chopped
- Salt and ground black pepper, to taste
- 1/2 teaspoon mustard seeds
- 2 large-sized zucchini cut the ends off, halved
- 2 ripe tomatoes, puréed
- 1/2 cup water

Directions
1. Press the "Sauté" button to heat up the Instant Pot. Now, heat the olive oil and sauté the onions and garlic until tender and fragrant.

2. Transfer the sautéed onion and garlic to a mixing bowl. Add the fish, cheese, cilantro, salt, black pepper, and mustard seeds.
3. Core out your zucchini with a spoon to make little "boats". Stuff these zucchini boats with the tuna mixture.
4. Mix the puréed tomatoes with water; now, pour this mixture over the stuffed zucchini.
5. Secure the lid. Choose "Manual" mode and High pressure; cook for 5 minutes.
6. Once cooking is complete, use a quick pressure release; carefully remove the lid. Serve garnished with some additional cheese, if desired. Bon appétit!

NORWEGIAN SALMON STEAKS WITH GARLIC YOGURT

Preparation Time: 10 minutes
Servings 4
Nutrition Values: 364 Calories; 21.2g Fat; 4.2g Total Carbs; 37.2g Protein; 3.3g Sugars
Ingredients
- 2 tablespoons olive oil
- 4 salmon steaks
- Coarse sea salt and ground black pepper, to taste

Garlic Yogurt:
1 (8-ounce) container full-fat Greek yogurt
2 tablespoons mayonnaise
1/3 teaspoon Dijon mustard
2 cloves garlic, minced

Directions
1. Start by adding 1 cup of water and a steamer rack to the Instant Pot.
2. Now, massage olive oil into the fish; generously season with salt and black pepper on all sides. Place the fish on the steamer rack.
3. Secure the lid. Choose "Manual" mode and High pressure; cook for 4 minutes. Once cooking is complete, use a quick pressure release; carefully remove the lid.
4. Then, make the garlic yogurt by whisking Greek yogurt, mayonnaise, Dijon mustard, and garlic.
5. Serve salmon steaks with the garlic yogurt on the side. Bon appétit!

HOT CHANTERELLES AND SCAMPI BOIL

Preparation Time: 10 minutes
Servings 4
Nutrition Values: 281 Calories; 13.6g Fat; 6.1g Total Carbs; 23.6g Protein; 0.9g Sugars
Ingredients
- 12 ounces lager beer
- 1 tablespoon Creole seasoning
- 1/2 teaspoon paprika
- 1/3 teaspoon dried dill weed
- Sea salt and ground black pepper, to taste
- 1 shallot, chopped
- 2 cloves garlic, crushed
- 1/2 teaspoon Sriracha
- 1/2 pound chanterelles, sliced
- 1 pound scampi, deveined

Directions
1. Simply throw all of the above ingredients into your Instant Pot.
2. Secure the lid. Choose "Manual" mode and Low pressure; cook for 2 minutes. Once cooking is complete, use a quick pressure release; carefully remove the lid.
3. Serve with fresh cucumbers and radishes on the side.

REFRESHING SEAFOOD BOWL

Preparation Time: 15 minutes
Servings 6
Nutrition Values: 280 Calories; 14g Fat; 6g Total Carbs; 32g Protein; 2.8g Sugars
Ingredients
- 1 ½ pounds shrimp, peeled and deveined
- 1/2 pound calamari, cleaned
- 1/2 pound lobster
- 2 bay leaves
- 2 rosemary sprigs
- 2 thyme sprigs
- 4 garlic cloves, halved
- 1/2 cup fresh lemon juice
- Sea salt and ground black pepper, to taste
- 3 ripe tomatoes, puréed
- 1/2 cup olives, pitted and halved
- 2 tablespoons fresh coriander, chopped
- 2 tablespoons fresh parsley, chopped
- 3 tablespoons extra-virgin olive oil
- 3 chili peppers, deveined and minced
- 1/2 cup red onion, chopped
- 1 avocado, pitted and sliced

Directions
1. Add shrimp, calamari, lobster, bay leaves, rosemary, thyme, and garlic to your Instant Pot. Pour in 1 cup of water.
2. Secure the lid. Choose "Manual" mode and Low pressure; cook for 3 minutes. Once cooking is complete, use a quick pressure release; carefully remove the lid.
3. Drain the seafood and transfer to a serving

bowl.
4. In a mixing bowl, thoroughly combine lemon juice, salt, black pepper, tomatoes, olives, coriander, parsley, olive oil, chili peppers, and red onion.
5. Transfer this mixture to the serving bowl with the seafood. Stir to combine well; serve well-chilled, garnished with avocado. Bon appétit!

TRADITIONAL TIGER PRAWNS WITH BUTTER SAUCE

Preparation Time: 10 minutes
Servings 6

Nutrition Values: 246 Calories; 16.1g Fat; 1.8g Total Carbs; 23.3g Protein; 0.6g Sugars

Ingredients

- 1 ½ pounds raw tiger prawns, peeled and deveined
- 1/4 cup rice wine vinegar
- 1 stick butter
- 1 teaspoon cumin seeds
- 1/2 teaspoon fennel seeds
- 1/2 teaspoon mustard seeds
- 1 teaspoon dried rosemary
- 1 teaspoon garlic paste
- 1 teaspoon red pepper flakes, crushed
- Salt and ground black pepper, to taste
- 2 tablespoons dry sherry
- 2 tablespoons fresh parsley, chopped
- 2 tablespoons fresh cilantro, chopped
- 2 tablespoons fresh lemon juice

Directions

1. Toss the prawns and rice wine vinegar into your Instant Pot. Pour in 1 cup of water.
2. Secure the lid. Choose "Manual" mode and Low pressure; cook for 2 minutes. Once cooking is complete, use a quick pressure release; carefully remove the lid. Drain tiger prawns and reserve.
3. Then, wipe down the Instant Pot with a damp cloth. Press the "Sauté" button to heat up the Instant Pot; then, warm the butter.
4. Now, sauté cumin seeds, fennel seeds, mustard seeds, rosemary, and garlic paste for 40 seconds, stirring continuously.
5. Now, add the reserved prawns, along with red pepper, salt, black pepper, dry sherry, parsley, cilantro, and lemon juice. Serve immediately and enjoy!

SIMPLE PARTY SEAFOOD DIP

Preparation Time: 10 minutes
Servings 8

Nutrition Values: 151 Calories; 8.3g Fat; 2.6g Total Carbs; 15.6g Protein; 0.7g Sugars

Ingredients

- 1/2 pound shrimp
- 1/2 pound crab
- 1/2 cup apple cider vinegar
- 1/2 cup water
- 1/4 cup heavy cream
- 1/2 tablespoon lime juice
- 2 tablespoons shallots, chopped
- 1 teaspoon garlic, minced
- Kosher salt and white pepper, to taste
- 1/2 teaspoon dried rosemary
- 1/2 teaspoon dried oregano
- 1/2 teaspoon cayenne pepper
- 10 ounces Ricotta cheese

Directions

1. Place the shrimp, crab, vinegar and water in your Instant Pot.
2. Secure the lid. Choose "Manual" mode and Low pressure; cook for 3 minutes. Once cooking is complete, use a quick pressure release; carefully remove the lid.
3. Then, process all of the remaining ingredients in your blender. Add the cooked shrimp and crab. Continue blending until your desired consistency is achieved.
4. Spoon the dip into a nice serving bowl. Serve with vegetable dippers and enjoy!

RED CURRY PERCH FILLETS

Preparation Time: 10 minutes
Servings 4

Nutrition Values: 135 Calories; 4.1g Fat; 1.3g Total Carbs; 22.3g Protein; 0.6g Sugars

Ingredients

- 1 cup water
- 1 large-sized lemon, sliced
- 2 sprigs rosemary
- 1 pound perch fillets
- Sea salt and ground black pepper, to taste
- 1 teaspoon cayenne pepper
- 1 tablespoon red curry paste
- 1 tablespoons butter

Directions

1. Pour 1 cup of water into the Instant Pot; add the lemon slices and rosemary; place a metal trivet inside.
2. Now, sprinkle the perch fillets with salt, black pepper, andcayenne pepper. Spread red curry paste and butter over the fillets.
3. Lower the fish onto the trivet.

4. Secure the lid. Choose "Manual" mode and Low pressure; cook for 6 minutes. Once cooking is complete, use a quick pressure release; carefully remove the lid.
5. Serve with your favorite keto sides. Bon appétit!

MILKY MACKEREL SOUP

Preparation Time: 10 minutes

Servings 4

Nutrition Values: 332 Calories; 20.3g Fat; 7g Total Carbs; 29.1g Protein; 6g Sugars

Ingredients

- 1 tablespoon olive oil
- 1 yellow onion, chopped
- 2 garlic cloves, minced
- 1 teaspoon grated ginger
- 1 pound mackerel fillets, sliced
- 1 ½ cups milk
- 2 cups chicken stock
- 1/2 cup double cream
- 1 tablespoon butter

Directions

1. Press the "Sauté" button to heat up the Instant Pot. Now, heat the olive oil. Once hot, sauté the onion until softened.
2. Then, sauté the garlic and ginger for 30 to 40 seconds more.
3. Add the remaining ingredients and stir to combine.
4. Secure the lid. Choose "Manual" mode and High pressure; cook for 6 minutes. Once cooking is complete, use a quick pressure release; carefully remove the lid. Bon appétit!

BLUEFISH IN SPECIAL SAUCE

Preparation Time: 10 minutes

Servings 4

Nutrition Values: 204 Calories; 7.9g Fat; 4.4g Total Carbs; 23.5g Protein; 2.3g Sugars

Ingredients

- 2 teaspoons butter
- 1/2 yellow onion, chopped
- 1 garlic clove, minced
- 1 pound bluefish fillets
- Sea salt and ground black pepper, to taste
- 1/4 cup vermouth
- 1 tablespoon rice vinegar
- 2 teaspoons tamari
- 1 teaspoon fresh tarragon leaves, chopped

Directions

1. Press the "Sauté" button to heat up the Instant Pot. Now, melt the butter. Once hot, sauté the onion until softened.
2. Add garlic and sauté for a further minute or until aromatic. Stir in the remaining ingredients.
3. Secure the lid. Choose "Manual" mode and Low pressure; cook for 3 minutes. Once cooking is complete, use a quick pressure release; carefully remove the lid. Bon appétit!

GROUPER WITH CREMINI MUSHROOMS AND SAUSAGE

Preparation Time: 15 minutes

Servings 4

Nutrition Values: 431 Calories; 13.7g Fat; 5.9g Total Carbs; 62.4g Protein; 2.3g Sugars

Ingredients

- 2 tablespoons butter
- 1/2 pound smoked turkey sausage, casing removed
- 1 pound Cremini mushrooms, sliced
- 2 garlic cloves, minced
- 4 grouper fillets
- Sea salt, to taste
- 1/2 teaspoon black peppercorns, freshly cracked
- 1/2 cup dry white wine
- 1 tablespoon fresh lime juice
- 2 tablespoons fresh cilantro, chopped

Directions

1. Press the "Sauté" button to heat up the Instant Pot. Now, melt the butter. Once hot, cook the sausage until nice and browned on all sides; reserve.
2. Then, cook Cremini mushrooms in pan drippings for about 3 minutes or until fragrant.
3. Add the garlic and continue to sauté an additional 30 seconds. Now, add the fish, salt, black peppercorns, and wine. Return the sausage back to the Instant Pot.
4. Secure the lid. Choose "Manual" mode and Low pressure; cook for 3 minutes. Once cooking is complete, use a quick pressure release; carefully remove the lid. Bon appétit!
5. Afterwards, divide your dish among serving plates and drizzle fresh lime juice over each serving. Serve garnished with fresh cilantro. Bon appétit!

EASY KING CRAB WITH MUSHROOMS

Preparation Time: 10 minutes

Servings 6

Nutrition Values: 176 Calories; 8.5g Fat; 2.4g Total Carbs; 22.3g Protein; 1.1g Sugars

Ingredients

- 1 ½ pounds king crab legs, halved
- 1/2 stick butter, softened
- 10 ounces baby Bella mushrooms
- 2 garlic cloves, minced
- 1 lemon, sliced

Directions

1. Start by adding 1 cup water and a steamer basket to your Instant Pot.
2. Now, add the king crab legs to the steamer basket.
3. Secure the lid. Choose "Manual" mode and Low pressure; cook for 3 minutes. Once cooking is complete, use a quick pressure release; carefully remove the lid.
4. Wipe down the Instant Pot with a damp cloth; then, warm the butter. Once hot, cook baby Bella mushrooms with minced garlic for 2 to 3 minutes.
5. Spoon the mushrooms sauce over prepared king crab legs and serve with lemon. Bon appétit!

SEAFOOD JAMBALAYA

Servings: 3
Preparation Time: 20 minutes'
Cooking Time: 4 hrs. 45 min

Ingredients

- 4 oz. catfish (cut into 1-inch cubes)
- 4 oz. shrimp (peeled and deveined)
- 1 tablespoon olive oil
- 2 bacon slices, chopped
- 1 1/5 cups vegetable broth
- ¾ cup sliced celery stalk
- ¼ teaspoon minced garlic
- ½ cup chopped onion
- 1 cup canned diced tomatoes
- 1 cup uncooked long-grain white rice
- ½ tablespoon Cajun seasoning
- ¼ teaspoon dried thyme
- ¼ teaspoon cayenne pepper
- ½ teaspoon dried oregano
- Salt and freshly ground black pepper, to taste

Directions

1. Select the "Sauté" function on your Instant Pot and add the oil into it.
2. Put the onion, garlic, celery, and bacon to the pot and cook for 10 minutes.
3. Add all the remaining ingredients to the pot except seafood.
4. Stir well, then secure the cooker lid.
5. Select the "Slow Cook" function on a medium mode.
6. Keep the pressure release handle on "venting" position. Cook for 4 hours.
7. Once done, remove the lid and add the seafood to the gravy.
8. Secure the lid again, keep the pressure handle in the venting position.
9. Cook for another 45 minutes then serve.

Nutrition Values:
Calories: 505
Carbohydrate: 58.6g
Protein: 27.4g
Fat: 16.8g
Sugar: 3.1g
Sodium: 818mg

SHRIMP CREOLE

Servings: 4
Preparation Time: 20 minutes
Cooking Time: 7 hrs. 10 min

Ingredients

- 1 lb. shrimp (peeled and deveined)
- 1 tablespoon olive oil
- 1 (28 oz.) can crush whole tomatoes
- 1 cup celery stalk (sliced)
- ¾ cup chopped white onion
- ½ cup green bell pepper (chopped)
- 1 (8 oz.) can tomato sauce
- ½ teaspoon minced garlic
- ¼ teaspoon ground black pepper
- 1 tablespoon Worcestershire sauce
- 4 drops hot pepper sauce
- Salt, to taste
- White rice for serving

Directions

1. Put the oil to the Instant Pot along with all the ingredients except the shrimp.
2. Secure the cooker lid and keep the pressure handle valve turned to the venting position.
3. Select the "Slow Cook" function on your cooker and set it on medium heat.
4. Let the mixture cook for 6 hours.
5. Remove the lid afterwards and add the shrimp to the pot.
6. Stir and let the shrimp cook for another 1 hour on "Slow Cook" function.
7. Keep the lid covered with pressure release handle in the venting position.
8. To serve, pour the juicy shrimp creole over steaming white rice.

Nutrition Values:

Calories: 146
Carbohydrate: 13.5g
Protein: 19.5g
Fat: 1.7g
Sugar: 0.9g
Sodium: 894mg

SALMON CASSEROLE

Servings: 4
Preparation Time: 20 minutes
Cooking Time: 8 hours

Ingredients

- ½ tablespoon olive oil
- 8 oz. cream of mushroom soup
- ¼ cup water
- 3 medium potatoes (peeled and sliced)
- 3 tablespoons flour
- 1 (16 oz.) can salmon (drained and flaked)
- ½ cup chopped scallion
- ¼ teaspoon ground nutmeg
- Salt and freshly ground black pepper, to taste

Directions

1. Pour mushroom soup and water in a separate bowl and mix them well.
2. Add the olive oil to the Instant Pot and grease it lightly.
3. Place half of the potatoes in the pot and sprinkle salt, pepper, and half of the flour over it.
4. Now add a layer of half of the salmon over potatoes, then a layer of half of the scallions.
5. Repeat these layers and pour mushroom soup mix on top.
6. Top it with nutmeg evenly.
7. Secure the lid and set its pressure release handle to the venting position.
8. Select the "Slow Cook" function with "Medium" heat on your Instant Pot.
9. Let it cook for 8 hours then serve.

Nutrition Values:

Calories: 235
Carbohydrate: 27.5g
Protein: 18g
Fat: 6.3g
Sugar: 1.2g
Sodium: 310mg

TUNA CHOWDER

Servings: 3
Preparation Time: 20 minutes
Cooking Time: 7 hours

Ingredients

- 6 oz. water-packed tuna (drained chunks)
- 1 (8 oz.) can diced tomatoes with juice
- ½ teaspoon crushed dried thyme
- ½ cup chopped celery
- ½ cup chopped onion
- ½ cup peeled and roughly shredded carrot
- 7 oz. chicken broth
- ½ teaspoon.cayenne pepper
- ½ teaspoon.freshly ground black pepper
- Salt to taste
- 1 chopped medium red potato

Directions

1. Add all the ingredients except tuna to the Instant Pot and mix them well.
2. Secure the lid with its pressure release handle on the venting position.
3. Select the "Slow Cook" function with "Medium" heat for 7 hours.
4. Remove the lid after 7 hours and add the tuna chunks to the pot.
5. Cover the lid immediately and let tuna stay in the steaming hot gravy for 5 minutes.
6. Serve the sizzling hot chowder immediately.

Nutrition Values:

Calories: 158
Carbohydrate: 18.7g
Protein: 18.3g
Fat: 1.2g
Sugar: 4.4g
Sodium: 772mg

SALMON SOUP

Servings: 3
Preparation Time: 20 minutes
Cooking Time: 17 minutes

Ingredients

- 1 lb. salmon fillets
- 1 tablespoon coconut oil
- 1 cup carrots, peeled and chopped
- ½ cup celery stalk, chopped
- ½ cup yellow onion, chopped
- 1 cup cauliflower, chopped
- 2 cups homemade chicken broth
- Salt and freshly ground black pepper, to taste
- 2 tablespoons fresh parsley for topping, chopped

Directions

1. Add 1 cup of water to the Instant Pot, then place the trivet in it.
2. Arrange a single layer of salmon fillets over the trivet.
3. Secure the lid and turn the pressure release handle to the "Sealed" position.
4. Select the "Manual" function on your cooker

to high pressure for 9 minutes
5. After the beep, release the steam with 'Quick release'.
6. Remove the salmon, trivet, and water from the pot.
7. Dice down salmon into edible chunks
8. Now add the coconut oil to the Instant Pot and select the "Sauté" function for cooking.
9. Add the celery, carrots, and onions to the pot and cook for 5 minutes with occasional stirring.
10. 1Add the chicken broth and cauliflower to the pot then secure the lid.
11. 1Select the "Manual" settings with high pressure for 8 minutes.
12. 1Once it beeps, do a Natural release.
13. 1Remove the lid and add the salmon chunks along with salt and pepper to the soup.
14. 1Serve with parsley sprinkled on top.

Nutrition Values:
Calories: 284
Carbohydrate: 41.3g
Protein: 132.8g
Fat: 16.4g
Sugar: 23.8g
Sodium: 508mg

SALMON CURRY

Servings: 8
Preparation Time: 10 minutes
Cooking Time: 12 minutes

Ingredients

- 3 lbs. salmon fillets (cut into pieces)
- 2 tablespoons olive oil
- 2 Serrano peppers, chopped
- 1 teaspoon ground turmeric
- 4 tablespoons curry powder
- 4 teaspoons ground cumin
- 4 curry leaves
- 4 teaspoons ground coriander
- 2 small yellow onions, chopped
- 2 teaspoons red chili powder
- 4 garlic cloves, minced
- 4 cups unsweetened coconut milk
- 2 ½ cups tomatoes, chopped
- 2 tablespoons fresh lemon juice
- Fresh cilantro leaves to garnish

Directions

1. Put the oil and curry leaves to the insert of the Instant Pot. Select the "Sauté" function to cook for 30 secs.
2. Add the garlic and onions to the pot, cook for 5 minutes.
3. Stir in all the spices and cook for another 1 minute.
4. Put the fish, Serrano pepper, coconut milk, and tomatoes while cooking.
5. Cover and lock the lid. Seal the pressure release valve.
6. Select the "Manual" function at low pressure for 5 minutes.
7. After the beep, do a "Natural" release to release all the steam.
8. Remove the lid and squeeze in lemon juice.
9. Garnish with fresh cilantro leaves and serve.

Nutrition Values:
Calories: 559
Carbohydrate: 12.2g
Protein: 36.9g
Fat: 43.2g
Sugar: 6.5g
Sodium: 106mg

SALMON F4ILLETS

Servings: 3
Preparation Time: 10 minutes
Cooking Time: 03 minutes

Ingredients

- 1 cup water
- 3 lemon slices
- 1 (5-oz.) salmon fillet
- 1 teaspoon fresh lemon juice
- Salt and ground black pepper, to taste
- Fresh cilantro to garnish

Directions

1. Add the water to the Instant pot and place a trivet inside.
2. In a shallow bowl, place the salmon fillet. Sprinkle salt and pepper over it.
3. Squeeze some lemon juice on top then place a lemon slice over the salmon fillet.
4. Cover the lid and lock it. Set its pressure release handle to "Sealing" position.
5. Use "Steam" function on your cooker for 3 minutes to cook.
6. After the beep, do a Quick release and release the steam.
7. Remove the lid, then serve with the lemon slice and fresh cilantro on top.

Nutrition Values:
Calories: 63
Carbohydrate: 0.2g
Protein: 9.2g
Fat: 2.9g
Sugar: 0.1g
Sodium: 48mg

BUTTER-DIPPED LOBSTERS

Servings: 4
Preparation Time: 20 minutes
Cooking Time: 03 Min

Ingredients

- 1 cup water.
- 4 lbs. lobster tails, cut in half
- 4 tablespoons unsalted butter, melted
- Salt and black pepper to taste

Directions

1. Pour 1 cup of water into the insert of Instant pot and place trivet inside it.
2. Place all the lobster tails over the trivet with their shell side down.
3. Cover the lid and lock it. Select the "Manual" function at low pressure for 3 minutes.
4. After the beep, press cancel and do a Quick release.
5. Remove the lid and trivet from the pot.
6. Transfer the lobster to a serving plate.
7. Pour the melted butter over lobster tails to add more flavor.
8. Sprinkle some salt and pepper on top, then serve.

Nutrition Values:

Calories: 507
Carbohydrate: 0g (Zero gram)
Protein: 86.3g
Fat: 15.3g
Sugar: 0g
Sodium: 1240mg

FISH CURRY DELIGHT

Servings: 8
Preparation Time: 05 minutes
Cooking Time: 12 Min

Ingredients

- 3 lbs. cod fillets, cut into bite-sized pieces
- 2 tablespoons olive oil
- 4 curry leaves
- 4 medium onions, chopped
- 2 tablespoons fresh ginger, grated finely
- 4 garlic cloves, minced
- 4 tablespoons curry powder
- 4 teaspoons ground cumin
- 4 teaspoons ground coriander
- 2 teaspoons red chili powder
- 1 teaspoon ground turmeric
- 4 cups unsweetened coconut milk
- 2 ½ cups tomatoes, chopped
- 2 Serrano peppers, seeded and chopped
- 2 tablespoons fresh lemon juice

Directions

1. Add the oil to the Instant Pot and select "Sauté" function for cooking.
2. Add the curry leaves and cook for 30 seconds. Stir the onion, garlic, and ginger into the pot and cook 5 minutes.
3. Add all the spices to the mixture and cook for another 1 ½ minutes.
4. Hit "Cancel" then add the coconut milk, Serrano pepper, tomatoes, and fish to the pot.
5. Secure the lid and select the "Manual" settings with low pressure and 5 minutes cooking time.
6. After the beep, do a Quick release and remove the lid.
7. Drizzle lemon juice over the curry then stir.
8. Serve immediately.

Nutrition Values:

Calories: 758
Carbohydrate: 47.3g
Protein: 29.8g
Fat: 54.1g
Sugar: 8.2g
Sodium: 940mg

SHRIMP CURRY

Servings: 8
Preparation Time: 05 minutes
Cooking Time: 09 minutes

Ingredients

- 2 tablespoons olive oil
- 1 ½ medium onion, chopped
- 1 ½ teaspoons ground cumin
- 2 teaspoons red chili powder
- 2 teaspoons ground turmeric
- 3 medium white rose potatoes, diced
- 6 medium tomatoes, chopped
- 2 lbs. medium shrimp, peeled and deveined
- 1 ½ tablespoons fresh lemon juice
- Salt to taste
- ½ cup fresh cilantro, chopped

Directions

1. Select the "Sauté" function on your Instant Pot. Add the oil and onions then cook for 2 minutes.
2. Add the tomatoes, potatoes, cilantro, lemon juice and all the spices into the pot and secure the lid.
3. Select the "Manual" function at medium pressure for 5 minutes.
4. Do a natural release then remove the lid. Stir shrimp into the pot.
5. Secure the lid again then set the "Manual" function with high pressure for 2 minutes.

6. After the beep, use "Natural" release and let it stand for 10 minutes.
7. Remove the lid and serve hot.

Nutrition Values:
Calories: 227
Carbohydrate: 19.2g
Protein: 27.1g
Fat: 5.4g
Sugar: 4.4g
Sodium: 298mg

SEAFOOD GUMBO

Servings: 4
Preparation Time: 10 minutes
Cooking Time: 22 minutes

Ingredients
- 4 tablespoons olive oil, divided
- 1 red bell pepper, seeded and chopped
- ½ onion, chopped
- 1 ½ celery stalks, chopped
- 2 garlic cloves, minced
- 1 smoked sausage, chopped
- 1 tablespoon dried thyme, crushed
- Freshly ground black pepper, to taste
- 3½ cups low-sodium chicken broth, divided
- 1/4 cup all-purpose flour
- ½ lb. crabmeat
- ½ lb. large shrimp, peeled and deveined
- ½ lb. scallops

Directions
1. Select the "Sauté" function on your Instant Pot, then add 2 tablespoons oil, onion, celery, bell pepper, garlic and cook for 5 minutes.
2. Hit "cancel" then stir in 3 cups chicken broth, black pepper, sausage, and thyme.
3. Secure the cooker lid then select the "Manual" function with medium pressure for 10 minutes.
4. After the beep, do a Quick release then remove the lid.
5. Meanwhile, add the remaining oil to a skillet and set it on a medium-low heat. Add the flour to oil then cook for 5 minutes while stirring constantly.
6. Turn off the heat, then stir in remaining chicken broth to the flour. Mix well to avoid lumps.
7. Now add this flour mixture and the Seafood to the Instant Pot and secure the lid.
8. Cook on the "Manual" function at medium pressure for 2 minutes.
9. After the beep, do a Quick release then remove the lid and serve immediately.

Nutrition Values:
Calories: 429
Carbohydrate: 25.4g
Protein: 35g
Fat: 20.3g
Sugar: 5.8g
Sodium: 968mg

SAFFRON CHILI COD

Preparation time: 5 minutes
Cooking time: 12 minutes
Servings: 4

Ingredients:
- 4 cod fillets, boneless and skinless
- 3 garlic cloves, minced
- 1 teaspoon turmeric powder
- 1 tablespoon chili paste
- 1 cup tomato passata

Directions:
1. In your instant pot, combine the cod with the rest of the ingredients, put the lid on and cook on High for 12 minutes.
2. Release the pressure fast for 5 minutes, divide everything between plates and serve.

Nutrition Value: calories 244, fat 12, fiber 1.6, carbs 4.5, protein 14.6

SALMON AND ENDIVES

Preparation time: 10 minutes
Cooking time: 15 minutes
Servings: 4

Ingredients:
- 4 salmon fillets, boneless
- 1 cup tomato passata
- 1 shallot, sliced
- 2 endives, trimmed and halved
- 1 tablespoon balsamic vinegar
- A pinch of salt and black pepper
- 1 tablespoon parsley, chopped

Directions:
1. In your instant pot, combine the salmon with the rest of the ingredients, put the lid on and cook on High for 15 minutes.
2. Release the pressure naturally for 10 minutes, divide the mix between plates and serve.

Nutrition Value: calories 251, fat 11.1, fiber 1, carbs 3.4, protein 35.4

CHILI TUNA

Preparation time: 5 minutes
Cooking time: 15 minutes
Servings: 4

Ingredients:

- 1 pound tuna, skinless, boneless and cubed
- Juice of 1 lemon
- 1 tablespoon chili powder
- 1 cup tomato passata
- A pinch of salt and black pepper
- 1 shallot, chopped
- 1 tablespoon chives, chopped
- 1 tablespoon cilantro, chopped

Directions:
1. In your instant pot, combine the tuna with the lemon juice and the rest of the ingredients, put the lid on and cook on High for 15 minutes.
2. Release the pressure fast for 5 minutes, divide the chili into bowls and serve.

Nutrition Value: calories 232, fat 9.6, fiber 1.6, carbs 4.4, protein 31.2

MACKEREL AND SHRIMP MIX

Preparation time: 5 minutes
Cooking time: 12 minutes
Servings: 6

Ingredients:
- 1 pound shrimp, peeled and deveined
- 1 pound mackerel, skinless, boneless and cubed
- 1 cup radishes, cubed
- ½ cup chicken stock
- 2 garlic cloves, minced
- 1 tablespoon olive oil
- 1 cup tomato passata

Directions:
1. Set instant pot on Sauté mode, add the oil, heat it up, add the radishes and the garlic and sauté for 2 minutes.
2. Add the rest of the ingredients, put the lid on and cook on High for 10 minutes.
3. Release the pressure fast for 5 minutes, divide the mix into bowls and serve.

Nutrition Value: calories 332, fat 17.4, fiber 0.9, carbs 4.4, protein 36.4

MACKEREL AND BASIL SAUCE

Preparation time: 10 minutes
Cooking time: 15 minutes
Servings: 4

Ingredients:
- 1 cup veggie stock
- 2 chili peppers, chopped
- 2 tablespoons olive oil
- 1 pound mackerel, skinless, boneless and cubed
- 2 teaspoons red pepper flakes
- A pinch of salt and black pepper
- ½ cup basil, chopped

Directions:
1. Set your instant pot on Sauté mode, add the oil, heat it up, add the chili peppers and the pepper flakes and cook for 2 minutes.
2. Add the rest of the ingredients, put the lid on and cook on High for 12 minutes.
3. Release the pressure naturally for 10 minutes, divide everything between plates and serve.

Nutrition Value: calories 362, fat 14.7, fiber 0.4, carbs 0.8, protein 27.5

OREGANO TUNA

Preparation time: 10 minutes
Cooking time: 12 minutes
Servings: 4

Ingredients:
- 1 pound tuna, skinless, boneless and cubed
- 1 cup black olives, pitted and sliced
- 2 tablespoon avocado oil
- 1 shallot, chopped
- 14 ounces tomatoes, chopped
- 2 tablespoons oregano, chopped

Directions:
1. Set your instant pot on Sauté mode, add the oil, heat it up, add the shallot and sauté for 2 minutes.
2. Add the tuna and the rest of the ingredients, put the lid on and cook on High for 10 minutes.
3. Release the pressure naturally for 10 minutes, divide the mix between plates and serve.

Nutrition Value: calories 284, fat 14.1, fiber 3.5, carbs 6.7, protein 31.4

CREAMY SHRIMP AND RADISH MIX

Preparation time: 5 minutes
Cooking time: 6 minutes
Servings: 4

Ingredients:
- 1 and ½ pound shrimp, peeled and deveined
- 1 cup red radishes, sliced
- ½ cup black olives, pitted
- 2 spring onions, chopped
- 1 and ½ cups coconut cream
- 1 tablespoon cilantro, chopped
- 1 tablespoon sweet paprika

Directions:
1. In your instant pot, combine the shrimp with the rest of the ingredients, put the lid on and cook on High for 6 minutes.
2. Release the pressure fast for 5 minutes, divide

the mix into bowls and serve.

Nutrition Value: calories 301, fat 5.9, fiber 1.9, carbs 6.4, protein 52.4

MARJORAM TUNA

Preparation time: 10 minutes
Cooking time: 15 minutes
Servings: 4

Ingredients:
- 1 and ½ pounds tuna, skinless, boneless and cubed
- 2 spring onions, chopped
- 1 tablespoon avocado oil
- 3 garlic cloves, minced
- ½ cup basil, chopped
- ½ cup chicken stock
- 2 tablespoons tomato passata
- 1 tablespoon marjoram, chopped
- A pinch of salt and black pepper

Directions:
1. Set your instant pot on Sauté mode, add the oil, heat it up, add the garlic and the spring onions, stir and sauté for 3 minutes.
2. Add the rest of the ingredients, put the lid on and cook on High for 12 minutes.
3. Release the pressure naturally for 10 minutes, divide the mix between plates and serve.

Nutrition Value: calories 345, fat 16.9, fiber 0.7, carbs 2.4, protein 26.6

BACON TROUT MIX

Preparation time: 10 minutes
Cooking time: 15 minutes
Servings: 4

Ingredients:
- 1 cup bacon, cooked and crumbled
- 4 trout fillets, boneless and skinless
- 10 ounces tomato passata
- 2 tablespoons cilantro, chopped
- 1 shallot, chopped
- 1 tablespoon olive oil
- 1 tablespoon lemon juice

Directions:
1. Set your instant pot on Sauté mode, add the oil, heat it up, add the shallot and sauté for 2 minutes.
2. Add the rest of the ingredients, put the lid on and cook on High for 13 minutes.
3. Release the pressure naturally for 10 minutes, divide the mix between plates and serve.

Nutrition Value: calories 166, fat 8.9, fiber 1.1, carbs 3.8, protein 17.5

TUNA AND FENNEL MIX

Preparation time: 10 minutes
Cooking time: 15 minutes
Servings: 4

Ingredients:
- 1 tablespoon avocado oil
- 1 pound tuna, skinless, boneless and cubed
- 2 tuna fillets, boneless, skinless and cubed
- 3 garlic cloves, minced
- ¼ cup parsley, chopped
- ½ cup chicken stock
- 2 fennel bulbs, sliced
- 1 tablespoon sweet paprika

Directions:
1. Set the instant pot on Sauté mode, add the oil, heat it up, add the garlic and cook for 2 minutes.
2. Add the tuna, fennel and the rest of the ingredients, put the lid on and cook on High for 13 minutes,
3. Release the pressure naturally for 10 minutes, divide everything between plates and serve.

Nutrition Value: calories 263, fat 10.2, fiber 2.4, carbs 4.8, protein 23.5

TILAPIA SALAD

Preparation time: 5 minutes
Cooking time: 12 minutes
Servings: 4

Ingredients:
- 1 and ½ pounds tilapia fillets, boneless, skinless and cubed
- 1 cup black olives, pitted
- 1 cup zucchinis, cubed
- 1 cup baby spinach
- 1 tablespoon olive oil
- 1 tablespoon balsamic vinegar
- A pinch of salt and black pepper
- 2 tomatoes, cubed
- ½ cup chicken stock
- 1 tablespoon lemon juice
- 1 tablespoon sweet paprika

Directions:
1. In your instant pot, combine the fish with the olives, zucchinis, tomatoes, stock, paprika, salt and pepper, toss, put the lid on and cook on High for 12 minutes.
2. Release the pressure fast for 5 minutes, transfer the mix to a bowl, add the remaining ingredients, toss and serve.

Nutrition Value: calories 187, fat 8.6, fiber 3, carbs 6.9, protein 22.8

SALMON AND DILL SAUCE

Preparation time: 10 minutes
Cooking time: 20 minutes
Servings: 6

Ingredients:
- 6 salmon fillets, boneless
- ½ teaspoon lemon pepper
- 1 spring onion, chopped
- Juice of ½ lemon
- A pinch of salt and black pepper
- 1 tablespoon chives, chopped
- ½ cup avocado mayonnaise
- ½ cup heavy cream
- 1 teaspoon dill, chopped

Directions:
1. Set the instant pot on Sauté mode, add the cream, dill and the rest of the ingredients except the salmon and the mayonnaise, whisk and cook for 5 minutes.
2. Add the fish, put the lid on and cook on High for 15 minutes.
3. Release the pressure naturally for 10 minutes, add the avocado mayonnaise, toss gently, divide everything between plates and serve.

Nutrition Value: calories 399, fat 22.1, fiber 0.2, carbs 1.1, protein 23.8

TILAPIA AND OLIVES SALSA

Preparation time: 10 minutes
Cooking time: 15 minutes
Servings: 4

Ingredients:
- 4 tilapia fillets, boneless
- 1 tablespoon olive oil
- A pinch of salt and black pepper
- 12 ounces tomato passata
- 2 tablespoon sweet red pepper, chopped
- 2 tablespoon green onions, chopped
- ½ tablespoons Italian seasoning
- 1 and ½ cups black olives, pitted
- 1 tablespoon balsamic vinegar

Directions:
1. Set the instant pot on Sauté mode, add the oil, heat it up, add the fish and cook for 2 minutes on each side.
2. Add salt, pepper and the tomato passata, put the lid on and cook on High for 10 minutes.
3. Release the pressure naturally for 10 minutes and divide the fish between plates.
4. In a bowl, mix the red pepper with the remaining ingredients, toss, divide next to the fish and serve.

Nutrition Value: calories 155, fat 4.6, fiber 2.5, carbs 3.4, protein 7.4

CATFISH AND AVOCADO MIX

Preparation time: 10 minutes
Cooking time: 16 minutes
Servings: 4

Ingredients:
- 4 catfish fillets, boneless
- 2 teaspoons olive oil
- 2 tablespoons lime juice
- 2 tablespoons cilantro, chopped
- A pinch of salt and black pepper
- 2 teaspoons sweet paprika
- 1/3 cup spring onions, chopped
- 2 teaspoons oregano, dried
- 2 teaspoons cumin, dried
- ½ cup tomato passata
- 1 avocado, peeled, pitted and cubed

Directions:
1. Set the instant pot on Sauté mode, add the oil, heat it up, add the onions and cook for 2 minutes.
2. Add the fish and cook for 1 minute on each side.
3. Add the rest of the ingredients, put the lid on and cook on High for 12 minutes more.
4. Release the pressure naturally for 10 minutes, divide everything between plates and serve.

Nutrition Value: calories 353, fat 23.4, fiber 2.6, carbs 6.4, protein 15.3

TILAPIA AND CAPERS MIX

Preparation time: 10 minutes
Cooking time: 15 minutes
Servings: 4

Ingredients:
- 4 tilapia fillets, boneless
- 3 tablespoons lemon juice
- 2 tablespoons ghee, melted
- A pinch of salt and black pepper
- ½ teaspoon oregano, dried
- 2 tablespoons capers, drained and chopped
- 1 teaspoon sweet paprika
- ½ teaspoon garlic powder
- ½ cup chicken stock

Directions:
1. Set the instant pot on Sauté mode, add the ghee, melt it, add the fish and sear for 2 minutes on each side.
2. Add salt, pepper and the rest of the ingredients, put the lid on and cook on High

3. Release the pressure naturally for 10 minutes, divide the mix between plates and serve.

Nutrition Value: calories 173, fat 7.2, fiber 0.5, carbs 2.3, protein 4.7

GLAZED SALMON

Preparation time: 10 minutes
Cooking time: 15 minutes
Servings: 4

Ingredients:
- 4 salmon fillets, boneless
- A pinch of salt and black pepper
- 4 teaspoons mustard
- 1 tablespoon coconut aminos
- 1 teaspoon balsamic vinegar
- 3 tablespoons swerve

Directions:
1. Set the instant pot on Sauté mode, add the mustard, the aminos and the rest of the ingredients except the salmon, whisk well and cook for 3 minutes.
2. Add the salmon, put the lid on and cook on High for 12 minutes.
3. Release the pressure naturally for 10 minutes, divide the salmon between plates, drizzle the glaze all over and serve.

Nutrition Value: calories 251, fat 11.9, fiber 0.5, carbs 1.2, protein 35.4

SPICY TILAPIA AND KALE

Preparation time: 10 minutes
Cooking time: 20 minutes
Servings: 4

Ingredients:
- 4 tilapia fillets, boneless
- A pinch of salt and black pepper
- 3 tablespoons olive oil
- 2 garlic cloves, minced
- 1 teaspoon fennel seed
- 14 ounces canned tomatoes, crushed
- 1 bunch kale, chopped
- ½ teaspoon red pepper flakes

Directions:
1. Set the instant pot on Sauté mode, add the oil, heat it up, add the garlic and fennel seed and cook for 3 minutes.
2. Add the rest of the ingredients except the fish, toss and sauté for 4 minutes more.
3. Add the fish, put the lid on and cook on High for 12 minutes.
4. Release the pressure naturally for 10 minutes, divide the mix between plates and serve.

Nutrition Value: calories 138, fat 11.2, fiber 1.5, carbs 4.8, protein 6.3

LIME GLAZED SALMON

Preparation time: 10 minutes
Cooking time: 15 minutes
Servings: 4

Ingredients:
- 4 salmon fillets, boneless
- A pinch of salt and black pepper
- 1 tablespoon ginger, grated
- 1 tablespoon coconut aminos
- 1 tablespoon sesame seeds
- 1 teaspoon lime zest, grated
- 1 tablespoon lime juice
- ½ cup chicken stock

Directions:
1. Set the instant pot on Sauté mode, add the stock, lime juice and the rest of the ingredients except the salmon and the sesame seeds, whisk and cook for 3 minutes.
2. Add the salmon, put the lid on and cook on High for 12 minutes.
3. Release the pressure naturally for 10 minutes, divide the salmon mix between plates, sprinkle the sesame seeds on top and serve.

POULTRY

LEMONGRASS TURKEY
Preparation time: 10 minutes
Cooking time: 25 minutes
Servings: 4
Ingredients:
- 1 bunch lemongrass, chopped
- 4 garlic cloves, minced
- 2 tablespoons balsamic vinegar
- 1 tablespoon oregano, chopped
- 1 cup coconut milk
- 2 turkey breasts, skinless, boneless and cubed
- A pinch of salt and black pepper
- ¼ cup cilantro, chopped

Directions:
1. In your food processor, mix the lemongrass with the rest of the ingredients except the turkey and the coconut milk and pulse well.
2. In your instant pot, combine the turkey with the lemongrass mix and the coconut milk, put the lid on and cook on High for 25 minutes.
3. Release the pressure naturally for 10 minutes, divide everything between plates and serve with the cilantro sprinkled on top.

Nutrition Value: calories 263, fat 12, fiber 3, carbs 6, protein 14

CILANTRO STUFFED CHICKEN BREAST
Preparation time: 10 minutes
Cooking time: 25 minutes
Servings: 4
Ingredients:
- 2 chicken breasts, skinless, boneless, halved and flattened
- 1 cup cilantro, chopped
- 1 teaspoon sweet paprika
- 2 spring onions, chopped
- A pinch of salt and black pepper
- 1 cup tomato sauce
- 1 tablespoon olive oil

Directions:
1. Arrange the chicken breasts on a working surface, divide the cilantro, onion and paprika on each and season with salt and pepper.
2. Roll each chicken breast half and secure with a toothpick.
3. Set the instant pot on Sauté mode, add the oil, heat it up, add the stuffed chicken and sear for 2 minutes on each side.
4. Add the tomato sauce, put the lid on and cook on High for 20 minutes.
5. Release the pressure naturally for 10 minutes, divide everything between plates and serve.

Nutrition Value: calories 162, fat 8, fiber 2, carbs 5, protein 9

TURKEY BITES AND MUSTARD SAUCE
Preparation time: 10 minutes
Cooking time: 25 minutes
Servings: 4
Ingredients:
- 2 tablespoons olive oil
- 1 big turkey breast, skinless, boneless and cubed
- ¾ cup chicken stock
- ¼ cup lime juice
- 3 tablespoons Dijon mustard
- 2 tablespoons sweet paprika
- 1 tablespoon oregano, chopped
- A pinch of salt and black pepper

Directions:
1. Set your instant pot on sauté mode, add the oil, heat it up, add the meat and brown for 5 minutes.
2. Add the stock and the rest of the ingredients except the oregano, toss well, put the lid on and cook on High for 20 minutes.
3. Release the pressure naturally for 10 minutes, divide the mix between plates, sprinkle the oregano on top and serve.

Nutrition Value: calories 200, fat 9, fiber 2, carbs 5, protein 10

ORANGE AND OREGANO CHICKEN
Preparation time: 10 minutes
Cooking time: 20 minutes
Servings: 4
Ingredients:
- 2 chicken breasts, skinless, boneless and halved
- 1 cup orange juice
- ½ cup chicken stock
- 1 tablespoon oregano, chopped
- A pinch of salt and black pepper
- 1 teaspoon chili powder

Directions:
1. In your instant pot, combine the chicken with the orange juice and the rest of the ingredients, put the lid on and cook on High

for 20 minutes.
2. Release the pressure naturally for 10 minutes, divide the chicken and the orange sauce between plates and serve.

Nutrition Value: calories 200, fat 7, fiber 2, carbs 6, protein 11

CINNAMON AND TURMERIC CHICKEN

Preparation time: 5 minutes
Cooking time: 20 minutes
Servings: 4

Ingredients:
- 2 chicken breasts, skinless, boneless and cubed
- 2 tablespoons olive oil
- ½ teaspoon turmeric, ground
- ½ teaspoon cinnamon, ground
- 1 teaspoon sweet paprika
- 1 red onion, chopped
- 2 tablespoons tomato paste
- 1 cup chicken stock
- ½ cup parsley, chopped

Directions:
1. Set your instant pot on Sauté mode, add the oil, heat it up, add the onion and the meat and brown for 5 minutes.
2. Add the rest of the ingredients except the parsley, toss, put the lid on and cook on High for 15 minutes.
3. Release the pressure fast for 5 minutes, divide the chicken mix between plates, sprinkle the parsley on top and serve.

Nutrition Value: calories 210, fat 8, fiber 2, carbs 6, protein 11

Mozzarella Chicken Thighs

Preparation time: 10 minutes
Cooking time: 20 minutes
Servings: 4

Ingredients:
- 1 cup chicken stock
- A pinch of salt and black pepper
- 8 chicken thighs, boneless and skinless
- 1 yellow onion, chopped
- 1 tablespoon hot paprika
- 1 tablespoon chives, chopped
- 1 cup mozzarella, shredded
- 1 tablespoon olive oil

Directions:
1. Set your instant pot on Sauté mode, add the oil, heat it up, add the onion and the chicken thighs and brown for 5 minutes.
2. Add the rest of the ingredients except the chives and mozzarella, put the lid on and cook on High for 15 minutes.
3. Release the pressure fast for 5 minutes, sprinkle the chives and the mozzarella all over and leave the mix aside for 5 minutes more.
4. Divide everything between plates and serve.

Nutrition Value: calories 220, fat 8, fiber 2, carbs 5, protein 11

SWEET BASIL AND PAPRIKA CHICKEN

Preparation time: 10 minutes
Cooking time: 25 minutes
Servings: 4

Ingredients:
- 2 chicken breasts, skinless, boneless and halved
- Salt and black pepper to the taste
- 2 tablespoons coconut sugar
- 2 teaspoons sweet paprika
- ½ cup chicken stock
- 1 tablespoon basil, chopped

Directions:
1. Set the instant pot on Sauté mode, add the sugar and the rest of the ingredients except the chicken, stir and simmer for 5 minutes.
2. Whisk the mix again, add the chicken breasts, toss a bit, put the lid on and cook on High for 20 minutes.
3. Release the pressure naturally for 10 minutes, divide the mix between plates and serve.

Nutrition Value: calories 192, fat 12, fiber 3, carbs 5, protein 12

THAI CHILI CHICKEN

Preparation time: 10 minutes
Cooking time: 20 minutes
Servings: 4

Ingredients:
- 2 chicken breasts, skinless, boneless and halved
- 1 cup lime juice
- 2 tablespoons avocado oil
- 2 Thai chilies, minced
- 1 teaspoon ginger, grated
- 2 teaspoons cilantro, chopped
- 1 cup chicken stock

Directions:
1. Set the instant pot on Sauté mode, add the oil, heat it up, add the chilies and the ginger and cook for 2 minutes.
2. Add the chicken and brown for 3 minutes more.
3. Add the rest of the ingredients, put the lid on and cook on High for 15 minutes.

4. Release the pressure naturally for 10 minutes, divide the mix between plates and serve.

Nutrition Value: calories 200, fat 7, fiber 1, carbs 5, protein 12

CUMIN AND CARDAMOM TURKEY

Preparation time: 10 minutes
Cooking time: 20 minutes
Servings: 4

Ingredients:
- 1 turkey breast, skinless, boneless and cubed
- A pinch of salt and black pepper
- 1 cup chicken stock
- 1 yellow onion, chopped
- 3 garlic cloves, minced
- 1 and ½ teaspoons cumin, ground
- 1 teaspoon cardamom, ground
- 1 tablespoon chives, chopped

Directions:
1. In your instant pot, combine the turkey with salt, pepper, the stock and the rest of the ingredients except the chives, put the lid on and cook on High for 20 minutes.
2. Release the pressure naturally for 10 minutes, divide the mix between plates and serve.

Nutrition Value: calories 231, fat 7, fiber 2, carbs 6, protein 12

TURKEY AND EGGPLANT MIX

Preparation time: 10 minutes
Cooking time: 20 minutes
Servings: 4

Ingredients:
- 1 big turkey breast, skinless, boneless and cubed
- A pinch of salt and black pepper
- 1 big eggplant, roughly cubed
- 2 tablespoons avocado oil
- 1 red onion, chopped
- 10 ounces tomato sauce
- 1 tablespoon oregano, dried
- 1 teaspoon basil, dried

Directions:
1. Set your instant pot on Sauté mode, add the oil, heat it up, add the onion and the turkey and brown for 5 minutes.
2. Add the eggplant and the rest of the ingredients, put the lid on and cook on High for 15 minutes.
3. Release the pressure naturally for 10 minutes, divide everything between plates and serve.

Nutrition Value: calories 252, fat 12, fiber 4, carbs 7, protein 13

SALSA CHICKEN BURRITO BOWLS

Preparation time: 10 minutes
Cooking time: 7 minutes
Total time: 17 minutes

Ingredients:
- 2 lbs. of boneless chicken breasts
- Chili powder
- Salt and pepper
- 1 cup salsa – any of your favorite salsa
- Sour cream, scallions, cheese, for topping

Directions:
1. Place the chicken into the bottom of your Pressure Cooker.
2. Generously season each side with chili powder, salt and pepper. Pour salsa evenly over chicken.
3. Close and lock the lid in place and ensure that the valve is in sealing position.
4. Select Manual function to cook on High Pressure for about 7 minutes.
5. When the time is up, use a quick pressure release.
6. Carefully open the lid and remove the chicken from your Pressure Cooker.
7. Shred the chicken on a cutting board and top with cooking liquid.
8. Give everything a good stir to distribute evenly in individual serving bowls.
9. Top with desired ingredients and serve immediately.

MEDITERRANEAN CHICKEN ORZO

Preparation time: 15 minutes
Cooking time: 3 minutes
Total time: 18 minutes
Servings: 6

Ingredients:
- 6 boneless skinless chicken thighs (about 1 - ½ lbs.), cut into 1-inch pieces
- 2 cups of reduced-sodium chicken broth
- 2 medium tomatoes, chopped
- 1 cup of sliced pitted green olives, drained
- 1 cup of sliced pitted ripe olives, drained
- 1 large carrot, halved lengthwise and chopped
- 1 small red onion, finely chopped
- 1 tbsp. of grated lemon zest
- 3 tbsp. of lemon juice
- 2 tbsp. of butter
- 1 tbsp. of Herbs de Provence
- 1 cup of uncooked orzo pasta

Directions:
1. Combine together the first 11 ingredients in

your 6 quart electric pressure cooker.
2. Close and lock the lid in place and ensure that the valve is in sealing position. Select Manual function to cook on High Pressure for about 8 minutes.
3. When the time is up, use a quick pressure release. Carefully open the lid and add the orzo. Close and lock the lid again and ensure that the vent is in closed position.
4. Select Manual function to cook on Low Pressure for about 3 minutes. When the time is up, use a natural pressure release for about 4 minutes.
5. Quick release any remaining pressure and allow it to sit for about 8 minutes before serving.
6. Serve and enjoy!

HONEY GARLIC CHICKEN

Preparation time: 5 minutes
Cooking time: 30 minutes
Total time: 35 minutes
Servings: 7

Ingredients:
- 1 tbsp. sesame seed oil
- 1/3 cup of honey
- 4 cloves garlic, minced
- salt and fresh ground pepper, to taste
- ½ cup of salt less ketchup
- ½ tsp. dried oregano
- 2 tbsp. chopped fresh parsley
- 6 bone-in, skinless chicken thighs
- ½ tbsp. toasted sesame seeds, for garnish
- sliced green onions
- ½ cup low sodium soy sauce

Directions:
1. In a medium bowl, mix together the honey, minced garlic, soy sauce, ketchup, oregano and parsley and set aside.
2. Set the Instant Pot to sauté mode and heat the pot. Add sesame oil to the pot. Add the chicken thighs with salt and pepper and cook for about 3 minutes per side.
3. Add the prepared honey-garlic sauce to the Instant Pot. Close and lock the lid in place and ensure that the valve is in sealing position. Press the manual button to cook on high pressure for about 20 minutes.
4. When the time is up, use a natural pressure release for about 10 minutes. Carefully open the lid once the pressure has been released.
5. Add the chicken on a serving plate and scoop the sauce over the chicken. Garnish with toasted sesame seeds and green onions.
6. Serve immediately and enjoy!

KUN PAO CHICKEN

Preparation time: 7 minutes
Cooking time: 25 minutes
Total time: 32 minutes
Servings: 5

Ingredients:
For the chicken:
- Green onion to garnish
- 1 zucchini minced
- 1/2 red bell pepper diced
- 1/2 cup of onion chopped red or white
- 3 1/2 garlic cloves diced
- 2 tbsp. vegetable oil
- 1 cup of cashews or peanuts
- 1 ½ lbs. Chicken skinless chicken breast

For the sauce:
- 1/4 tsp. ground black pepper
- 2/3 cup of garlic coconut amino
- 1/2 tsp. red pepper flakes
- 1/2 tsp. ground ginger

Directions:
1. Add the oil to Instant Pot and fry chicken until it gets brownish.
2. Add all vegetables and stir. Add sauces. Close and lock the lid in place and ensure that the valve is in sealing position.
3. Press the manual function to cook on low pressure for about 25 minutes.
4. When the time is up, use a natural pressure release for about 7 minutes.
5. Carefully remove the lid and give everything a good stir.
6. Serve and enjoy!

BUTTERY LEMON CHICKEN

Preparation time: 7 minutes
Cooking time: 10 minutes
Total time: 17 minutes
Servings: 5

Ingredients:
- 2 lbs. chicken breast or thighs
- 2 tbsp. ghee or butter
- 1 onion, diced
- 1 cup organic chicken broth
- 3 cloves diced garlic
- 1 tsp. salt
- 1 tsp. paprika
- ½ tsp. pepper
- 1 tsp. dried parsley

- ½ cup lemon juice, 2 lemons
- 3 tsp. arrowroot flour

Cooking Instructions
1. Add the Instant Pot on sauté mode and add butter to melt.
2. Add the onion, garlic, paprika, parsley, and pepper and fry for about 2-3 minutes.
3. Using the same setting put the chicken and fry until it becomes brownish. Put chicken brother, lemon juice, and salt over chicken and stir.
4. Close and lock the lid in place and ensure that the valve is in sealing position. Press the manual key to cook on high pressure for about 8 minutes.
5. When the time is up, use a natural pressure release for about 10 minutes. Remove the chicken from the Instant Pot, but leave the sauce in the pan.
6. Gently pour arrowroot flour to thicken the sauce.
7. Serve and enjoy!

TACO RANCH CHICKEN CHILI

Servings: 4
Preparation time: 10 minutes
Cooking time: 35 minutes
Total time: 45 minutes

Ingredients:
- 3 (16 ounces) cans of Bush's White Chili Beans (don't drain)
- 1 (10 ounces) can Rotel (don't drain)
- 1 (1.25 ounces) packet reduced sodium taco seasoning
- 1 (1 ounces) packet ranch seasoning mix
- 1 pound of chicken breasts
- Optional toppings: lime wedges, sour cream, cilantro

Directions:
1. In a medium bowl, mix together white chili beans, Rotel, taco seasoning, ranch seasoning and chicken breasts.
2. Add the mixture into the bottom of your Instant Pot.
3. Close and lock the lid in place and ensure that the valve is in sealing position.
4. Select Manual function to cook on High Pressure for about 15 minutes.
5. When the time is up, use a quick pressure release.
6. Carefully open the lid and remove the chicken to a cutting board.
7. Shred the chicken and add back to the pot. Give everything a good stir to combine.
8. Serve with your desired optional and enjoy!

KOREAN CHICKEN MEATBALLS

Preparation time: 5 minutes
Cooking time: 20 minutes
Total time: 25 minutes
Servings: 5

Ingredients:
- 2 egg
- 2 lb. ground chicken
- 1 1/2 tsp. olive oil
- 2 garlic cloves, minced
- 1 tbsp. grated ginger (not packed)
- 1 tsp. red pepper flakes
- 1/2 tbsp. sesame oil
- 1/2 cup of panko crumbs
- 1/2 cup of Korean BBQ Sauce
- 1/3 tsp. salt

Directions:
1. Mix all the ingredients together except for the panko crumbs, Korean BBQ sauce, and green onions.
2. Add the panko crumbs over the chicken, mix and let the panko soak into the chicken mixture for 7 minutes.
3. Make about 10 balls, put the olive oil to the bottom of the Instant Pot and then put the chicken to the Instant Pot.
4. Close and lock the lid in place and ensure that the valve is in sealing position.
5. Press the manual function to cook on high pressure for about 20 minutes.
6. When the time is up, use a natural pressure release for about 8 minutes.
7. Prepare the Korean BBQ Sauce while the balls are cooking.
8. Serve and enjoy!

GROUND TURKEY LENTIL CHILI

Preparation time: 25 minutes
Cooking time: 20 minutes
Total time: 45 minutes
Servings: 5

Ingredients:
- 1 (10 oz.) can tomato sauce
- 2 lb. ground turkey
- 2 diced garlic cloves
- 2 tbsp. tomato paste
- 1/2 tsp. pepper
- 1 1/2 tsp. salt
- 1 ½ cup of dry green lentils
- 2 cups of water
- 1 (12 oz.) can petite diced tomatoes

- 1 (4 oz.) can diced green chili
- 2 tsp. chili powder
- 1 tsp. cumin
- 1 medium yellow onion, diced

Directions:
1. Switch your Instant Pot on to Sauté function. Fry the ground turkey to brown.
2. Add the minced onions, garlic, tomato paste and salt and cook until meat is browned and onions are soften.
3. Add the lentils, water, tomato sauce, diced tomatoes, green chili, chili powder, cumin and pepper. Close and lock the lid in place and ensure that the valve is in sealing position.
4. Press the manual key to cook on high pressure for about 15 minutes. When the time is up, use a natural pressure release for about 15 minutes.
5. Carefully remove the lid and scoop the chili into plates. Top with a dollop of sour cream and some diced green onions.
6. Serve and enjoy!

HONEY SESAME CHICKEN
Servings: 6
Preparation time: 12 minutes
Cooking time: 3 minutes
Total time: 15 minutes

Ingredients:
- 4 large boneless skinless chicken breasts, diced (about 2 pounds)
- Freshly ground pepper and salt
- 1 tbsp. of vegetable oil
- ½ cup of diced onion
- 2 cloves garlic, minced
- ½ cup of soy sauce
- ¼ cup of ketchup
- 2 tsp. of sesame oil
- ½ cup of honey
- ¼ tsp. of red pepper flakes
- 2 tbsp. of cornstarch
- 3 tbsp. of water
- 2 green onions, chopped
- Sesame seeds, toasted

Directions:
1. Generously seasons the chicken with the freshly ground pepper.
2. Preheat your Pressure Cooker on Sauté function and add the oil. Add the onion, garlic, and chicken to the pot.
3. Sauté stirring frequently until the onion is softened for about 3 minutes. Add the soy sauce, ketchup, and red pepper flakes.
4. Give everything a good stir to combine. Close and lock the lid in place and ensure that the valve is in sealing position.
5. Select Manual function to cook on High Pressure for about 3 minutes. When the time is up, do a quick pressure release.
6. Carefully open the lid and add the sesame oil and honey. Give everything in your Pressure Cooker a good stir to combine.
7. In a medium bowl, slowly add the cornstarch to dissolve in water and add to the pot.
8. Select the Sauté function and simmer until sauce thickens. Stir in green onions. Taste and adjust the seasoning with more salt.
9. Serve over rice sprinkled with sesame seeds and enjoy!

GREEN CHILI CHICKEN ENCHILADA SOUP
Preparation time: 7 minutes
Cooking time: 25 minutes
Total time: 32 minutes
Servings: 7

Ingredients:
- 1 cup of thick and chunky salsa Verde
- 1 tbsp. cumin
- 2 ½ chicken breast halves (frozen or fresh)
- 4 ½ cups water
- 2 tsp. Better Than Bouillon Chicken Base
- 2 tbsp. lime juice
- 1 10 oz. can green chili enchilada sauce
- 1 5 oz. can green chili
- 1 ½ tsp. chili powder
- Salt and pepper
- 1 tsp. garlic powder
- ½ cup of long grain brown rice, uncooked
- 1 13 oz. can seasoned white beans, drained
- 1 ½ cups of frozen sweet white corn
- 4 oz. cream cheese
- 1 tsp. onion powder
- Optional toppings: tortilla chips, grated cheese, sour cream, jalapenos, and cilantro

Directions:
1. Add the chicken, water, bouillon, enchilada sauce, green chili, salsa and cumin into the bottom of your Instant Pot.
2. Add the chili powder, onion powder, garlic powder, rice and beans to the Instant Pot. Give everything a good mix.
3. Close and lock the lid in place and ensure that the valve is in sealing position. Press the manual setting to cook on high pressure for about 25 minutes.

4. When the time is up, use a natural pressure release for about 15 minutes. Carefully open the lid. Place the chicken on a cutting board and shred.
5. Place them back to the pot. Sprinkle the corn and cream cheese until the cream cheese is melted.
6. Add the lime juice and stir. Add Salt and pepper to taste. Scoop into plates and add toppings of your choice.
7. Serve and enjoy!

ROOT BEER CHICKEN WINGS

Preparation time: 12 minutes
Cooking time: 18 minutes
Total time: 30 minutes

Ingredients:
- 5 lbs. of chicken wings, frozen or thawed
- 1 can of root beer, we used Saranac
- ¼ cup of brown sugar
- ¼ cup of root beer

Directions:
1. Add the chicken wings into the bottom of your Instant Pot.
2. Pour in a full can or bottle of root beer.
3. Close and lock the lid in place and ensure that the valve is in sealing position.
4. Select Manual function to cook on High Pressure for about 18 minutes.
5. When the time is up, do a quick release. Carefully open the lid and remove the chicken wings.
6. Mix together the ¼ cup of brown sugar and ¼ cup of soda.
7. Brush the wings with the mixture and place in the broiler to broil for about 2 minutes.
8. Serve and enjoy!

GARLIC SESAME CHICKEN

Servings: 4
Preparation time: 10 minutes
Cooking time: 25 minutes
Total time: 35 minutes

Ingredients:
- 2 pounds of boneless and skinless chicken thighs cut into 1-2 inch pieces
- 2 tbsp. of sesame oil
- ¼ cup of low sodium soy sauce
- 1 tbsp. of minced garlic
- 1 tbsp. of ginger, grated
- 1/3 cup of brown sugar
- ½ cup of low sodium chicken broth
- 1 tbsp. of rice vinegar
- ¼ cup of water
- ¼ tsp. of red pepper flakes

Cornstarch Slurry:
- 2 tbsp. of water
- 2 tbsp. of cornstarch

Garnish:
- 2 green onions, sliced
- Sesame seeds

Directions:
1. Add all the first 10 ingredients into the bottom of your Instant Pot.
2. Close and lock the lid in place and ensure that the valve is in sealing position.
3. Select Manual function to cook on High Pressure for about 5 minutes.
4. When the time is up, use a natural pressure release for about 10 minutes.
5. Carefully open the lid and press the Sauté function, on LOW.
6. In a medium bowl, combine together 2 tbsp. of cornstarch with 2 tbsp. of water, whisk until well combined with no lumps.
7. Pour the mixture in the Instant Pot and give everything a good stir to combine.
8. Cook on Sauté setting for a couple of minutes, stirring gently, until the sauce thickens for about 5 minutes.
9. If you desire a thicker sauce, mix in additional 1 tbsp. of cornstarch with 1 tbsp. of juice and add the mixture to the pot.
10. 1Allow the chicken to stand for about 5 to 7 minutes to thicken the sauce.
11. Garnish with fresh chopped green onions and sesame seeds.
12. 1Serve over rice and enjoy!

BBQ CHICKEN WITH POTATOES

Preparation time: 10 minutes
Cooking time: 15 minutes
Total time: 25 minutes

Ingredients:
- lb. of frozen chicken, if fresh
- 1 cup of favorite BBQ sauce
- ½ cup of water
- 1 tbsp. of Italian seasoning
- 1 tbsp. of minced garlic
- 2-3 large potatoes, chopped
- 1 large red onion, sliced

Directions:
1. Add all ingredients into the bottom of your Instant Pot.
2. Secure the lid in place. Select Poultry function to cook for 15 minutes.
3. When the timer beeps, do a natural pressure

release for 10 minutes. Carefully open the lid and remove the chicken.
4. Shred the chicken with two forks and add back into the pot. Give everything a good stir to until chicken is covered in sauce.
5. Serve and enjoy!

APPLE BALSAMIC CHICKEN
Preparation time: 15 minutes
Cooking time: 15 minutes
Total time: 30 minutes
Servings: 4

Ingredients:
- ½ cup of chicken broth
- ¼ cup of apple cider or juice
- ¼ cup of balsamic vinegar
- tbsp. of lemon juice
- ½ tsp. of salt
- ½ tsp. of garlic powder
- ½ tsp. of dried thyme
- ½ tsp. of paprika
- ½ tsp. of pepper
- bone-in chicken thighs (about 1-1/2 pounds), skin removed
- 2 tbsp. of butter
- 2 tbsp. of all-purpose flour

Directions:
1. In a medium bowl, combine together the first nine ingredients.
2. Add the chicken in your 6 quart electric pressure cooker and pour the broth mixture over meat.
3. Close and lock the lid in place and ensure that the valve is in sealing position. Select Manual function to cook on High Pressure for about 10 minutes.
4. When the time is up, use a natural pressure release for about 10 minutes, then quick release any remaining pressure.
5. Carefully open the lid and remove the chicken. Skim fat from cooking liquid. Melt the butter in a small saucepan and whisk in flour until smooth.
6. Slowly add the cooking liquid. Cook and stir until sauce is thickened for about 2 to 3 minutes. Serve with chicken and enjoy!

BUTTER CHICKEN
Preparation time: 10 minutes
Cooking time: 8 minutes
Total time: 18 minutes

Ingredients:
- 2 tbsp. of ghee
- 1 onion, diced
- tsp. of minced garlic
- 1 tsp. of minced ginger
- 1 ½ lbs. of skinless and boneless chicken thighs, cut into quarters

Spices:
- 1 tsp. of coriander powder
- 1 tsp. of garam masala
- 1 tsp. of paprika
- 1 tsp. of salt
- 1 tsp. of turmeric
- ¼ tsp. of black pepper
- ¼ tsp. of cayenne
- ¼ tsp. of ground cumin
- 1 (15 oz.) can tomato sauce

Add Later:
- 2 green bell peppers, chopped in large pieces
- ½ cup of heavy cream or full-fat coconut milk
- Pinch of dried fenugreek leaves (kasoorimethi)
- Cilantro, garnish

Directions:
1. Press the Sauté function on your Instant Pot and add the ghee and onions.
2. Stir-fry the onions for 6 to 7 minutes or until the onions start to brown. Add the garlic, ginger and chicken.
3. Stir-fry the chicken for 6 to 7 minutes or until the chicken is no longer pink.
4. Add the spices and mix thoroughly. Stir in the tomato sauce.
5. Close and lock the lid in place and ensure that the valve is in sealing position.
6. Select Manual function to cook on High Pressure for about 8 minutes.
7. When the time is up, use a quick pressure release.
8. Carefully open the lid. Press the Sauté function and add the bell peppers.
9. Cook the contents until they soften. Stir in the cream and fenugreek leaves. Garnish with cilantro if desired.
10. 1Serve and enjoy!

CHICKEN CORN CHOWDER
Preparation time: 10 minutes
Cooking time: 15 minutes
Total time: 25 minutes

Ingredients:
- 1 pound of chicken tenderloins, cubed
- 2 tablespoons of butter
    - cups of potatoes, peeled and diced (We used 1 large and 3 small

potatoes)
- 32 ounces chicken stock
- 12 ounces bag frozen corn (We used Birds Eye Steam fresh)
- 1 cup of frozen carrots
- ¼ cup of onion, diced
- ½ teaspoon of parsley flakes
- 1 cup of milk
- 2 ounces of cream cheese
- ½ cup of real shredded bacon (We used Oscar Mayer)

Directions:
1. Press the sauté function on your Instant Pot and add the butter.
2. Add the chicken and cook until brown. Add the potatoes, chicken stock, corn, carrots, onion, and parsley to the pot.
3. Secure the lid in place and ensure that the valve is in sealing position. Select Manual, High Pressure for 15 minutes.
4. When the timer beeps, do a quick pressure release. Carefully open the lid and add the milk, cream cheese and bacon.
5. Set to sauté and stir until cream cheese is completely blended in. Add a little corn starch to make the soup thicker.
6. Serve with shredded cheddar on top if desired.

CHICKEN TIKKA MASALA

Preparation time: 20 minutes
Cooking time: 20 minutes
Total time: 40 minutes
Servings: 8

Ingredients:
- 2 tbsp. of olive oil
- ½ large onion, finely chopped
- 4-1/2 tsp. of minced fresh gingerroot
- 4 garlic cloves, minced
- 1 tbsp. of garam masala
- 2-1/2 tsp. of salt
- 1-1/2 tsp. of ground cumin
- 1 tsp. of paprika
- ¾ tsp. of pepper
- ½ tsp. of cayenne pepper
- ¼ tsp. of ground cinnamon
- 2-1/2 lbs. of boneless skinless chicken breasts, cut into 1-1/2-inch cubes
- 1 can (29 oz.) tomato puree
- 1/3 cup of water
- 1 jalapeno pepper, halved and seeded
- 1 bay leaf
- 1 tbsp. of cornstarch
- 1-1/2 cups (12 oz.) plain yogurt
- Hot cooked basmati rice
- Chopped fresh cilantro, optional

Directions:
1. Press the Sauté function in your 6 quart electric pressure cooker, adjust for medium heat and add oil.
2. Add the onion and cook until tender. Add the ginger and garlic and cook for about 1 minute.
3. Stir in seasonings and cook for additional 30 seconds. Add the chicken, tomato puree, water, jalapeno and bay leaf.
4. Close and lock the lid in place and ensure that the valve is in sealing position. Select Manual function to cook on High Pressure for about 10 minutes.
5. When the time is up, use a quick pressure release. Carefully open the lid and discard the bay leaf.
6. Select the Sauté function and adjust for medium heat; bring mixture to a boil. In a medium bowl, mix together the cornstarch and yogurt until smooth.
7. Slowly stir the mixture into the sauce. Cook and stir until sauce is thickened for about 3 minutes.
8. Serve with rice and sprinkle with cilantro if desired.

WHITE CHICKEN CHILI

Preparation time: 10 minutes
Cooking time: 5 minutes
Total time: 15 minutes
Servings: 6

Ingredients:
- 1 chicken breast cubed, about 2 cups
- 3 tablespoons of olive oil
- 1 tablespoon of minced garlic
- 14-16 ounces chicken broth use less if you want it thicker
- 1 small can diced chilies
- 1 cup of canned corn drained
- 1 jar salsa verde, 16 ounces
- 2 cans white beans
- 1 tablespoon of cornstarch

Salt to taste
- Toppings: sour cream, avocado
- Spicy jack cheese shredded
- ½ onion, diced

Directions:
1. Turn your Instant Pot to sauté and add your olive oil. Add the garlic, and onions. Sauté until onions are softened slightly.

2. Add the cubed chicken and cook for about 3 minutes. Press the Cancel function and add the salsa verde, broth, chilies, white beans, corn and a pinch of salt.
3. Secure the lid in place. Select Manual, High Pressure for 5 minutes. When the timer beeps, do a quick pressure release and carefully open the lid.
4. In a medium bowl, add a small ladle full of chili liquid with cornstarch and stir. Add the mixture into your pot and stir to thicken. Give everything a good stir.
5. Serve topped with spicy jack cheese, avocado and sour cream!!

CHICKEN CACCIATORE

Preparation time: 10 minutes
Cooking time: 3 minutes
Total time: 13 minutes
Servings: 6

Ingredients:
- 1 jar spaghetti sauce 24 ounces
- 4 chicken breasts boneless skinless, cut into bite size pieces
- ½ onion
- 3 bell peppers
- ½ teaspoon of chili powder
- 1 teaspoon of garlic salt
- ½ cup of water

Directions:
1. Cube the chicken and add them into the bottom of your Instant Pot.
2. Pour spaghetti sauce over the chicken. Add the ½ cup of water into your jar, place on top and shake to get rest of the sauce out of jar.
3. Pour the on top of chicken. Cut bell peppers and onion into strips and add into your Instant Pot.
4. Sprinkle with chili powder and garlic salt over. Give everything a good stir to combine. Secure the lid in place.
5. Select Manual, High Pressure for 3 minutes. When the timer beeps, do a quick pressure release.
6. Carefully open the lid and give everything a good stir.
7. Serve over rice and enjoy!

SPICY CHICKEN

Preparation Time: 18 minutes
Servings: 4

Ingredients:
- 3 large boneless; skinless chicken breasts
- 1/2 an onion; chopped..
- 1 can full-fat coconut milk
- 3 cloves garlic; minced
- 1½ tsp. black pepper
- 1 tsp. turmeric
- 1/2 cup of water
- 1 tbsp. olive oil
- 2 tsp. smoked paprika
- 1½ tsp. ground cumin
- Sea salt to taste

Directions:
1. Place the chicken and water in the instant pot. Cover with the lid and lock
2. Use manual settings for high pressure and set timer to 15minutes
3. When the timer beeps; use natural release pressure to release the steam
4. Remove the chicken from the pot and shred it using two forks
5. Add the oil onion and garlic to the instant pot; keeping the *Sauté* mode on.
6. Let the Ingredients cook for 3 minutes; stirring constantly
7. Turn the *Sauté* function off then add the shredded chicken, cumin, turmeric, coconut milk, smoked paprika, black pepper and salt to the pot
8. Mix all the Ingredients well with the chicken. Serve with steaming boiled rice

CHICKEN AND GRAPE TOMATOES

Preparation Time: 35 minutes
Servings: 2

Ingredients:
- 2/3 lb. boneless; skinless chicken breast
- 3 cups of cold water
- 1/2 tsp salt
- 1 tbsp. Dijon mustard
- 1 tbsp. honey
- 1 tbsp. balsamic vinegar
- 3 cloves garlic; finely minced
- 3 tbsp. olive oil
- Grape tomatoes; cut in half
- Field greens,

Directions:
1. Take a large bowl and put two cups of water and the chicken pieces into it. Let it refrigerate for 45 minutes,
2. Pour 1 cup of water into the instant pot and place a trivet over it.
3. Place the chicken pieces on the trivet and select *Manual* function to set high pressure for 5 minutes

4. After it beeps sound; release the steam naturally then let the chicken stay for 5 minutes
5. Meanwhile; put the Dijon mustard, olive oil, garlic, balsamic vinegar and honey into a bowl and mix them all together
6. Slice the chicken and add the field greens and tomatoes, Pour the honey mixture over the chicken and serve

CHICKEN DUMPLINGS

Preparation Time: 35 minutes
Servings: 6

Ingredients:

- 2 lb. chicken breasts, skinless and bone-in
- 4 carrots; chopped.
- 2 cups flour
- 3 celery stalks; chopped.
- 3/4 cup chicken stock
- 1 yellow onion; chopped.
- 1/2 tsp. thyme; dried
- 2 eggs
- 2/3 cup milk
- 1 tbsp. chives
- 1 tbsp. baking powder
- Salt and black pepper to the taste

Directions:

1. In your instant pot; add chicken, onion, carrots, celery, stock, thyme, salt and pepper; then stir well. seal the instant pot lid and cook on Low for 15 minutes
2. Quick release the pressure, transfer chicken to a bowl and keep warm for now.
3. In a bowl, mix eggs with salt, milk and baking powder and stir
4. Add flour gradually and stir very well
5. Set instant pot to Simmer mode and bring the liquid inside to a boil.
6. Shape dumplings from eggs mix, drop them into stock, seal the instant pot lid and cook at High for 7 minutes.
7. Shred chicken and add to the pot after you've released the pressure; then stir well. divide everything among plates and serve with chives sprinkled on top

CHICKEN TACOS

Preparation Time: 35 minutes
Servings: 12

Ingredients:

- 4 skinless; boneless chicken breasts

For Mojo:
- 1/4 cup olive oil
- 2/3 cup fresh lime juice
- 1/4 tsp. ground black pepper
- 2/3 cup orange juice
- 2 tsp. ground cumin
- 8 garlic cloves; minced
- 1 tbsp. dried oregano
- 1 tbsp. grated orange peel
- 2 tsp. kosher salt
- 1/2 cup chopped fresh cilantro

For Serving:
- 1/2 cup red onion; finely diced
- 12 organic corn tortillas
- Chopped cilantro.
- 1 avocado; sliced

Directions:

1. Put all the Ingredients of mojo into a small bowl and mix together
2. Put the chicken in the pot and pour the mojo mix over it
3. Cover with the cooker lid and select the *poultry* function with 20 minutes on the timer.
4. When it beeps; use *Natural Release* for 10 minutes then *Quick Release* to remove all the steam.
5. Remove the lid carefully. Shred the chicken inside the pot using two forks.
6. To make the chicken crispier, broil it in an oven for 8 minutes, Serve it with tacos, onion, avocado and fresh cilantro on top.

BBQ CHICKEN WINGS

Preparation Time: 25 minutes
Servings: 6

Ingredients:

- 3/4 cup favorite barbecue sauce
- 2 lb. chicken wings
- 2 tbsp. seasoned salt
- 1/4 cup hot sauce
- 3/4 cup cold water

Directions:

1. Place chicken wings in a medium-sized bowl and add seasoned salt to it
2. Toss the wings in the bowl to add more flavor
3. Put the seasoned chicken wings in an instant pot and add the barbecue sauce to it
4. Add 1 cup of water to the pot then secure the lid
5. Select the *Manual* function on the pressure cooker and set to high pressure with 10 minutes cooking time,
6. After it beeps sound; release the steam

carefully with *Quick Release*
7. Remove the lid and let the wings stay for 2 minutes.
8. Now stir the sauce in with the chicken wings to enrich their flavor. Serve the dish with red pepper slices and celery sticks

CLASSIC TURKEY CHEESE GNOCCHI

Preparation Time: 30 minutes
Servings: 6

Ingredients:
- 1 lb. turkey boneless pieces,
- 2 cups fresh spinach chopped.
- 2 cups mozzarella cheese shredded
- 1/2 cup parmesan cheese shredded
- 2 tbsp. olive oil
- 1/2 tsp. black pepper
- 1/4 cup shallots chopped.
- 2 cloves garlic minced
- 1/4 cup sun-dried tomatoes,
- 1 cup cream
- 2 cups chicken broth
- 2 lb. gnocchi
- 1/2 tsp. salt

Directions:
1. Select the *Sauté* option on your instant pot. Pour in the oil and heat
2. Add the turkey, with salt and pepper. Let it cook for 3 minutes on each side.
3. Now add the garlic tomatoes and the shallots to the pot. Cook for 2 minutes while stirring.
4. Add the cream and chicken broth to the pot. Secure the cooker lid
5. Select *Manual* settings at high pressure for 10 minutes
6. When it beeps; release the steam naturally then remove the lid
7. Add the gnocchi to the mixture
8. Select the *Sauté* function and let it all cook for 5 minutes until gnocchi is tender
9. Switch off the appliance then add the cheese to the pot. Serve immediately.

TURKEY STUFFED TACOS

Preparation Time: 25 minutes
Servings: 6

Ingredients:
- 3/4 lb. chopped white turkey meat
- 1/2 bottle of any dark beer
- 2 tbsp. olive oil
- 1 medium onion
- 1 tsp. cumin
- 3 cloves garlic
- 1 jalapeno pepper; diced
- 4 diced tomatoes
- 8 taco shells
- Salt and pepper to taste

Toppings:
- Tomatoes
- Salsa
- Lettuce
- Cheddar cheese

Directions:
1. Put the olive oil, chopped onion and garlic into the instant pot
2. Select the *Sauté* function and let it cook for 5 minutes
3. Add the jalapeno pepper and chopped turkey to the pot
4. Let it cook for 5 minutes
5. Now add the salt, pepper, cumin and diced tomatoes
6. After 5 minutes more cooking, pour in the beer
7. Now cover the lid and lock it properly. Select the *Manual* function - 5 minutes at high pressure
8. When it beeps; use the *Natural Release* to release all the steam
9. Remove the cooker lid but leave the prepared filling to one side, To serve; stuff the filling in a taco wrap and add cheese on top.

RICH TASTE KUNG PAO TURKEY

Preparation Time: 25 minutes
Servings: 4

Ingredients:
Turkey marinade:
- 2 tbsp. soy sauce
- 2 tbsp. cornstarch
- 2 tbsp. red wine vinegar
- 3 cloves garlic minced
- 1 tbsp. sesame oil
- Salt and pepper to taste

Main ingredients:
- 1½ lb. turkey breast cut into cubes
- 1 large yellow bell pepper; chopped.
- 1 cucumber; chopped.
- 1/2 cup pistachios
- green onions; chopped.
- 3 tbsp. olive oil
- 5 cloves of garlic; minced
- Salt and pepper to taste

Sauce:
- 2 tbsp. red wine vinegar

- 4 tbsp. soy sauce
- 2 tbsp. hot and spicy ketchup
- 1 tbsp. chili garlic sauce
- 1 tbsp. brown sugar
- 1/2 cup water
- 2 tbsp. cornstarch

Directions:
1. Put all the Ingredients for the marinade into a large bowl and mix
2. Add the turkey pieces to the marinade, Let them soak for 20 minutes
3. Pour the olive oil into the instant pot and select the *Sauté* function.
4. Add the minced garlic and let it cook for 30 seconds.
5. Now add the marinated turkey and let it cook for 10 minutes
6. Add all the vegetables, except green onions, to the pot.
7. Allow the dish to cook for 3 minutes then add all the Ingredients for the sauce.
8. Keep cooking until the sauce thickens
9. Stir the pistachios and green onions into the turkey sauce, Switch off the instant pot and serve.

TURKEY WITH GARLIC HERB SAUCE

Preparation Time: 25 minutes
Servings: 4

Ingredients:
- 4 turkey thighs with skin and bones
- 2 tsp. fresh oregano; chopped.
- 2 tbsp. olive oil
- cloves garlic; minced
- 1/2 cup sherry; or dry red wine
- 1/2 cup chicken broth
- 2 tsp. fresh thyme; chopped.
- Salt and pepper to taste

Directions:
1. Add salt and pepper seasoning to the turkey thighs.
2. Select the *Sauté* function on the instant pot and add the olive oil to it
3. Place the turkey thighs in the pot and let them cook for 5 minutes on both sides.
4. Remove the turkey thighs when they turn golden brown
5. Now; put the oil, garlic, thyme and oregano into the pot and *Sauté* for 2 minutes
6. Add the sherry (or wine)the chicken broth and fried turkey thighs to the pot
7. Close the instant pot lid and select the *Manual* function, high pressure for 20 minutes
8. When it beeps; use the *Natural Release* to vent the steam. Serve with fresh herbs sprinkled on top.

BRAISED DUCK AND POTATOES RECIPE

Preparation Time: 30 minutes
Servings: 4

Ingredients:
- 1 duck, cut into small chunks
- 4 tbsp. soy sauce
- 4 tbsp. sherry wine
- 1/4 cup water
- 1 potato; cut into cubes
- 1-inch ginger root; sliced
- 4 garlic cloves; minced.
- 4 tbsp. sugar
- 2 green onions; roughly chopped
- A pinch of salt
- Black pepper to the taste

Directions:
1. Set your instant pot on Sauté mode; add duck pieces, stir and brown them for a few minutes
2. Add garlic, ginger, green onions, soy sauce, sugar, wine, a pinch of salt, black pepper and water; then stir well. close the lid; set the pot to Poultry mode and cook for 18 minutes
3. Quick release the pressure, carefully open the lid; add potatoes; then stir well. Seal the Instant Pot lid and cook at High for 5 minutes.
4. Quick release the pressure, divide braised duck among plates and serve

TACO BOWLS

Preparation Time: 25 minutes
Servings: 6

Ingredients:
- 5 chicken breasts (boneless, skinless)
- 1 (12 oz.) bag frozen corn
- 3 cups uncooked jasmine rice; rinsed
- 3 cups chicken broth
- 1 (15 oz.) can black beans
- 1/2 cup shredded cheddar cheese
- 1 (15.5 oz.) jar salsa
- 2 tbsp. taco seasoning
- cilantro
- sour cream

Directions:
1. Pour one cup of chicken broth into the instant pot.
2. Add the chicken rice, taco seasoning, salsa,

corns and beans to the pot
3. Select the *Manual* function on your cooker; setting it to high pressure and 12 minutes cooking time
4. Let it cook until it beeps.
5. Use *Quick Release* to vent the steam
6. Remove the lid when pressure is completely released
7. Shred the chicken in the pot. Serve it with cheddar cheese, sour cream and cilantro on top

STUFFED CHICKEN BREAST
Preparation Time: 40 minutes
Servings: 2
Ingredients:
- 2 chicken breasts, skinless and boneless and butterflied
- 1-piece ham; halved and cooked
- 2 cup water
- 4 mozzarella cheese slices
- 16 bacon strips
- 6 asparagus spears
- Salt and black pepper to taste

Directions:
1. In a bowl; mix chicken breasts with salt and 1 cup water, stir, cover and keep in the fridge for 30 minutes
2. Pat dry chicken breasts and place them on a working surface
3. Add 2 slices of mozzarella, 1-piece ham and 3 asparagus pieces on each.
4. Add salt and pepper and roll up each chicken breast
5. Place 8 bacon strips on a working surface, add chicken and wrap it in bacon.
6. Repeat this with the rest of the bacon strips and the other chicken breast.
7. Put rolls in the steamer basket of the pot, add 1 cup water in the pot; cover and cook at High for 10 minutes.
8. Release the pressure quick, pat dry rolls with paper towels and leave them on a plate
9. Set your instant pot on Sauté mode; add chicken rolls and brown them for a few minutes. Divide among plates and serve

SCAMPI CHICKEN
Preparation Time: 20 minutes
Servings: 6
Ingredients:
- 3 chicken breasts; cut into strips
- 1/2 red onion sliced
- 1/2 tsp. pepper
- 1/2 cup chicken broth
- 1/2 tsp. garlic powder
- 1/2 tsp. Italian seasoning
- 1 yellow bell pepper sliced
- 1 red bell pepper sliced
- 3 cloves of garlic minced
- 1 cup white wine
- 1/2 cup parmesan cheese
- 2 tbsp. olive oil
- 1/2 cup flour
- 1 tsp. salt

Directions:
1. Select the *Sauté* function on your instant pot pressure cooker. Allow it to preheat for 5 minutes.
2. Meanwhile put the flour, salt and pepper into a shallow container. Add the chicken strips to the dry mix and dredge it through to get an even coating
3. Now put the oil into the preheated cooker and place chicken in it.
4. Let it cook for 3 minutes; from each side, until it turns golden brown
5. Add the peppers, garlic cloves, onions, chicken broth and wine
6. Cover with the cooker lid. Using the *Manual* function, set the timer for 5 minutes and cook at high pressure,
7. When it beeps; do a *Quick Release* then open the lid.
8. Add parmesan cheese to the pot immediately. Stir it well in. Serve over pasta

POTATOES WITH BBQ CHICKEN
Preparation Time: 35 minutes
Servings: 6
Ingredients:
- 2 lb. chicken breasts
- 1 tbsp. minced garlic
- 2 - 3 large potatoes; chopped.
- 1 cup BBQ sauce
- 1 large; red onion, sliced
- 1/2 cup water
- 1 tbsp. Italian seasoning

Directions:
1. Place all the Ingredients in the instant pot
2. Cover with the cooker lid and lock.
3. Select the *poultry* function on the cooker and set it for 15 minutes cooking time
4. After it's done; use the *Natural Release* for 10 minutes to discharge the steam
5. Remove the lid and shred the chicken with

two forks
6. Stir the sauce well to simmer the shredded chicken into it. Serve immediately

CHICKEN CURRY WITH HONEY
Preparation Time: 31 minutes
Servings: 4
Ingredients:
- 1½ lb. boneless; skinless chicken thighs or breasts
- 1½ tsp. hot curry powder
- 1/4 cup yellow mustard
- 1/4 tsp. cayenne pepper
- 1/4 cup unsalted butter; melted
- 1 tsp. salt
- 1/2 cup honey

Directions:
1. Put the mustard, curry powder, honey, cayenne pepper, salt and melted butter into the inner pot.
2. Mix all the Ingredients well. Place the pot in the cooker with the trivet
3. Place the chicken pieces on the trivet
4. Use *Manual* settings to set the cooker to high pressure for 18 minutes.
5. After cooking is complete, use the *Natural Release* for 10 minutes to vent the steam
6. Remove the chicken and trivet. Shred the pieces and put them to one side
7. Leave the remaining Ingredients in the pot and set the sauté option for 5 minutes
8. Boil the sauce until it thickens
9. Pour the sauce over the shredded chicken and stir well. Serve with boiled rice

DELICIOUS CHICKEN SANDWICHES
Preparation Time: 25 minutes
Servings: 8
Ingredients:
- 20 oz. canned pineapple and its juice; chopped.
- 12 oz. canned orange juice
- 15 oz. canned peaches and their juice
- 6 chicken breasts; skinless and boneless
- 1 tsp. soy sauce
- 2 tbsp. lemon juice
- 1 tbsp. cornstarch
- 1/4 cup brown sugar
- 8 hamburger buns
- 8 grilled pineapple slices; for serving

Directions:
1. In a bowl, mix orange juice with soy sauce, lemon juice, canned pineapples pieces, peaches and sugar and stir well
2. Pour half of this mix in your instant pot; add chicken and pour the rest of the sauce over meat.
3. Cover the pot and cook at High for 12 minutes
4. Quick release the pressure, take the chicken and put on a cutting board
5. Shred meat and leave aside for now.
6. In a bowl; mix cornstarch with 1 tablespoon cooking juice and stir well.
7. Transfer the sauce to a pot, add cornstarch mix and chicken, stir and cook for a few more minutes.
8. Divide this chicken mix on hamburger buns; top with grilled pineapple pieces and serve

CHICKEN NOODLE PHO RECIPE
Preparation Time: 25 minutes
Servings: 4
Ingredients:
Broth:
- 2 lb. chicken pieces; bones-in
- 3 whole cloves
- 1 tbsp. coriander seeds
- 1½ tbsp. fish sauce
- 2 tsp. maple syrup
- 1 small Fuji apple; sliced
- 1 large yellow onion; sliced
- 4 cups just-boiled water
- 3/4 cup chopped cilantro sprigs
- 2¼ tsp. sea salt
- 2-inch ginger; sliced

Bowls:
- oz. flat rice noodles; boiled
- 1/4 cup chopped fresh cilantro; leafy tops only
- 1/2 small yellow onions; thinly sliced
- 2 thinly sliced green onions; green parts
- Freshly ground black pepper.

Directions:
1. Select the *Sauté* function on your instant pot and add the coriander seeds and the cloves.
2. Let them roast for 60 seconds then add 4 cups of water chicken, salt, apple, cilantro and salt
3. Close the instant pot lid and set the cooker on *Manual* to cook for 15 minutes at high pressure
4. When it beeps; use *Natural Release* for 20 minutes to vent all the steam
5. Remove the chicken from the broth. Pull the meat from the bones and put it aside as thin

slices
6. Strain the remaining chicken broth and discard all the solids.
7. Place all the vegetables boiled noodles and chicken slices in a serving bowl. Pour the hot broth into the bowl; sprinkle black pepper and serve immediately

SPECIAL TURKEY MEATBALLS

Preparation Time: 50 minutes
Servings: 8

Ingredients:

- 1 lb. turkey meat; ground.
- one egg; whisked
- 3 dried shiitake mushrooms; soaked in water, drained and chopped.
- 2 tbsp. cornstarch mixed with 2 tbsp. water
- 4 garlic cloves; minced.
- 1/4 cup parsley; chopped.
- 1/4 cup milk
- 1/4 cup parmesan cheese; grated
- 1/2 cup panko bread crumbs
- 1 yellow onion; minced.
- 1 cup chicken stock
- 2 tbsp. extra virgin olive oil
- 2 tsp. soy sauce
- 1 tsp. fish sauce
- 2 tbsp. butter
- 1 tsp. oregano; dried
- cremini mushrooms; chopped.
- Salt and black pepper to the taste
- A splash of sherry wine

Directions:

1. In a bowl; mix turkey meat with parmesan cheese, salt, pepper to the taste, yellow onion, garlic, bread crumbs, parsley, oregano, egg, milk, 1 tsp. soy sauce and 1 tsp. fish sauce, stir very well and shape 16 meatballs
2. Heat up a pan with 1 tablespoon oil over medium high heat, add meatballs, brown them for 1 minutes on each side and transfer them to a plate.
3. Pour chicken stock into the pan, stir and take off heat
4. Set your instant pot on Sauté mode; add 1 tablespoon oil and 2 tablespoon butter and heat them up.
5. Add cremini mushrooms, salt, and pepper; stir and cook for 10 minutes.
6. Add dried mushrooms, sherry wine and the rest of the soy sauce and stir well.
7. Add meatballs, seal the instant pot lid and cook at High for 6 minutes
8. Quick release the pressure, carefully open the lid; add cornstarch mix, stir well, divide everything between plates and serve.

CRACK CHICKEN RECIPE

Preparation Time: 30 minutes
Servings: 6

Ingredients:

- 4 chicken breasts
- 1 packet ranch dressing mix
- 1 lb. bacon; diced, raw
- 8 oz. cream cheese
- 1/2 cup chicken broth
- 1 cup mayonnaise
- 2 cups shredded cheddar cheese
- 1/4 cup chopped green onions

Directions:

1. Select the *Sauté* function on your instant pot. Put chopped bacon into the pot and cook for 5 minutes,
2. Clean the pot then add the chicken breasts and cream cheese.
3. Add the chicken broth to the pot
4. Secure the lid. Select *Manual* function and set to high pressure with 15 minutes on the timer.
5. When it beeps; release the steam over 5 minutes using *Natural Release*
6. Use the *Quick Release* to discharge any remaining steam.
7. Remove the lid and take the chicken out of the pot
8. Shred the chicken and put it aside.
9. Use the *Sauté* function to cook the remaining cream cheese, Keep stirring until it thickens.
10. Stir in the mayonnaise the shredded chicken, cheese, green onions and bacon. Serve and enjoy

GREEN CHILLI ADOBO CHICKEN

Servings: 6
Preparation Time: 6 minutes'
Cooking Time: 25 minutes

Ingredients

- 6 boneless, skinless chicken breasts
- ½ cup water
- 1 tablespoon turmeric
- 1 tablespoon GOYA Adobo all-purpose seasoning with pepper
- two cups diced tomatoes
- 1 cup diced green chillies

- White rice or fill tacos to serve

Directions
1. Place the chicken breasts in the inner pot.
2. Add the Adobo seasoning pepper to the chicken. Sprinkle on both sides.
3. Add the diced tomatoes to the chicken.
4. Pour half-cup of water over the chicken.
5. Cover and lock the lid. Use manual settings and set the time to 25 minutes.
6. When cooking is complete at the beep, use 'natural release' to vent the steam for 15 minutes.
7. Use 'quick release' option to vent all the remaining steam.
8. Remove the pot and shred the chicken inside using two forks.
9. Serve with rice, or fill the tacos with the shredded chicken.

Nutrition Values:
Calories: 204
Carbohydrate: 7.6g
Protein: 32.9g
Fat: 4.2g
Sugar: 2.2g
Sodium: 735mg

CHICKEN CURRY WITH HONEY

Servings: 4
Preparation Time: 6 minutes
Cooking Time: 25 minutes

Ingredients
- ¼ cup yellow mustard
- ¼ cup unsalted butter, melted
- ¼ teaspoon cayenne pepper
- 1½ lbs boneless, skinless chicken thighs or breasts
- 1½ teaspoons hot curry powder
- 1 teaspoon salt
- ½ cup honey
- Boiled rice to serve

Directions
1. Put the mustard, curry powder, honey, cayenne pepper, salt, and melted butter into the inner pot.
2. Mix all the ingredients well. Place the pot in the cooker with the trivet.
3. Place the chicken pieces on the trivet.
4. Use 'manual' settings to set the cooker at high pressure for 18 minutes.
5. After cooking is complete, use the 'natural release' for 10 minutes to vent the steam.
6. Remove the chicken and trivet. Shred the pieces and put them to one side.
7. Leave the remaining ingredients in the pot and set the sauté option for 5 minutes.
8. Boil the sauce until it thickens.
9. Pour the sauce over the shredded chicken and stir well.
10. 1Serve with boiled rice.

Nutrition Values:
Calories: 1895
Carbohydrate: 41.3g
Protein: 132.8g
Fat: 133.6g
Sugar: 34.9g
Sodium: 894mg

CHICKEN BOWL WITH SMOKED PAPRIKA

Servings: 6
Preparation Time: 10 minutes
Cooking Time: 10 minutes

Ingredients
- 1 teaspoon olive oil
- 3 strips bacon, chopped
- 1 small onion, chopped
- 2 garlic cloves, minced.
- 1 small red bell pepper, chopped
- 2 teaspoons smoked paprika
- 1 teaspoon salt
- 1 (12 oz.) can of beer.
- 1½ lb chicken breasts cut into small pieces
- 1 cup white rice
- 2 strips bacon, cooked (topping)

Directions
1. Put the oil and bacon in the pot. Sauté it, without covering the lid, for 3 minutes.
2. Add the bell pepper to the oil and bacon and sauté for 3 more minutes.
3. Add the chopped onion and garlic and sauté for 2 minutes.
4. Add all the seasoning to the pot and turn off the 'sauté' function.
5. Add the beer to the mixture. Mix all the ingredients well.
6. Add the chicken and rice to the pot and select 'manual settings'.
7. Set to high pressure for 10 minutes and leave it to cook.
8. Use 'quick release' to vent all the steam, then remove the lid.
9. Serve the dish with the bacon strips on top.

Nutrition Values:
Calories: 524
Carbohydrate: 29.3g
Protein: 68.5g
Fat: 10.3g

Sugar: 1.2g
Sodium: 310mg

CHICKEN DUMPLINGS

Servings: 4
Preparation Time: 10 minutes
Cooking Time: 10 minutes

Ingredients

- 1 cup water
- 2 cups chicken broth
- 1½ lbs chicken breast, cubed
- 1 cup chopped carrots
- 1 teaspoon olive oil
- 1 cup frozen peas
- 2 teaspoons oregano
- 1 teaspoon onion powder
- 1 tube (16 oz. refrigerated biscuits
- 1 teaspoon basil
- ½ teaspoon salt
- 2 cloves minced garlic
- ½ teaspoon pepper

Directions

1. Press the biscuits to flatten them, then cut them into 2-inch strips with a sharp knife.
2. Put the olive oil, onion powder, oregano, chicken, garlic, salt, pepper and basil into the pot and mix them well.
3. Select the 'sauté' function on your pressure cooker and allow it to cook until the chicken turns brown.
4. Cancel the 'sauté' function when the cooking is finished.
5. Add the water, peas, carrots and chicken broth to the pot. Add the biscuits then stir well.
6. Cover with the lid and lock it.
7. Select the 'manual' function, and set the timer for 5 minutes.
8. After the beep, use the 'natural release' for 10 minutes to vent all the steam.
9. Press 'cancel' to turn the cooker off, then remove the lid.
10. 1Serve the cooked chicken in a bowl.

Nutrition Values:

Calories: 610
Carbohydrate: 13.6g
Protein: 100.5g
Fat: 12.1g
Sugar: 4.4g
Sodium: 717mg

SESAME CHICKEN TERIYAKI

Servings: 4
Preparation Time: 10 minutes
Cooking Time: 10 minutes

Ingredients

- 1 lb boneless, skinless chicken breasts.
- ½ cup soy sauce
- 1/3 cup honey
- 2 tablespoons apple cider vinegar.
- 1 teaspoon sesame oil
- 2 garlic cloves, minced
- 2 teaspoons minced ginger
- 2 tablespoons corn starch
- 3 tablespoons water
- Garnish: sliced green onions, sesame seeds

Directions

1. Place the chicken in the pressure cooker pot.
2. In a separate small bowl, mix the soy sauce, sesame oil, ginger, garlic, vinegar and honey. Mix the ingredients well.
3. Pour the prepared mixture over the chicken in the pot.
4. Close the cooker lid and lock it.
5. Select the 'manual' function and set on high pressure for 5 minutes. Let it cook.
6. When the completion beep sounds, use the 'natural release' to vent all the pressure. This should take around 15 minutes.
7. Remove the chicken from the pot and shred it using two forks. Put it to one side.
8. Select the 'sauté function and add the cornstarch and water to the remaining mixture.
9. Cook the sauce while stirring until it thickens.
10. 1Now add the chicken to the sauce and mix well.
11. 1Serve it with sprinkled sesame seeds and green onions on top.

Nutrition Values:

Calories: 645
Carbohydrate: 30.9g
Protein: 97.2g
Fat: 12.4g
Sugar: 23.8g
Sodium: 1427mg

CHICKEN WITH LETTUCE WRAP

Servings: 4
Preparation Time: 10 minutes
Cooking Time: 10 minutes

Ingredients

- 1 tablespoon olive oil
- 1 clove garlic, minced
- 1 medium onion, chopped.
- 2 cups chicken broth
- 7 oz. sliced mushrooms
- Large lettuce leaves

- ½ cup buffalo wing sauce
- 1/3 cup low sodium soy sauce
- 2 lbs boneless, skinless chicken breast
- ½ cup shredded carrots

Directions
1. Turn your instant pot to 'sauté' setting and add the oil and then onions. Add in the chicken, brown them for around 5 minutes.
2. Add in the mushrooms, garlic, chicken broth, wing sauce, and soy sauce. Stir them well
3. Cover the pot and secure the lid. Make sure valve is set to sealing. Set the manual button to 4 minutes on high pressure.
4. Once done, let the pot sit there for 10 minutes. Then remove the valve to venting and remove the lid.
5. Stir a bit. Prepare the lettuce leaves.
6. Shred the chicken while still in the pot using two forks.
7. Pour the chicken and sauce over the lettuce leaves.
8. Garnish the dish with the shredded carrots and then serve.

Nutrition Values:
Calories: 564
Carbohydrate: 6.2g
Protein: 99.2g
Fat: 11.9g
Sugar: 4.3g
Sodium: 823mg

CHICKEN WITH BLACK BEANS

Servings: 4
Preparation Time: 10 minutes
Cooking Time: 6 minutes

Ingredients
- 1 small onion chopped
- 4 cups diced tomatoes with juice
- 2 lbs boneless, skinless chicken breasts
- 1 tablespoon chipotle peppers
- ½ cup water
- 1 cup jasmine rice (uncooked)
- ½ lime, juiced
- 2 teaspoons sea salt.
- ½ teaspoon ground black pepper
- 2 tablespoons butter.
- 1 can organic black beans drained and rinsed
- 2 cups cheddar chesses for serving, shredded

Directions
1. Put the chicken, tomatoes, peppers, water, rice, salt, lemon juice, butter and onion in your instant pot.
2. Use 'manual' settings on high pressure for 6 minutes.
3. Let it cook until the cooker beeps.
4. Use the 'quick pressure release' to vent the steam.
5. Add the black beans to the chicken then stir well.
6. Add the salt and pepper to taste.
7. Serve with shredded cheese on top.

Nutrition Values:
Calories: 447
Carbohydrate: 15.2g
Protein: 66.2g
Fat: 11.7g
Sugar: 3.9g
Sodium: 188mg

STEAMED GARLIC CHICKEN BREASTS

Servings: 3
Preparation Time: 5 minutes
Cooking time: 9 minutes

Ingredients
- ¼ teaspoon garlic powder
- 2 lbs. boneless chicken breasts
- 1 teaspoon black pepper
- ⅛ teaspoon dried oregano
- ⅛ teaspoon dried basil
- 1 tablespoon olive oil
- 1 cup water
- Salt to taste
- For serving: lime wedges, sprinkled oregano, and basil

Directions
1. Add the oil to the pot and select the 'sauté' function. Let it heat up without the lid on.
2. Sprinkle seasonings on both sides of the chicken.
3. Put the seasoned chicken into the pot with the oil, and cook each side for 3-4 minutes until they turn golden brown.
4. Add the water to the pot then set the trivet in the pot.
5. Place the chicken pieces on the trivet.
6. Select 'manual' settings on high pressure for 5 minutes. Let it cook.
7. Use the 'natural release', after the beep, to release the steam. Use 'quick release' afterwards to make sure all the steam has been vented.
8. Remove the lid. Transfer the chicken to a platter.
9. Wait 5 minutes and serve with lime wedges, sprinkled oregano, and basil on top.

Nutrition Values:

Calories: 155
Carbohydrate: 0.3g
Protein: 21.3g
Fat: 7.2g
Sugar: 4.3g
Sodium: 62mg

CHICKEN WITH CASHEW BUTTER

Servings: 5
Preparation Time: 5 minutes
Cooking Time: 07 minutes

Ingredients

- 2 lbs chicken breasts
- ¼ cup rice vinegar
- ½ cup smooth cashew butter
- 1 cup jasmine rice (uncooked)
- ¼ cup Soy Sauce
- 1 tablespoon chilli sauce
- ½ cup chicken broth
- ¼ cup honey
- 3 cloves garlic minced
- 3 tablespoons fresh cilantro for topping (chopped)
- 3 tablespoons cashews for topping (chopped)

Directions

3

1. Cut the chicken breasts into small, 2-inch chunks. Put the pieces in the cooker pot.
2. Put the cashew butter, honey, rice, soy sauce, chilli sauce, vinegar, chicken broth and garlic in a separate bowl and mix all the ingredients well.
3. Pour the butter mixture over the chicken pieces. Then cover with the lid.
4. After securing the lid select 'manual' function on high pressure for 7 minutes
5. Let it cook till it beeps. Then use the 'quick release' method to vent the steam.
6. Serve the chicken on a platter with the chopped cashews and fresh cilantro on top.

Nutrition Values:

Calories: 640
Carbohydrate: 26.3g
Protein: 69.9g
Fat: 27.6g
Sugar: 13.7g
Sodium: 754mg

LIME CHICKEN WITH CHILLIES

Servings: 5
Preparation Time: 5 minutes
Cooking Time: 15 minutes

Ingredients

- 2 lbs. boneless skinless chicken breasts
- 1 teaspoon sea salt
- ¼ teaspoon black pepper
- 1 onion, chopped
- 2 tablespoons olive oil.
- 4 garlic cloves, minced
- ½ cup organic chicken broth
- 1 teaspoon dried parsley
- 1½ teaspoons chili powder
- 2 medium (or large) sized limes, juiced
- 4 teaspoons arrowroot flour - optional

Directions

1. Add the oil and chopped onions in the instant pot. Select the 'sauté' function to cook onions for 5 minutes or until turns light brown.
2. Add all the remaining ingredients to the pot. Stir until the chicken is well coated.
3. Cover the pot and secure the lid. Make sure valve is set to sealing. Cook at high pressure for 10 minutes.
4. Once done, let the pressure naturally release for 10 minutes. Then vent the pressure valve to release the remaining steam. Check if the sauce is thicken enough.
5. If not, add the dissolved arrowroot flour into the sauce to increase the thickness.
6. Transfer the cooked chicken onto a platter and serve immediately.

Nutrition Values:

Calories: 697
Carbohydrate: 2.9g
Protein: 127.3g
Fat: 46.1g
Sugar: 0.7
Sodium: 501mg

MEAT

EASY CARIBBEAN BEEF

Preparation Time: 5 Mins
Total Time: 60 Mins
Servings: 4

Ingredients:
- 2 pounds Beef Roast
- 1 tsp Thyme
- 1 tsp grated Ginger
- 1 tsp Garlic Powder
- 6-8 Whole Cloves
- ¼ tsp Pepper
- 1 cup Water

Direction
1. Combine all of the herbs and spices and rub the mixture into the beef.
2. Stick the cloves into the meat and then place the meat inside the IP.
3. Pour the water around not over! the meat.
4. Put the lid on.
5. Seal and set the IP to MANUAL.
6. Cook on HIGH for 45 minutes.
7. Release the pressure quickly.
8. Shred with two forks and serve as desired.
9. Enjoy!

Nutrition Values:
Calories 700
Total Fats 12g
Carbs: 1.3g
Protein 55g
Dietary Fiber: 0.2g

MARJORAM LEG OF LAMB

Preparation Time: 5 Mins
Total Time: 80 Mins
Servings: 4

Ingredients:
- 6 pounds Leg of Lamb
- 1 Bay Leaf
- ½ tsp Sage
- 2 tsp Marjoram
- 2 Garlic Cloves, minced
- 2 tbsp Arrowroot
- 1 ½ tbsp Olive Oil
- 1 ½ cups Homemade Chicken Broth

Direction
1. Set your Instant Pot to SAUTE and heat the oil in it.
2. Combine the garlic and herbs and rub into the meat.
3. Add the lamb in the Instant Pot and sear until brown on all sides.
4. Pour the chicken broth over the meat and place the bay leaf inside.
5. Close the lid, seal, and set the IP to MEAT/STEW.
6. Cook for 60 minutes and then release the pressure quickly.
7. Open the lid and whisk in the arrowroot.
8. Set the IP to SAUTE and cook until thickened.
9. Serve and enjoy!

Nutrition Values:
Calories 620
Total Fats 26g
Carbs: 3g
Protein 55g
Dietary Fiber: 0g

TOMATO BRISKET

Preparation Time: 5 Mins
Total Time: 6 hours and 20 Mins
Servings: 6

Ingredients:
- 1 cup Beef Stock
- 3 pounds Beef Brisket
- 28 ounces canned diced Tomatoes
- 4 Garlic Cloves, minced
- 1 Onion, chopped
- 2 tbsp Olive Oil

Direction
1. Heat half of the oil in the IP on SAUTE.
2. Add the beef and sear it on all sides until it becomes brown.
3. Transfer to a plate.
4. Add the remaining oil.
5. When hot, add the onions and cook for 3 minutes.
6. Add the garlic and cook for 1 more minute.
7. Add the tomatoes and broth.
8. Return the meat to the IP and close the lid.
9. Set the IP to SLOW COOK and cook for 6 hours on LOW.
10. Do a quick pressure release.
11. Serve and enjoy!

Nutrition Values:
Calories 505
Total Fats 19g
Carbs: 10g
Protein 70g

Dietary Fiber: 2g

DIJON MEATLOAF

Preparation Time: 5 Mins
Total Time: 45 Mins
Servings: 4

Ingredients:
- 1 pound Ground Beef
- 2 tbsp organic Dijon Mustard
- 1 Egg
- 1 small Onion, diced
- ½ cup Almond Flour
- ½ tsp Garlic Powder
- ½ tsp Thyme
- ¼ cup Tomato Sauce
- 1 cup Water

Direction
1. Pour the water into the IP and lower the trivet.
2. In a large bowl, place the remaining ingredients.
3. Mix with your hand until incorporated.
4. Grease a loaf pan and press the meatloaf mixture in it.
5. Place the loaf pan on the trivet and close the lid.
6. Seal the pot and choose MANUAL.
7. Cook for 35 minutes.
8. Do a quick pressure release.
9. Serve and enjoy!

Nutrition Values:
Calories 410
Total Fats 10g
Carbs: 38g
Protein 41g
Dietary Fiber: 3g

PORK CHOPS WITH BRUSSEL SPROUTS

Preparation Time: 5 Mins
Total Time: 35 Mins
Servings: 4

Ingredients:
- 1 pound Pork Chops
- 1 cup sliced Carrots
- 1 tbsp Arrowroot
- 1 cup Homemade Chicken Stock
- 2 cups Brussel Sprouts
- ½ tsp Thyme
- 2 Garlic Cloves, minced
- 1 cup sliced Onions
- 1 tbsp Ghee
- Pinch of Pepper

Direction
1. Set your Instant Pot to SAUTE and add the ghee.
2. When melted, add the pork chops and cook until they become browned. Transfer to a plate.
3. Add the onions and cook for 3 minutes.
4. Add the garlic and cook for another minute.
5. Pour the broth over and return the chops to the pot.
6. Close the lid and set the IP to MANUAL.
7. Cook for 15 minutes on HIGH.
8. Do a quick pressure release and open the lid.
9. Stir in the carrots and Brussel sprouts and close the lid again.
10. Cook on HIGH for 3 minutes.
11. Do a quick pressure release and transfer the pork and veggies to a plate.
12. Whisk the arrowroot into the pot and cook on SAUTE until thickened.
13. Drizzle the sauce over the pork and veggies.
14. Serve and enjoy!

Nutrition Values:
Calories 440
Total Fats 32g
Carbs: 12g
Protein 28g
Dietary Fiber: 2g

SHREDDED CHIPOTLE PORK

Preparation Time: 5 Mins
Total Time: 40 Mins
Servings: 4

Ingredients:
- 1 ½ pounds Pork Shoulder
- 2 Chipotle Peppers, diced
- ½ tsp Cumin
- ½ tsp Garlic Powder
- ½ tsp Paprika
- ¼ tsp Pepper
- 1 cup Homemade Beef Broth
- 1 Onion, sliced

Direction
1. Season the pork well with the spices and place it in the Instant Pot.
2. Arrange the onion slices and peppers on top and pour the broth over.
3. Close the lid and set the IP to MEAT/STEW.
4. Cook for 55 minutes.
5. Let the float valve drop on its own and then open the lid.
6. Let the pork sit for 10 minutes before serving.
7. Enjoy!

Nutrition Values:
Calories 580

Total Fats 40g
Carbs: 2g
Protein 49g
Dietary Fiber: 1g

FLAVORFUL BRAISED CHUCK

Preparation Time: 5 Mins
Total Time: 80 Mins
Servings: 4

Ingredients:
- 1 cup Homemade Beef Broth
- 2 Rosemary Sprigs
- 1 Thyme Sprig
- 1 Onion, sliced
- 2 pounds Chuck Roast
- 2 tsp minced Garlic
- 2 tbsp Ghee
- Pinch of Cumin
- Pinch of Black Pepper

Direction
1. Set your Instant Pot to SAUTE and melt the coconut oil in it.
2. Add the onions and saute for 3 minutes.
3. Stir in the garlic and cook for another minute.
4. Add the beef and sear it on all sides, until is lightly browned.
5. Pour the broth over and add the herbs.
6. Close the lid and set the IP to MANUAL.
7. Cook on HIGH for 50-6 minutes, depending on your desired doneness.
8. Do a natural pressure release.
9. Serve and enjoy!

Nutrition Values:
Calories 660
Total Fats 50g
Carbs: 3g
Protein 47g
Dietary Fiber: 0.5g

BALSAMIC BEEF ROAST

Preparation Time: 5 Mins
Total Time: 65 Mins
Servings: 6

Ingredients:
- 1 cup Homemade Beef Broth
- 1 tbsp Olive Oil
- 4 tbsp Balsamic Vinegar
- 3 pounds Beef Roast
- 1 tbsp Coconut Oil, melted
- ½ tsp Thyme
- ½ tsp Garlic Powder
- ¼ tsp Onion Powder
- Pinch of Pepper

Direction
1. Heat the olive oil in your Instant Pot on SAUTE.
2. Add the beef and sear on all sides until it becomes browned.
3. Whisk together the remaining ingredients and pour the mixture over the beef.
4. Close the lid and set the IP to MANUAL.
5. Cook on HIGH for 40 minutes.
6. Do a natural pressure release.
7. Serve and enjoy!

Nutrition Values:
Calories 530
Total Fats 23g
Carbs: 0.5g
Protein 75g
Dietary Fiber: 0g

LAMB WITH TOMATOES AND ZUCCHINI

Preparation Time: 5 Mins
Total Time: 3 hours and 40 Mins
Servings: 4

Ingredients:
- 1 pound Lamb, cut into cubes
- 1 tbsp Ghee
- 2 Large Tomatoes, diced
- 1 Zucchini, diced
- ½ Yellow Onion, diced
- 2 Carrots, sliced
- ½ cup Coconut Milk
- 1 tsp minced Garlic
- ½ tsp ground Ginger

Direction
1. In a bowl, combine the coconut milk, lamb, ginger, and garlic.
2. Cover and let sit in the fridge for 3 hours.
3. Dump the lamb along with the coconut milk into the IP.
4. Add the tomatoes, carrots, onion, and ghee, and close the lid.
5. Set the IP to MANUAL and cook on HIGH for 20 minutes.
6. Open the lid with a quick pressure release and stir in the zucchini.
7. Set the IP to SAUTE and cook for 5 minutes.
8. Serve and enjoy!

Nutrition Values:
Calories 340
Total Fats 22g
Carbs: 12.5g
Protein 24g
Dietary Fiber: 3g

BASIL BEEF WITH YAMS

Preparation Time: 5 Mins
Total Time: 45 Mins
Servings: 6
Ingredients:
- 2 Yams, peeled and chopped
- 1 ½ cups Homemade Bone Broth
- 3 Garlic Cloves, minced
- 2 ½ pounds Beef, cut into cubes
- 1 Bell Pepper, chopped
- 1 Onion, diced
- ½ tbsp dried Basil
- 3 tbsp Tomato Paste
- 1 tbsp Olive Oil

Direction
1. Heat the olive oil in the Instant Pot on SAUTE.
2. Add the onions and peppers and cook for 3 minutes.
3. Add the garlic and cook for one more.
4. Place the beef inside and cook it until it becomes browned.
5. Stir in the remaining ingredients and close the lid.
6. Set the IP to MANUAL and cook on HIGH for 30 minutes.
7. Do a quick pressure release.
8. Serve and enjoy!

Nutrition Values:
Calories 390
Total Fats 28g
Carbs: 2g
Protein 43g
Dietary Fiber: 1g

COCONUT OIL PORK CHOPS

Preparation Time: 5 Mins
Total Time: 25 Mins
Servings: 6
Ingredients:
- 6 Pork Chops
- 1 cup Homemade Bone Broth
- 8 tbsp Coconut Oil
- 1 tbsp Olive Oil
- 1 tsp Whole30 Compliant Seasoning by choice

Direction
1. Season the pork chops with the seasoning.
2. Set the IP to SAUTE and heat the oil in it.
3. Add the pork chops and cook on both sides until they become browned.
4. Place the coconut oil on top and pour the broth over.
5. Close the lid and set the IP to MANUAL.
6. Cook for 12 minutes on HIGH.
7. Do a quick pressure release.
8. Serve and enjoy!

Nutrition Values:
Calories 430
Total Fats 38g
Carbs: 0g
Protein 22g
Dietary Fiber: 0g

CINNAMON AND ORANGE PORK SHOULDER

Preparation Time: 5 Mins
Total Time: 70 Mins
Servings: 10
Ingredients:
- 5 pounds Pork Shoulder
- 2 Bay Leaves
- 2 cups Fresh Orange Juice
- 2 Cinnamon Sticks
- 2 tbsp Olive Oil
- 1 Onion, chopped
- 1 Jalapeno Pepper, seeded and diced
- 2 tsp minced Garlic
- 1 tbsp Cumin
- 2 tsp Oregano
- ½ tsp Thyme
- ¼ tsp Garlic Powder
- ¼ tsp Pepper

Direction
1. Combine half of the oil and spices in a small bowl.
2. Rub the mixture into the meat.
3. Heat the remaining oil in the Instant Pot on SAUTE.
4. Add the meat and sear on all sides. Transfer to a plate.
5. Deglaze the pot with the orange juice and stir the remaining ingredients inside.
6. Add the pork shoulder and close the lid.
7. Set the Instant Pot on MANUAL.
8. Cook on HIGH for 40 minutes.
9. Let the pressure drop on its own.
10. Open the lid and transfer the meat to a cutting board.
11. Shred or slice and serve drizzled with the juices.
12. Enjoy!

Nutrition Values:
Calories 750
Total Fats 55g
Carbs: 14g
Protein 55g
Dietary Fiber: 3g

BEEF RIBS WITH BUTTON MUSHROOMS
Preparation Time: 5 Mins
Total Time: 40 Mins
Servings: 4
Ingredients:
- 2 pounds Beef Ribs
- 1 Onion, chopped
- 2 cups quartered Button Mushrooms
- 1 cup sliced Carrots
- 1 tsp minced Garlic
- 2 tbsp Olive Oil
- ¼ cup Tomato Sauce
- 2 ½ cups Homemade Bone Broth
- ¼ tsp Cumin
- ¼ tsp Pepper

Direction
1. Add the oil to the IP and set it to SAUTE.
2. When hot and sizzling, and the ribs and cook until they are browned.
3. Add the remaining ingredients and stir well to combine.
4. Close the lid and set the IP to MANUAL.
5. Cook on HIGH for 20 minutes.
6. Do a quick pressure release.
7. Serve and enjoy!

Nutrition Values:
Calories 525
Total Fats 29g
Carbs: 8g
Protein 533g
Dietary Fiber: 2.5g

CHILI BRAISED LAMB CHOPS
Preparation Time: 5 Mins
Total Time: 30 Mins
Servings: 4
Ingredients:
- 1 Onion, diced
- 1 tsp minced Garlic
- 1 tsp Olive Oil
- 4 Lamb Chops
- 2 tbsp Chili Powder
- 14 ounces canned diced Tomatoes
- 2 tbsp Chili Powder
- ½ cup Homemade Beef Broth

Direction
1. Set the Instant Pot to SAUTE and add the oil.
2. When hot, add the onions and cook for 3 minutes.
3. Stir in the chili powder and garlic and cook for an additional minute.
4. Place the lamb chops inside and brown them on all sides.
5. Add the tomatoes and broth and stir to combine.
6. Close the lid and set the IP to MANUAL.
7. Cook on HIGH for 15 minutes.
8. Do a quick pressure release.
9. Serve and enjoy!

Nutrition Values:
Calories 442
Total Fats 23g
Carbs: 1g
Protein 45g
Dietary Fiber: 0.5g

PORK WITH RUTABAGA AND APPLES
Preparation Time: 5 Mins
Total Time: 3 hours and 40 Mins
Servings: 4
Ingredients:
- 1 pound Pork Loin, cubed
- 1 tbsp Olive Oil
- 1 Onion, diced
- 1 ½ cup Homemade Beef Broth
- 2 Rutabagas, peeled and cubed
- 2 Apples, peeled and cubed
- 1 Celery Stalk, diced
- ½ tsp Cumin
- 1 tbsp dried Parsley
- ¼ tsp Thyme
- ½ cup sliced Leeks

Direction
1. Heat half of the oil in the IP on SAUTE.
2. Add the beef and cook until browned. Transfer to a plate.
3. Heat the remaining oil and add the onions, leeks, and celery.
4. Cook for 2-3 minutes.
5. Return the beef to the pot and stir in the herbs, spices, and broth.
6. Seal the IP and choose MANUAL.
7. Cook on HIGH for 10 minutes.
8. Do a quick pressure release and open the lid.
9. Stir in the apples and seal again.
10. Cook for another 5 minutes.
11. Do a quick pressure release and serve.
12. Enjoy!

Nutrition Values:
Calories 420
Total Fats 24g
Carbs: 2g
Protein 44g
Dietary Fiber: 1g

INSTANT POT ITALIAN BEEF

Preparation Time: 10 Mins
Total Time: 1H 40 Mins
Servings: 8

Ingredients:
- 3 pound grass-fed chuck roast
- 6 cloves garlic
- 1 tsp marjoram
- 1 tsp basil
- 1 tsp oregano
- 1/2 tsp ground ginger
- 1 tsp onion powder
- 2 tsp garlic powder
- 1 tsp salt
- 1/4 cup apple cider vinegar
- 1 cup Homemade beef broth

Direction
1. Cut slits in the roast with a sharp knife and then stuff with garlic cloves.
2. In a bowl, whisk together marjoram, basil, oregano, ground ginger, onion powder, garlic powder and salt until well blended; rub the seasoning all over the roast and place it in your instant pot.
3. Add vinegar and broth and lock lid; cook on high for 90 minutes.
4. Release pressure naturally and then shred meat with a fork.
5. Serve along with cooking juices.

Nutrition Values:
Calories 174
Total Fats 9.2g
Carbs: 1.9g
Protein 21g
Dietary Fiber: 0.3g

INSTANT POT BEEF AND SWEET POTATO STEW

Preparation Time: 10 Mins
Total Time: 35 Mins
Servings: 10

Ingredients:
- 2 pounds ground beef
- 3 cups Homemade beef stock
- 2 sweet potatoes, peeled and diced
- 1 clove garlic, minced
- 1 onion, diced
- 1 14-oz can petite minced tomatoes
- 2 14-oz cans tomato sauce
- 3-4 tbsp. chili powder
- ¼ tsp. oregano
- 2 tsp. salt
- ½ tsp. black pepper
- Cilantro, optional, for garnish

Direction
1. Brown the beef in a pan over medium heat; drain excess fat and then transfer it to an instant pot.
2. Stir in the remaining ingredients and lock lid; cook on high for 25 minutes and then release pressure naturally.
3. Garnish with cilantro and serve warm.

Nutrition Values:
Calories 240
Total Fats 6.4g
Carbs: 15.1g
Protein 30.3g
Dietary Fiber: 3.5g

HEALTHY INSTANT POT GROUND BEEF JALAPENO STEW

Preparation Time: 25 Mins
Total Time: 4H 25 Mins
Servings: 6

Ingredients:
- 1-1.5 pounds ground beef
- 1 red bell pepper, chopped
- 1 green bell pepper, chopped
- 2 jalapeños, finely diced
- 1 acorn squash, peeled and diced
- 2 zucchini, sliced
- 4 small carrots, sliced
- 3 green onions, thinly sliced
- 1 28 ounce can whole peeled tomatoes
- 4 tbsp. chili powder
- 1 6 ounce can tomato paste
- 1 14 ounce can tomato sauce

Direction
1. Brown ground beef in a pan over medium heat.
2. In an instant pot, combine the browned beef, bell peppers, Jalapeños, zucchinis, carrots, onions, and squash.
3. Add whole tomatoes and stir with a spatula to mix well.
4. Stir in chili powder along with the remaining ingredients and lock lid; cook on high for 25 minutes.
5. Serve over green salad.

Nutrition Values:
Calories 265
Total Fats 6.1 g
Carbs: 28.4g
Protein 27.9g
Dietary Fiber: 7.4g

TASTY PORK LOIN WITH GOAT-CHEESE SAUCE

Preparation Time: 20 minutes
Servings 6

Nutrition Values: 449 Calories; 27.5g Fat; 4.5g Total Carbs; 43.8g Protein; 2.3g Sugars

Ingredients
- 1 tablespoon grapeseed oil
- 2 pounds pork loin, sliced
- 2 garlic cloves, pressed
- 1 red onion, chopped
- 1 bell pepper, chopped
- 1 jalapeño pepper, finely chopped
- 1/2 cup vegetable stock
- 1/2 cup double cream
- 2 ounces Ricotta cheese
- 1/2 cup goat cheese
- 1/2 teaspoon dried basil
- 1/2 teaspoon dried marjoram
- 1/2 teaspoon celery seeds
- 1/3 teaspoon pepper
- Sea salt, to your liking

Directions
1. Press the "Sauté" button to heat up the Instant Pot. Heat the oil until sizzling. Now, sear the pork loin until slightly browned on both sides, approximately 3 minutes.
2. Add the garlic, onion, pepper, and vegetable stock to the Instant Pot.
3. Secure the lid. Choose the "Manual" setting and cook for 12 minutes under High pressure. Once cooking is complete, use a natural pressure release; carefully remove the lid.
4. Next, add the remaining ingredients and let it cook in the residual heat or until cheese is melted.
5. Add pork chops back to the cheese sauce and serve. Bon appétit!

TRADITIONAL PORK CHILI

Preparation Time: 10 minutes
Servings 6

Nutrition Values: 532 Calories; 37.6g Fat; 4.4g Total Carbs; 41.6g Protein; 1.8g Sugars

Ingredients
- 2 tablespoons lard
- 1/2 cup leeks, chopped
- 1 celery stick, cubed
- 2 breakfast pork sausages, casing removed and sliced
- 1 jalapeño pepper, seeded and minced
- 2 pounds ground pork
- 2 cloves garlic, minced
- 1 cup tomatoes, puréed
- 1 cup broth, preferably homemade
- 1 teaspoon coconut aminos
- 1 teaspoon mustard seeds
- 1 teaspoon ground coriander seed
- Seasoned salt and ground black pepper, to taste
- 2 tablespoons fresh cilantro leaves, roughly chopped
- 1/2 cup Cheddar cheese, shredded

Directions
1. Press the "Sauté" button to heat up the Instant Pot. Now, melt the lard. Once hot, cook the leeks and celery until softened.
2. Add the sausage, jalapeño pepper, pork, and garlic; cook an additional 2 minutes, stirring constantly.
3. Now, add puréed tomatoes, broth, coconut aminos, mustard seeds, coriander seeds, salt, and black pepper. Stir to combine and secure the lid.
4. Choose the "Manual" setting and cook for 5 minutes at High pressure. Once cooking is complete, use a natural pressure release; carefully remove the lid.
5. Serve your chili topped with fresh cilantro leaves and Cheddar cheese. Bon appétit!

WINTER PORK AND BACON SOUP

Preparation Time: 30 minutes
Servings 4

Nutrition Values: 361 Calories; 19.6g Fat; 6.2g Total Carbs; 37.8g Protein; 3.7g Sugars

Ingredients
- 1/2 pound bacon
- 1/2 pound pork stew meat
- 2 tablespoons butter
- 1/2 cup yellow onions, chopped
- 1 celery with leaves, chopped
- 2 garlic cloves, minced
- 1 cup white mushrooms, sliced
- 1/2 teaspoon dried rosemary
- 1/2 teaspoon dried thyme
- Sea salt, to taste
- 1/2 teaspoon ground black pepper
- 1/2 teaspoon cayenne pepper
- A pinch of hot paprika
- A pinch of grated nutmeg
- 3 ½ cups beef stock

- 6 ounces Ricotta cheese
- 1/2 cup double cream
- 1/3 cup parsley, roughly chopped

Directions
1. Press the "Sauté" button to heat up the Instant Pot. Once hot, cook the bacon until crisp; crumble with a fork and set aside.
2. Now, brown the pork stew meat for 2 to 4 minutes, stirring frequently; set aside.
3. Melt the butter; cook the onion and celery until softened. After that, add the garlic and sliced mushrooms; sauté until fragrant.
4. Add all seasonings and beef stock. Return the reserved pork to the Instant Pot.
5. Secure the lid. Choose the "Manual" setting and cook for 8 minutes at High pressure. Once cooking is complete, use a quick pressure release; carefully remove the lid.
6. Afterwards, add Ricotta cheese, cream and parsley. Cover with the lid and allow it to sit for 15 minutes. Top with reserved bacon and enjoy!

BURRITO BOWL WITH PORK
Preparation Time: 20 minutes
Servings 8
Nutrition Values: 434 Calories; 23.8g Fat; 5g Total Carbs; 45.2g Protein; 3.2g Sugars
Ingredients
- 2 teaspoons grapeseed oil
- 3 pounds pork tenderloin, cut into slices
- 1/2 teaspoon dried thyme
- 1/2 teaspoon dried marjoram
- 1 teaspoon ground cumin
- 1 teaspoon paprika
- Sea salt and ground black pepper, to taste
- 1 teaspoon granulated garlic
- 1 cup water
- 1 avocado, pitted, peeled and sliced

Salsa Sauce:
- 1 cup pureed tomatoes
- 2 bell peppers, deveined and chopped
- 1 teaspoon granulated garlic
- 1 minced jalapeño, chopped
- 1 cup onion, chopped
- 2 tablespoons fresh cilantro, minced
- 3 teaspoons lime juice

Directions
1. Press the "Sauté" button to heat up the Instant Pot. Once hot, add the oil; sear the pork until delicately browned on all sides.
2. Add the seasonings, garlic, and water to the Instant Pot.
3. Secure the lid. Choose the "Manual" setting and cook for 12 minutes at High pressure. Once cooking is complete, use a natural pressure release; carefully remove the lid.
4. Shred the pork with two forks and reserve.
5. In a mixing bowl, thoroughly combine all salsa ingredients. Spoon the salsa mixture over the prepared pork. Garnish with avocado slices and serve. Bon appétit!

PORK SHANK WITH CAULIFLOWER
Preparation Time: 55 minutes
Servings 6
Nutrition Values: 342 Calories; 20.1g Fat; 6.6g Total Carbs; 32.7g Protein; 1.9g Sugars
Ingredients
- 2 pounds pork shank, cubed
- Sea salt, to taste
- 2 teaspoons coconut oil
- 1 cup chicken stock
- 1 leek, sliced
- 4 cloves garlic, sliced
- 1/2 teaspoon cumin powder
- 1/2 teaspoon porcini powder
- 1/2 teaspoon oregano
- 1/2 teaspoon basil
- 4 cups cauliflower, broken into small florets
- 1/2 teaspoon salt
- 1/4 teaspoon ground black pepper
- 1/4 teaspoon red pepper flakes, crushed

Directions
1. Generously season the pork shank with sea salt.
2. Press the "Sauté" button to heat up the Instant Pot. Now, melt the coconut oil. Once hot, cook pork shank until delicately browned on all sides.
3. Add chicken stock, leeks, garlic, cumin powder, porcini powder, oregano, and basil to the Instant Pot.
4. Secure the lid. Choose the "Meat/Stew" setting and cook for 50 minutes under High pressure. Once cooking is complete, use a natural pressure release; carefully remove the lid. Reserve the cooked meat.
5. Add the remaining ingredients to the Instant Pot.
6. Secure the lid. Choose the "Manual" setting and cook for 3 minutes under Low pressure. Once cooking is complete, use a natural pressure release; carefully remove the lid.
7. Serve the cooked cauliflower with reserved

pork shank. Bon appétit!

ASIAN-STYLE SIRLOIN PORK ROAST

Preparation Time: 2 hours 35 minutes
Servings 4
Nutrition Values: 364 Calories; 13.8g Fat; 4g Total Carbs; 53.1g Protein; 1.2g Sugars
Ingredients
- 1 ½ pounds sirloin pork roast
- Salt and ground black pepper, to taste
- 1/2 cup leeks, sliced
- 2 garlic cloves, minced
- 1 tablespoon Shoyu sauce
- 2 tablespoons Ryorishu
- 1 tablespoon Mirin
- 2 teaspoons sesame oil
- 6 drops Stevia liquid concentrate
- 1 teaspoon cayenne pepper
- 1 cup water
- 2 tablespoons black sesame seeds
- 2 tablespoons fresh chives, chopped

Directions
1. Generously season the sirloin pork roast with sea salt and ground black pepper.
2. In a mixing bowl, thoroughly combine the leeks, garlic, Shoyu sauce, Ryorishu, mirin, sesame oil, Stevia, cayenne pepper, and water.
3. Place the pork in a mixing bowl and let it marinate for 2 hours in your refrigerator. Place the pork and 1 cup of marinade in the Instant Pot.
4. Secure the lid. Choose the "Meat/Stew" setting and cook for 30 minutes at High pressure. Once cooking is complete, use a natural pressure release; carefully remove the lid.
5. Take the pork out of the Instant Pot. Then, press the "Sauté" button; add the remaining marinade.
6. Let the cooking liquid cook until it has reduced and thickened. Slice the sirloin pork roast and place on individual serving plates.
7. Spoon the sauce over the meat; garnish with sesame seeds and fresh chives. Bon appétit!

PORK SAUSAGES PEPERONATA STYLE

Preparation Time: 15 minutes
Servings 4
Nutrition Values: 582 Calories; 49.3g Fat; 6.1g Total Carbs; 24.5g Protein; 2.4g Sugars
Ingredients
- 1 teaspoon olive oil
- 8 pork sausages, casing removed
- 1 green bell pepper, seeded and sliced
- 1 red bell pepper, seeded and sliced
- 1 jalapeño pepper, seeded and sliced
- 1 red onion, chopped
- 2 garlic cloves, minced
- 2 Roma tomatoes, puréed
- 1 cup roasted vegetable broth
- 1 tablespoon Italian seasoning
- 2 tablespoons fresh Italian parsley
- 2 tablespoons ripe olives, pitted and sliced

Directions
1. Press the "Sauté" button to heat up the Instant Pot. Once hot, add the oil; sear your sausages until no longer pink in center.
2. Add the other ingredients, except for the olives and parsley; stir to combine well.
3. Secure the lid. Choose the "Manual" setting and cook for 8 minutes at High pressure. Once cooking is complete, use a quick pressure release; carefully remove the lid.
4. Serve garnished with fresh parsley and olives. Bon appétit!

MEXICAN STYLE PORK STEAKS

Preparation Time: 15 minutes
Servings 6
Nutrition Values: 448 Calories; 29.2g Fat; 4.1g Total Carbs; 39.4g Protein; 1.8g Sugars
Ingredients
- 1 tablespoon lard
- 2 pounds pork steaks
- 1 bell pepper, seeded and sliced
- 1/2 cup shallots, chopped
- 2 garlic cloves, minced
- 1 cup chicken bone broth, preferably homemade
- 1/4 cup water
- 1/4 cup dry red wine
- Salt, to taste
- 1/4 teaspoon freshly ground black pepper, or more to taste
- Pico de Gallo:
- 1 tomato, chopped
- 1 chili pepper, seeded and minced
- 1/2 cup red onion, chopped
- 2 garlic cloves, minced
- 1 tablespoon fresh cilantro, finely chopped
- Sea salt, to taste

Directions
1. Press the "Sauté" button to heat up the Instant Pot. Melt the lard and sear the pork

steaks about 4 minutes or until delicately browned on both sides.
2. Add bell pepper, shallot, garlic, chicken bone broth, water, wine, salt, and black pepper to the Instant Pot.
3. Secure the lid. Choose the "Manual" setting and cook for 8 minutes at High pressure. Once cooking is complete, use a quick pressure release; carefully remove the lid.
4. Meanwhile, make your Pico de Gallo by mixing all of the above ingredients. Refrigerate until ready to serve.
5. Serve warm pork steaks with well-chilled Pico de Gallo on the side. Bon appétit!

CHEESY MEATLOAF WITH BACON

Preparation Time: 35 minutes
Servings 6

Nutrition Values: 468 Calories; 35.7g Fat; 1.6g Total Carbs; 33.6g Protein; 1.2g Sugars

Ingredients

- 1 ½ pounds ground pork
- 1/2 pound ground chuck
- 1/2 teaspoon sea salt
- 1/2 teaspoon ground black pepper
- 1 teaspoon red pepper flakes, crushed
- 1/2 teaspoon ground bay leaf
- 1 teaspoon brown mustard
- 2 eggs, whisked
- 2/3 cup cream cheese
- 6 thin slices bacon
- 1/3 cup tomatillo salsa

Directions

1. Prepare your Instant Pot by adding 1 ½ cups of water and metal rack to the bottom of the inner pot.
2. In a mixing dish, thoroughly combine ground meat, salt, black pepper, red pepper flakes, ground bay leaf, brown mustard, eggs, and cream cheese.
3. Shape the mixture into the meatloaf. Place the meatloaf in a baking pan.
4. Now, arrange bacon slices, crosswise over meatloaf, overlapping them slightly. Top with tomatillo salsa.
5. Secure the lid. Choose the "Manual" setting and cook for 30 minutes at High pressure. Once cooking is complete, use a quick pressure release; carefully remove the lid. Enjoy!

B.B.B - BABY BACK RIBS

Preparation Time: 25 minutes
Servings 4

Nutrition Values: 404 Calories; 27.7g Fat; 4.5g Total Carbs; 34.7g Protein; 1.8g Sugars

Ingredients

- 2 tomatoes, puréed
- 2 tablespoons rice vinegar
- 1 tablespoon stone ground mustard
- 1 cup water
- 1/2 teaspoon porcini powder
- 1 teaspoon celery seeds
- 1 teaspoon coriander seeds
- 1/2 teaspoon granulated garlic
- 1/2 teaspoon shallot powder
- 1/3 teaspoon ground black pepper
- 1 teaspoon hot paprika
- Sea salt, to taste
- 1 ½ pounds baby back ribs

Directions

1. Thoroughly combine all of the above ingredients in your Instant Pot.
2. Secure the lid. Choose the "Meat/Stew" setting and cook for 20 minutes at High pressure. Once cooking is complete, use a natural pressure release; carefully remove the lid.
3. Serve warm garnished with a fresh salad of choice. Enjoy!

STICKY PORK SPARE RIBS

Preparation Time: 25 minutes
Servings 4

Nutrition Values: 266 Calories; 9.7g Fat; 6.2g Total Carbs; 36.7g Protein; 2.9g Sugars

Ingredients

- 1 ½ pounds spare ribs
- 1 thin sliced fresh ginger, peeled
- 4 garlic cloves, halved
- 1 jalapeño pepper, thinly sliced
- 1 bay leaf
- 1/2 teaspoon black peppercorns
- 1 tablespoon tamarind paste
- 1 teaspoon shrimp paste
- Sea salt and ground black pepper, to taste
- 1/2 cup marinara sauce

Directions

1. Arrange spare ribs on the bottom of your Instant Pot. Add fresh ginger, garlic, jalapeño pepper, bay leaf, and peppercorns.
2. Next, mix the tamarind paste, shrimp paste, salt, black pepper, marinara sauce, and water. Pour this tamarind sauce over the ribs in the Instant Pot.

3. Add enough water to cover the spare ribs.
4. Secure the lid. Choose the "Manual" setting and cook for 20 minutes at High pressure. Once cooking is complete, use a quick pressure release; carefully remove the lid.
5. Serve warm and enjoy!

YUMMY STUFFED MEATBALLS

Preparation Time: 15 minutes
Servings 5

Nutrition Values: 440 Calories; 31.9g Fat; 2.1g Total Carbs; 34.7g Protein; 0.8g Sugars

Ingredients

- 1 pound ground pork
- 1/4 cup double cream
- 2 eggs, beaten
- 2 cloves garlic, minced
- 2 tablespoons green onions, minced
- 1 tablespoon fresh parsley, minced
- 1/4 teaspoon dried thyme
- 1/2 teaspoon dried marjoram
- 1/2 teaspoon ground black pepper
- 1 teaspoon kosher salt
- 10 (1-inch cubes of provolone cheese

Directions

1. Prepare your Instant Pot by adding 1 ½ cups of water and a steamer basket to the bottom of the inner pot.
2. Thoroughly combine all ingredients, except the cubes of provolone cheese, in a mixing bowl.
3. Shape the mixture into 10 patties by using oiled hands. Now, place a cube of provolone cheese in the center of each patty, wrap the meat around the cheese, and roll into a ball.
4. Now, arrange the meatballs in the steamer basket.
5. Secure the lid. Choose the "Manual" setting and cook for 6 minutes at High pressure. Once cooking is complete, use a quick pressure release; carefully remove the lid.
6. Serve immediately, garnished with low-carb salsa. Bon appétit!

TRADITIONAL PORK ROAST

Preparation Time: 40 minutes
Servings 6

Nutrition Values: 310 Calories; 14.4g Fat; 2.1g Total Carbs; 43.5g Protein; 0.7g Sugars

Ingredients

- 2 tablespoons unsalted butter
- 2 pounds sirloin pork roast, cubed
- 8 ounces Cremini mushrooms, thinlysliced
- 2 garlic cloves, minced
- 1 heaping tablespoon fresh parsley, chopped
- 1/2 cup roasted vegetable broth
- 2/3 cup water
- 2 tablespoons dry white wine
- 1/2 teaspoon dried sage
- 1/2 teaspoon dried basil
- 1 teaspoon dried oregano
- Sea salt and ground black pepper, to taste
- 1 teaspoon cayenne pepper
- 1/3 cup Castelvetrano olives, pitted and halved

Directions

1. Press the "Sauté" button to heat up the Instant Pot. Melt the butter and sear the pork about 3 minutes or until delicately browned on all sides; reserve.
2. In pan drippings, cook the mushrooms and garlic until tender and fragrant.
3. Add parsley, broth, water, wine, sage, basil, oregano, salt, black pepper, and cayenne pepper; gently stir to combine.
4. Secure the lid. Choose the "Meat/Stew" setting and cook for 35 minutes at High pressure.
5. Once cooking is complete, use a natural pressure release; carefully remove the lid. Serve garnished with Castelvetrano olives. Bon appétit!

PORK SOUP WITH TORTILLA

Preparation Time: 15 minutes
Servings 5

Nutrition Values: 425 Calories; 31.1g Fat; 6.6g Total Carbs; 30.2g Protein; 3.7g Sugars

Ingredients

- 1 ½ tablespoons olive oil
- 1 pound pork stew meat, cubed
- 1/2 cup double cream
- 1/2 cup canned fire-roasted tomatoes, diced
- Sea salt and ground black pepper, to taste
- 1/2 teaspoon red pepper flakes, crushed
- 4 cups water
- 2 tablespoons vegetable bouillon granules
- 2 tablespoons enchilada sauce
- 10 ounces Cotija cheese, crumbled
- 1 cup kale chips
- 2 tablespoons fresh cilantro, chopped
- 4 lime wedges, for serving

Directions

1. Press the "Sauté" button to heat up the

Instant Pot. Heat the olive oil and sear the pork about 3 minutes or until delicately browned on all sides.
2. Stir in double cream, fire-roasted tomatoes, salt, ground black pepper, red pepper flakes, water, vegetable bouillon granules, and enchilada sauce.
3. Secure the lid. Choose the "Manual" setting and cook for 8 minutes at High pressure. Once cooking is complete, use a quick pressure release; carefully remove the lid.
4. Now, add Cotija cheese and press the "Sauté" button again; let it simmer until cheese is melted.
5. Ladle into soup bowls; top each serving with kale chips and fresh cilantro.
6. Serve garnished with lemon wedges and enjoy!

PORK SHOULDER WITH HERB DIJON SAUCE

Preparation Time: 1 hour
Servings 4
Nutrition Values: 341 Calories; 23.4g Fat; 1.3g Total Carbs; 29g Protein; 0.6g Sugars
Ingredients
- 1 pound pork shoulder
- Sea salt and ground black pepper, to taste
- 1 teaspoon cayenne pepper
- 1 tablespoon lard, at room temperature
- 1 cup beef bone broth

Herb Dijon Sauce:
- 1/2 teaspoon dried thyme
- 1/2 teaspoon dried rosemary
- 1/2 teaspoon dried sage
- 1/3 cup double cream
- 1 teaspoon balsamic vinegar
- 2 teaspoons Dijon mustard

Directions
1. Generously season the pork shoulder with salt, pepper, and cayenne pepper.
2. Press the "Sauté" button to heat up the Instant Pot. Melt the lard and sear the pork for 5 minutes, turning occasionally.
3. Use the broth to deglaze the pan.
4. Secure the lid. Choose the "Manual" setting and cook for 50 minutes at High pressure. Once cooking is complete, use a natural pressure release; carefully remove the lid. Reserve the pork shoulder.
5. Press the "Sauté" button again. Now, add thyme, rosemary, sage, cream and vinegar. Let it simmer for a couple of minutes.
6. Afterwards, stir in Dijon mustard and add the reserved pork shoulder back to the Instant Pot. Now, cook an additional minute or so, until heated through. Bon appétit!

TRADITIONAL PORK TACO BOWL

Preparation Time: 15 minutes
Servings 6
Nutrition Values: 271 Calories; 11.2g Fat; 7g Total Carbs; 36.1g Protein; 4.2g Sugars
Ingredients
- 1 teaspoon olive oil
- 2 pounds lean ground pork
- 1 cup chicken bone stock
- 3 ounces dried guajillo chilies, seeded, roasted and minced
- 1/2 cup yellow onions, chopped
- 2 cloves garlic, chopped
- 1 teaspoon dried Mexican oregano
- 1/2 teaspoon ground coriander
- Sea salt and ground black pepper, to taste
- 1 teaspoon cayenne pepper
- 1/2 teaspoon sweet paprika
- 1 cup cherry tomatoes, halved
- 1 tablespoon fresh lime juice
- 1/2 cup Cheddar cheese, shredded

Directions
1. Press the "Sauté" button to heat up the Instant Pot. Heat the olive oil and brown the pork, crumbling with a spatula.
2. Use the chicken bone stock to deglaze the pan. Now, add dried guajillo chilies, yellow onions, garlic, Mexican oregano, ground coriander, salt, black pepper, cayenne pepper, sweet paprika, and tomatoes.
3. Secure the lid. Choose the "Manual" setting and cook for 5 minutes at High pressure. Once cooking is complete, use a natural pressure release; carefully remove the lid.
4. Ladle into soup bowls; drizzle with some fresh lime juice and top with shredded cheese. Bon appétit!

HEARTY COUNTRY-STYLE PORK LOIN RIBS

Preparation Time: 25 minutes
Servings 6
Nutrition Values: 335 Calories; 20.1g Fat; 4.7g Total Carbs; 29.9g Protein; 2g Sugars
Ingredients
- 2 pounds country-style pork loin ribs, bone-in
- Coarse salt and ground black pepper, to taste
- 1 tablespoon lard, at room temperature

- 1 teaspoon chili powder
- 1 teaspoon porcini powder
- 1/3 cup champagne
- 1 cup water
- 1 celery with leaves, diced
- 1 parsnip, quartered
- 1 brown onion, chopped
- 2 garlic cloves, crushed
- 1 teaspoon liquid smoke
- 1 tablespoon coconut aminos

Directions
1. Generously season the pork ribs with the salt and black pepper.
2. Press the "Sauté" button to heat up the Instant Pot. Melt the lard and sear the pork ribs for 2 to 3 minutes on each side.
3. Add the remaining ingredients. Secure the lid. Choose the "Meat/Stew" setting and cook for 20 minutes at High pressure.
4. Once cooking is complete, use a natural pressure release; carefully remove the lid. Serve with favorite keto sides. Enjoy!

INDIAN-STYLE PORK VINDALOO

Preparation Time: 20 minutes
Servings 6

Nutrition Values: 354 Calories; 19.3g Fat; 3.3g Total Carbs; 39.8g Protein; 1.1g Sugars

Ingredients
- 1 tablespoon olive oil
- 2 pounds pork loin, sliced into strips
- Sea salt, to taste
- 2 garlic cloves, minced
- 2 tablespoons coconut aminos
- 1 teaspoon oyster sauce
- 1 head cauliflower, broken into florets
- 1 teaspoon ground cardamom
- 3 cloves, whole
- 1/2 teaspoon mixed peppercorns
- 1 teaspoon brown mustard seeds
- 1 teaspoon cayenne pepper
- 1 cup water
- 2 tablespoons fresh cilantro, roughly chopped

Directions
1. Press the "Sauté" button to heat up the Instant Pot. Heat the oil and sear the pork loin for 3 to 4 minutes, stirring periodically.
2. Add the remaining ingredients, except for fresh cilantro.
3. Secure the lid. Choose the "Meat/Stew" setting and cook for 12 minutes at High pressure.
4. Once cooking is complete, use a natural pressure release; carefully remove the lid. Serve topped with fresh cilantro. Bon appétit!

THAI PORK SALAD

Preparation Time: 35 minutes
Servings 4

Nutrition Values: 279 Calories; 12.7g Fat; 5.9g Total Carbs; 32.5g Protein; 2.9g Sugars

Ingredients
- 1 pound pork loin roast
- 1/2 cup broth, preferably homemade
- 1/2 cup water
- 1/2 head cabbage, shredded
- 2 celery with leaves, chopped
- 4 spring onions, chopped
- 1 cup baby spinach
- 1 cup arugula
- 1 red chili, deseeded and finely chopped
- 2 teaspoons each sesame oil
- 1 teaspoon Thai fish sauce
- 2 teaspoons tamari sauce
- Fresh juice of 1 lemon

Directions
1. Add pork loin roast, broth and water to the Instant Pot that is previously greased with a nonstick cooking spray.
2. Secure the lid. Choose the "Meat/Stew" setting and cook for 30 minutes at High pressure. Once cooking is complete, use a natural pressure release; carefully remove the lid.
3. Allow the pork loin roast to cool completely. Shred the meat and transfer to a salad bowl.
4. Add the cabbage, celery, green onions, spinach, arugula, and chili.
5. Now, make the dressing by mixing sesame oil with Thai fish sauce, tamari sauce, and lemon juice. Whisk to combine well and dress your salad. Serve well-chilled. Bon appétit!

SMOKY PORK RIBS

Preparation Time: 4 hours 35 minutes
Servings 6

Nutrition Values: 368 Calories; 22.9g Fat; 6.1g Total Carbs; 32.1g Protein; 2.6g Sugars

Ingredients
- 1/4 cup fresh lime juice
- 1/3 cup sesame oil
- 1 tablespoon champagne vinegar
- 3/4 cup tomato sauce
- 1 long red chili, finely chopped

- 1/2 teaspoon coarse sea salt
- 2 teaspoons smoked paprika
- 2 garlic cloves, crushed
- 2 pounds American-style pork ribs
- 1 tablespoon olive oil

Directions
1. In a large ceramic dish, combine the lime juice, sesame oil, champagne vinegar, tomato sauce, red chili, sea salt, paprika, and garlic.
2. Add American-style pork ribs and let them marinate at least 4 hours in the refrigerator.
3. Remove the ribs from the marinade. Heat the olive oil and brown the ribs for 3 to 4 minutes. Add 1/2 of the marinade.
4. Secure the lid. Choose the "Meat/Stew" setting and cook for 20 minutes at High pressure. Once cooking is complete, use a natural pressure release; carefully remove the lid.
5. Then, strain remaining marinade into a small skillet and bring it to a boil over moderately high heat.
6. Then, immediately reduce heat to medium; allow it to simmer for 4 to 6 minutes or until reduced. Pour this sauce over your ribs and serve warm. Bon appétit!

EASY PORK TACO FRITTATA

Preparation Time: 35 minutes
Servings 6

Nutrition Values: 409 Calories; 31.6g Fat; 4.7g Total Carbs; 25.7g Protein; 2.7g Sugars
Ingredients
- 3 ounces Cottage cheese, at room temperature
- 1/4 cup double cream
- 2 eggs
- 1 teaspoon taco seasoning
- 6 ounces Cotija cheese, crumbled
- 3/4 pound ground pork
- 1 tablespoon taco seasoning
- 1/2 cup tomatoes, puréed
- 3 ounces chopped green chilies
- 6 ounces QuesoManchego cheese, shredded

Directions
1. Prepare your Instant Pot by adding 1 ½ cups of water and a metal rack to the bottom of the inner pot.
2. In a mixing bowl, thoroughly combine Cottage cheese, double cream, eggs, and tacoseasoning.
3. Lightly grease a casserole dish; spread the Cotija cheese over the bottom. Pour in the Cottage/ egg mixture as evenly as possible.
4. Lower the casserole dish onto the rack.
5. Secure the lid. Choose "Manual" mode and High pressure; cook for 20 minutes. Once cooking is complete, use a quick pressure release; carefully remove the lid.
6. In the meantime, heat a cast-iron skillet over a moderately high heat. Now, brown ground pork, crumbling it with a fork.
7. Add taco seasoning, tomato purée andgreen chilies. Spread this mixture over the prepared cheese crust.
8. Top with shredded QuesoManchego.
9. Secure the lid. Choose "Manual" mode and High pressure; cook for 10 minutes. Once cooking is complete, use a quick pressure release; carefully remove the lid. Serve and enjoy!

RUBY PORT-BRAISED PORK

Preparation Time: 20 minutes
Servings 4

Nutrition Values: 320 Calories; 10g Fat; 3.4g Total Carbs; 46.9g Protein; 0.9g Sugars
Ingredients
- 1 tablespoon grapeseed oil
- 1 ½ pounds pork tenderloins
- Sea salt and ground pepper, to your liking
- 1 teaspoon roasted garlic paste
- 1/2 cup ruby port
- 1 cup vegetable stock
- 1/2 cup scallions, chopped
- 1/4 teaspoon dried dill weed
- 1/2 teaspoon dried basil
- 1/4 teaspoon dried oregano
- 2 cups mustard greens

Directions
1. Press the "Sauté" button to heat up the Instant Pot. Heat the grapeseed oil until sizzling. Once hot, cook the pork until delicately browned on both sides.
2. Season with the salt and black pepper; add garlic paste, ruby port, vegetable stock, scallions, dill, basil, and oregano.
3. Secure the lid. Choose "Manual" mode and High pressure; cook for 12 minutes. Once cooking is complete, use a quick pressure release; carefully remove the lid.
4. Lastly, add mustard greens; cover your Instant Pot and let it sit until your greens are wilted. Taste, adjust the seasonings, and serve warm. Bon appétit!

BUFFALO PORK CHOWDER

Preparation Time: 20 minutes

Servings 4

Nutrition Values: 443 Calories; 32.7g Fat; 3.7g Total Carbs; 32.6g Protein; 1.9g Sugars

Ingredients
- 2 tablespoons butter
- 1 pound pork loin, boneless and cubed
- 1/2 cup celery, diced
- 1 tablespoon hot sauce
- 1/3 cup blue cheese powder
- Seasoned salt and ground black pepper, to taste
- 1/2 teaspoon onion powder
- 1/2 teaspoon garlic powder
- 1 teaspoon paprika
- 1/4 teaspoon dried dill weed
- 4 cups beef bone stock
- 1 cup heavy cream

Directions
1. Press the "Sauté" button to heat up the Instant Pot. Now, melt the butter and cook pork loin for 2 to 4 minutes, stirring frequently.
2. Add the celery, hot sauce, blue cheese powder, salt, pepper, onion powder, garlic powder, paprika, dill, and beef bone stock.
3. Secure the lid. Choose "Manual" mode and High pressure; cook for 12 minutes. Once cooking is complete, use a quick pressure release; carefully remove the lid.
4. Add heavy cream and press the "Sauté" button one more time. Let the soup simmer until thickened. Serve hot and enjoy!

GREEK-STYLE PORK CUTLETS

Preparation Time: 3 hours 15 minutes
Servings 6

Nutrition Values: 417 Calories; 25.7g Fat; 4.6g Total Carbs; 40.4g Protein; 1.5g Sugars

Ingredients
- 3 tablespoons olive oil
- 1 lemon, juiced
- 2 garlic cloves, finely minced
- 1 bunch of fresh cilantro leaves, chopped
- 1 tablespoons stone ground mustard
- 2 sprigs fresh rosemary, chopped
- 1 sprig lemon thyme, chopped
- 2 pounds pork cutlets, bone-in
- Coarse sea salt and ground black pepper, to taste
- 1/4 cup white rum
- 1 cup chicken stock
- 1/2 cup black olives, pitted and sliced

Directions
1. Add 2 tablespoons of olive oil, lemon juice, garlic, cilantro, mustard, rosemary, and lemon thyme to a ceramic dish.
2. Add bone-in pork cutlets and let them marinate at least 3 hours or overnight.
3. Press the "Sauté" button to heat up the Instant Pot. Now, heat the remaining tablespoon of olive oil and brown the pork for 2 to 4 minutes or until delicately browned on each side.
4. Season with salt and pepper to taste.
5. Deglaze the bottom of the inner pot with the white rum until it has almost all evaporated. Pour in the stock.
6. Secure the lid. Choose "Manual" mode and High pressure; cook for 8 minutes. Once cooking is complete, use a quick pressure release; carefully remove the lid.
7. Serve warm garnished with black olives. Bon appétit!

TRADITIONAL KIELBASA WITH SQUASH

Preparation Time: 15 minutes
Servings 4

Nutrition Values: 440 Calories; 36.9g Fat; 5.8g Total Carbs; 18.3g Protein; 3.5g Sugars

Ingredients
- 1 teaspoon olive oil
- 1 pound beef Polska Kielbasa, casing removed, sliced
- 1 pound summer squash, peeled and diced
- 1 red onion, chopped
- 1 celery, chopped
- 1 cup beef stock
- 1 cup tomato purée
- 1 tablespoon coconut aminos
- 1 teaspoon red pepper flakes, crushed
- Coarse sea salt and ground black pepper, to taste
- 1 cup Cremini mushrooms, sliced
- 1/2 cup chunky salsa

Directions
1. Press the "Sauté" button to heat up the Instant Pot; heat the olive oil. Once hot, cook kielbasa until no longer pink.
2. Add the squash, onion, celery, stock, tomato puréed, coconut aminos, red pepper flakes, salt, black pepper, and mushrooms to the Instant Pot.
3. Secure the lid. Choose "Manual" mode and High pressure; cook for 5 minutes. Once

cooking is complete, use a quick pressure release; carefully remove the lid.
4. Serve with a chunky salsa. Bon appétit!

RICH BEEF, BACON AND SPINACH CHILI

Preparation Time: 15 minutes
Servings 6
Nutrition Values: 392 Calories; 25.4g Fat; 5.8g Total Carbs; 33.6g Protein; 1.8g Sugars
Ingredients
- 1 ½ pounds ground beef
- 4 slices bacon, chopped
- 8 ounces tomato puréed
- 1 onion, chopped
- 2 garlic cloves, minced
- 2 cups chicken stock, preferably homemade
- 1/2 teaspoon ground cumin
- 1 teaspoon smoked paprika
- 1/2 teaspoon dried basil
- 1/2 teaspoon dried oregano
- Sea salt and ground black pepper, to taste
- 1 teaspoon red pepper flakes, crushed
- 2 bay leaves
- 1/4 teaspoon ground allspice
- 2 cups spinach, fresh or frozen

Directions
1. Press the "Sauté" button to heat up the Instant Pot. Once hot, cook ground beef and bacon for 2 to 3 minutes, crumbling them with a fork.
2. Add the remaining ingredients, except for spinach.
3. Secure the lid. Choose "Manual" mode and High pressure; cook for 6 minutes. Once cooking is complete, use a quick pressure release; carefully remove the lid.
4. Add spinach and cover with the lid. Let it sit until the spinach wilts. Ladle into individual bowls and serve warm. Bon appétit!

JUICY STEAK WITH RAINBOW NOODLES

Preparation Time: 45 minutes
Servings 6
Nutrition Values: 259 Calories; 12.2g Fat; 3g Total Carbs; 32.4g Protein; 1.2g Sugars
Ingredients
- 1 zucchini
- 1 carrot
- 1 yellow onion
- 2 tablespoons ghee
- Sea salt, to taste
- 2 pounds beef steak
- 2 large cloves garlic
- 1/3 teaspoon ground black pepper

Directions
1. Slice the zucchini, carrot, and yellow onion using a mandolin.
2. Preheat an oven to 390 degrees F. Grease a baking sheet with the ghee; toss the vegetables with salt and bake for 18 to 22 minutes, tossing once or twice.
3. Meanwhile, add the beef, garlic, and black pepper to your Instant Pot.
4. Secure the lid. Choose "Manual" mode and High pressure; cook for 20 minutes. Once cooking is complete, use a quick pressure release; carefully remove the lid. Salt the beef to taste.
5. Serve the prepared beef steak over roasted vegetable noodles and enjoy!

ZETTUCCINI WITH PEPPERONI AND ROMANO SAUCE

Preparation Time: 10 minutes
Servings 4
Nutrition Values: 437 Calories; 38.3g Fat; 2.6g Total Carbs; 19.5g Protein; 1.7g Sugars
Ingredients
- 2 zucchini
- 1/2 pound pepperoni, sliced
- 1/2 cup cream cheese
- Sea salt and ground black pepper, to taste
- 1/2 teaspoon red pepper flakes, crushed
- 1 teaspoon cayenne pepper
- 1/2 cup Romano cheese, grated

Directions
1. Slice the zucchini with a mandolin; add your zettuccini to the Instant Pot.
2. Now, stir in the pepperoni, cream cheese, salt, black pepper, red pepper, and cayenne pepper.
3. Secure the lid. Choose "Manual" mode and High pressure; cook for 5 minutes. Once cooking is complete, use a quick pressure release; carefully remove the lid.
4. Afterwards, stir in Romano cheese, cover and let it melt for a couple of minutes. Bon appétit!

TASTY BOTTOM EYE ROAST IN HOISIN SAUCE

Preparation Time: 45 minutes
Servings 8
Nutrition Values: 313 Calories; 17.3g Fat; 3.8g Total Carbs; 35.8g Protein; 2.3g Sugars
Ingredients

- 1 tablespoon tallow
- 3 pounds bottom eye roast
- Sea salt and ground black pepper, to taste
- 3 garlic cloves, halved

Hoisin Sauce:
- 3 tablespoons soy sauce
- 2 tablespoons peanut butter
- 1 tablespoon black vinegar
- 2 cloves garlic, minced
- 2 ½ tablespoons toasted sesame oil
- 1 teaspoon Chinese chili sauce
- 1/2 teaspoon Chinese five spice powder
- 1 tablespoon Splenda

Directions
1. Press the "Sauté" button to heat up the Instant Pot. Now, melt the tallow; once hot, cook the bottom eye roast for 2 to 3 minutes on each side. Season with salt and black pepper.
2. Then, make small slits along the surface of the beef cut and place garlic in them.
3. Secure the lid. Choose "Meat/Stew" mode and High pressure; cook for 40 minutes. Once cooking is complete, use a natural pressure release; carefully remove the lid.
4. Meanwhile, process all sauce ingredients in your blender; blitz until everything is well mixed.
5. Add the hoisin sauce to the Instant Pot; stir for a couple of minutes more. Serve immediately and enjoy!

WINTER GULASCH
Preparation Time: 30 minutes
Servings 8
Nutrition Values: 334 Calories; 15.3g Fat; 6g Total Carbs; 38.2g Protein; 2.3g Sugars
Ingredients
- 1 tablespoon olive oil
- 3 pounds rump roast, boneless and cubed
- Salt and ground black pepper, to taste
- 1 red onion, chopped
- 2 cloves garlic, minced
- 2 tomatoes, puréed
- 1 habanero pepper, seeded and sliced
- 1 green bell pepper, seeded and sliced
- 1 red bell peppers, seeded and sliced
- 2 cups chicken stock
- 1/2 cup dry red wine
- 1/2 teaspoon dried rosemary
- 1/2 teaspoon dried basil
- 1/2 teaspoon dried oregano
- 1/2 teaspoon caraway seed
- 1 tablespoon coconut aminos
- 1 cup sour cream, to serve

Directions
1. Press the "Sauté" button to heat up the Instant Pot. Now, heat the oil; once hot, cook the rump roast for 3 to 4 minutes.
2. Season with salt and black pepper to taste. Add a splash of wine to scrape up any browned bits from the bottom.
3. Add the onion, garlic, tomatoes, peppers, chicken stock, remaining wine, rosemary, basil, oregano, caraway seeds, and coconut aminos.
4. Secure the lid. Choose "Meat/Stew" mode and High pressure; cook for 25 minutes. Once cooking is complete, use a natural pressure release; carefully remove the lid.
5. Ladle into serving bowls; serve dolloped with sour cream. Bon appétit!

WINTER BEEF CHOWDER
Preparation Time: 30 minutes
Servings 6
Nutrition Values: 324 Calories; 17.9g Fat; 6.8g Total Carbs; 34.6g Protein; 1.9g Sugars
Ingredients
- 1 tablespoon grapeseed oil
- 2 pounds top chuck, trimmed, boneless and cubed
- 3 slices slab bacon, chopped
- 1/2 cup yellow onion, chopped
- 1 celery ribs, sliced
- 1 parsnip, sliced
- 4 teaspoons beef base
- 6 cups water
- 1/4 cup dry white wine
- 7 ounces tomato purée
- 1 head savoy cabbage
- Sea salt, to your liking
- 1 teaspoon dried juniper berries
- 1/2 teaspoon dried sage, crushed
- 1/2 teaspoon dried rosemary, leaves picked
- 1 teaspoon whole mixed peppercorns
- 2 sprigs parsley, roughly chopped

Directions
1. Press the "Sauté" button to heat up the Instant Pot. Now, heat the oil; once hot, cook the chuck for 2 to 3 minutes on each side.
2. Add the remaining ingredients and stir to combine well.

3. Secure the lid. Choose "Meat/Stew" mode and High pressure; cook for 25 minutes. Once cooking is complete, use a quick pressure release; carefully remove the lid.
4. Serve in individual bowls garnished with some extra fresh parsley if desired. Bon appétit!

ITALIAN-STYLE BEEF STEW

Preparation Time: 50 minutes
Servings 6
Nutrition Values: 324 Calories; 17.9g Fat; 6.8g Total Carbs; 34.6g Protein; 1.9g Sugars
Ingredients
- 1 tablespoon bacon grease
- 2 pounds chuck roast, trimmed and cubed
- 1 onion, diced
- 2 cloves garlic, sliced
- 4 ounces celery, diced
- 1 cup cabbage, diced
- 1 cup fennel, diced
- 1 carrot, sliced
- 1/2 cup tomato puree
- 4 cups broth, preferably homemade
- 2 tablespoons balsamic vinegar
- 2 bay leaves
- 1 teaspoon winter savory
- 1/2 teaspoon black peppercorns, crushed
- 1 teaspoon dried rosemary
- 1 teaspoon dried thyme
- Sea salt, to taste
- 2 tablespoons fresh basil, snipped

Directions
1. Press the "Sauté" button to heat up the Instant Pot. Now, melt the bacon grease; once hot, cook the chuck for 2 to 3 minutes on each side; reserve.
2. Add the onion and cook an additional 3 minutes or until it is translucent.
3. Add the vegetables to the Instant Pot. Then, stir in tomato puree, broth, balsamic vinegar, bay leaves, winter savory, black peppercorns, dried rosemary, thyme, and sea salt.
4. Secure the lid. Choose "Meat/Stew" mode and High pressure; cook for 40 minutes. Once cooking is complete, use a natural pressure release; carefully remove the lid.
5. Serve garnished with fresh basil. Bon appétit!

LEBERKÄSE WITH SAUERKRAUT

Preparation Time: 15 minutes
Servings 6
Nutrition Values: 382 Calories; 27.1g Fat; 6.1g Total Carbs; 24.5g Protein; 2.7g Sugars
Ingredients
- 2 pounds Leberkäse
- 18 ounces sauerkraut plus 1 cup sauerkraut juice
- 2 garlic cloves, minced
- 1 yellow onion, sliced
- 1 teaspoon dried thyme
- 1/2 cup water
- 1/2 cup chicken stock
- 1 bay leaf

Directions
1. Press the "Sauté" button to heat up the Instant Pot. Once hot, cook your Leberkäse for 2 to 3 minutes, turning periodically.
2. Place all ingredients in your Instant Pot.
3. Secure the lid. Choose "Manual" mode and High pressure; cook for 8 minutes. Once cooking is complete, use a quick pressure release; carefully remove the lid.
4. Discard bay leaf and serve warm. Bon appétit!

HOLIDAY BACON MEATLOAF

Preparation Time: 40 minutes
Servings 6
Nutrition Values: 589 Calories; 44.9g Fat; 6.9g Total Carbs; 38.6g Protein; 2.9g Sugars
Ingredients
- 1 ½ pounds ground chuck
- 1/2 cup heavy whipping cream
- 1 cup cheddar cheese, shredded
- Sea salt and ground black pepper, to taste
- 1 tablespoon dried parsley
- 1 shallot, chopped
- 1 cup mushrooms, diced
- 2 eggs, whisked
- 1 teaspoon fresh thyme
- 1/2 teaspoon dried rosemary
- 1 teaspoon dried marjoram
- 1/2 teaspoon caraway seeds
- 1 teaspoon mustard powder
- 16 long slices bacon
- 1/2 cup tomato chili sauce

Directions
1. Prepare your Instant Pot by adding 1 ½ cups of water and a metal rack to the bottom of the inner pot.
2. In a mixing bowl, thoroughly combine all ingredients, except for bacon and tomato chili sauce.
3. Shape the mixture into a loaf. Place the bacon slices on the top. Weave the bacon (under,

4. Place the meatloaf in a lightly greased baking pan; lower the baking pan onto the rack.
   5. Secure the lid. Choose "Manual" mode and High pressure; cook for 23 minutes. Once cooking is complete, use a quick pressure release; carefully remove the lid.
   6. Spread the tomato chili sauce over the meatloaf. Place the meatloaf under the broiler for 6 to 7 minutes. Allow your meatloaf to sit for 10 minutes before slicing. Bon appétit!

GRANDMA'S CHEESEBURGER SOUP

Preparation Time: 20 minutes
Servings 4
Nutrition Values: 571 Calories; 39g Fat; 3.6g Total Carbs; 48.4g Protein; 1.6g Sugars
Ingredients
- 2 slices bacon, chopped
- 1 pound ground chuck
- 1 teaspoon ghee, room temperature
- Salt and ground black pepper, to taste
- 4 cups vegetable stock, preferably homemade
- 2 garlic cloves, minced
- 1/2 cup scallions, chopped
- 1 teaspoon mustard seeds
- 1 teaspoon paprika
- 1 teaspoon chili powder
- 1/2 cup tomato puree
- 1 bay leaf
- 1 ½ cups Monterey-Jack cheese, shredded
- 2 ounces sour cream
- 1 small handful fresh parsley, roughly chopped

Directions
   1. Press the "Sauté" button to heat up the Instant Pot. Once hot, cook the bacon and ground beef for 2 to 3 minutes, crumbling them with a fork.
   2. Add the ghee, salt, black pepper, vegetable stock, garlic, scallions, mustard seeds, paprika, chili powder, tomato puree, and bay leaf.
   3. Secure the lid. Choose "Manual" mode and High pressure; cook for 8 minutes. Once cooking is complete, use a natural pressure release; carefully remove the lid.
   4. After that, add Monterey-Jack cheese and sour cream; seal the lid and let it stand for at least 5 minutes.
   5. Serve warm in individual bowls garnished with fresh parsley. Bon appétit!

BEST BURGERS WITH KALE AND CHEESE

Preparation Time: 15 minutes
Servings 6
Nutrition Values: 323 Calories; 20.3g Fat; 5.8g Total Carbs; 29.9g Protein; 0.6g Sugars
Ingredients
- 1 pound ground beef
- 1/2 pound beef sausage, crumbled
- 1 ½ cups kale, chopped
- 1/4 cup scallions, chopped
- 2 garlic cloves, minced
- 1/2 Romano cheese, grated
- 1/3 cup blue cheese, crumbled
- Salt and ground black pepper, to taste
- 1 teaspoon crushed dried sage
- 1/2 teaspoon oregano
- 1/2 teaspoon dried basil
- 1 tablespoon olive oil

Directions
   1. Place 1 ½ cups of water and a steamer basket in your Instant Pot.
   2. Mix all ingredients until everything is well incorporated.
   3. Shape the mixture into 6 equal sized patties. Place the burgers on the steamer basket.
   4. Secure the lid. Choose "Manual" mode and High pressure; cook for 6 minutes. Once cooking is complete, use a quick pressure release; carefully remove the lid. Bon appétit!

MODERN BEEF STROGANOFF

Preparation Time: 20 minutes
Servings 6
Nutrition Values: 347 Calories; 20.7g Fat; 5.9g Total Carbs; 33.5g Protein; 2.2g Sugars
Ingredients
- 1 tablespoon lard
- 1 ½ pounds beef stew meat, cubed
- 1 yellow onion, chopped
- 2 garlic cloves, chopped
- 1 red bell pepper, chopped
- Kosher salt and freshly ground black pepper, to taste
- 1/2 teaspoon dried rosemary
- 1/2 teaspoon dried thyme
- 2 cups mushrooms, chopped
- 2 ½ cups broth, preferably homemade
- 1 (10-ounce) box frozen chopped spinach, thawed and squeezed dry
- 1 cup sour cream
- 4 slices Muenster cheese

Directions
   1. Press the "Sauté" button to heat up the

Instant Pot. Now, melt the lard; once hot, cook the beef for 3 to 4 minutes.
2. Add the onion, garlic, bell pepper, salt, black pepper, rosemary, thyme, mushrooms, and broth.
3. Secure the lid. Choose "Manual" mode and High pressure; cook for 10 minutes. Once cooking is complete, use a quick pressure release; carefully remove the lid.
4. Lastly, stir in the spinach, sour cream and cheese. Let it stand in the residual heat until everything is well incorporated. Ladle into soup bowls and serve warm. Bon appétit!

HOT BROCCOLI, LEEK AND BEEF CHOWDER

Preparation Time: 20 minutes
Servings 6
Nutrition Values: 373 Calories; 29.2g Fat; 5.7g Total Carbs; 21.2g Protein; 2.4g Sugars
Ingredients
- 1 tablespoon olive oil
- 1 ½ pounds beef stew meat
- 1/2 cup leeks
- 1 cup broccoli, chopped into florets
- 1 carrot, chopped
- 1 celery with leaves, chopped
- 1 cup tomatoes, puréed
- 4 ½ cups roasted vegetable stock
- 1 teaspoon garlic powder
- 1 teaspoon dried basil
- 1 (1-inch) piece ginger root, grated
- 1 teaspoon Sriracha

Directions
1. Press the "Sauté" button to heat up the Instant Pot. Now, heat the oil; once hot, cook the beef for 3 to 4 minutes; reserve.
2. Now, sauté the leeks in pan drippings until tender and fragrant. Add the remaining ingredients, including the reserved beef.
3. Secure the lid. Choose "Manual" mode and High pressure; cook for 15 minutes. Once cooking is complete, use a quick pressure release; carefully remove the lid.
4. Ladle into individual bowls and garnish with some extra leek leaves if desired. Bon appétit!

STEW WITH SMOKED CHEDDAR CHEESE AND RED WINE

Preparation Time: 30 minutes
Servings 6
Nutrition Values: 381 Calories; 16.7g Fat; 4.5g Total Carbs; 49.2g Protein; 1.8g Sugars
Ingredients
- 1 tablespoon tallow, at room temperature
- 2 pounds bottom round roast, trimmed and diced
- Coarse sea salt and ground black pepper, to taste
- 1 tablespoon Montreal steak seasoning
- 1 banana shallot, chopped
- 1 carrot, chopped
- 1 celery, chopped
- 1/2 cup dry red wine
- 2 cups beef stock
- 2 bay leaves
- 1 cup smoked cheddar cheese, grated

Directions
1. Press the "Sauté" button to heat up the Instant Pot. Now, melt the tallow; once hot, cook the bottom round roast for 3 to 4 minutes. Season with salt and black pepper.
2. Now, add Montreal steak seasoning, shallot, carrot, celery, wine, beef stock, and bay leaves to your Instant Pot.
3. Secure the lid. Choose "Meat/Stew" mode and High pressure; cook for 25 minutes. Once cooking is complete, use a quick pressure release; carefully remove the lid.
4. Divide the stew among 6 serving bowls; top each serving with grated cheese and serve warm. Bon appétit!

FILET MIGNON IN BEER SAUCE

Preparation Time: 20 minutes
Servings 4
Nutrition Values: 499 Calories; 38g Fat; 5.6g Total Carbs; 32.1g Protein; 1.9g Sugars
Ingredients
- 2 tablespoons sesame oil
- 4 (8-ounce) filet mignon steaks
- 1 onion, diced
- 2 garlic cloves, minced
- 1/2 teaspoon dried rosemary
- 1 teaspoon cayenne pepper
- Sea salt and ground black pepper, to taste
- 1/3 cup ale beer
- 1 cup stock, preferably homemade

Directions
1. Press the "Sauté" button to heat up the Instant Pot. Heat the sesame oil. Once hot, cook filet mignon steaks for 2 to 3 minutes per side.
2. Now, add the remaining ingredients and secure the lid.

3. Secure the lid. Choose "Manual" mode and High pressure; cook for 12 minutes. Once cooking is complete, use a natural pressure release; carefully remove the lid.
4. Serve with a fresh salad of choice. Bon appétit!

FRENCH-STYLE BEEF SHANKS

Preparation Time: 35 minutes
Servings 8
Nutrition Values: 210 Calories; 6.6g Fat; 4.2g Total Carbs; 31.1g Protein; 0g Sugars
Ingredients
- 2 teaspoons lard, room temperature
- 2 ½ pounds beef shanks, 1 ½-inch wide
- 1 ½ cups beef broth
- 1 teaspoon Dijon mustard
- 1/2 teaspoon cayenne pepper
- 1/4 teaspoon freshly cracked black pepper
- 1 teaspoon salt
- 1 bay leaf
- 1/2 teaspoon dried marjoram, crushed
- 1/2 teaspoon caraway seeds
- 1 teaspoon dried sage, crushed
- 2 sprigs mint, roughly chopped

Directions
1. Press the "Sauté" button to heat up the Instant Pot. Melt the lard. Once hot, sear the beef shanks for 2 to 3 minutes per side.
2. Add the remaining ingredients, except for the mint.
3. Secure the lid. Choose "Meat/Stew" mode and High pressure; cook for 30 minutes. Once cooking is complete, use a quick pressure release; carefully remove the lid.
4. Serve garnished with fresh mint and enjoy!

GREEK-STYLE BEEF CURRY

Preparation Time: 30 minutes
Servings 6
Nutrition Values: 375 Calories; 17.7g Fat; 5.4g Total Carbs; 43.9g Protein; 1.9g Sugars
Ingredients
- 2 tablespoons olive oil
- 2 ½ pounds beef steaks, cubed
- Sea salt and ground black pepper, to taste
- 1/2 teaspoon red pepper flakes, crushed
- 1 shallot, chopped
- 2 garlic cloves, minced
- 1 habanero pepper, minced
- 1 ½ teaspoons red curry paste
- 1/4 teaspoon ground cinnamon
- 1 ½ tablespoons rice vinegar
- 1 ½ cups chicken stock, preferably homemade
- 1 cup canned coconut milk, unsweetened
- 1/2 cup yogurt
- A small handful coriander, chopped

Directions
1. Press the "Sauté" button to heat up the Instant Pot. Now, heat the olive oil. Once hot, sear the beef steaks for 3 to 4 minutes, stirring periodically; season with salt, black pepper, and red pepper; reserve.
2. Then, cook the shallot, garlic and habanero pepper in pan drippings until fragrant.
3. Add red curry paste, cinnamon, vinegar, and chicken stock.
4. Secure the lid. Choose "Manual" mode and High pressure; cook for 18 minutes. Once cooking is complete, use a quick pressure release; carefully remove the lid.
5. Then, add coconut milk and yogurt. Stir to combine well and press the "Sauté" button one more time; let it simmer until thoroughly heated.
6. Serve in individual bowls, garnished with fresh coriander. Bon appétit!

BEEF SHORT RIBS WITH CILANTRO CREAM

Preparation Time: 25 minutes
Servings 8
Nutrition Values: 346 Calories; 24.1g Fat; 2.1g Total Carbs; 31g Protein; 1.1g Sugars
Ingredients
- 1 tablespoon sesame oil
- 2 ½ pounds beef short ribs
- 1/2 teaspoon red pepper flakes, crushed
- Sea salt and ground black pepper, to taste

Cilantro Cream:
- 1 cup cream cheese, softened
- 1/3 cup sour cream
- A pinch of celery salt
- A pinch of paprika
- 1 teaspoon garlic powder
- 1 bunch fresh cilantro, chopped
- 1 tablespoon fresh lime juice

Directions
1. Press the "Sauté" button to heat up the Instant Pot. Now, heat the sesame oil. Sear the ribs until nicely browned on all sides.
2. Season the ribs with red pepper, salt, and black pepper.
3. Secure the lid. Choose "Manual" mode and

High pressure; cook for 20 minutes. Once cooking is complete, use a quick pressure release; carefully remove the lid.
4. Meanwhile, mix all ingredients for the cilantro cream. Place in the refrigerator until ready to serve. Serve warm ribs with the chilled cilantro cream on the side. Bon appétit!
5. Bean, Rice & Grains

MEXICAN GREEN RICE

Preparation time: 10 minutes
Cooking time: 8 minutes
Servings: 10

Ingredients:
- 3 ½ cups of water or chicken stock
- 1 cup of tightly packed fresh cilantro leaves
- 1 large Poblano chili, seeded and roughly chopped
- 1 green onion, cut into pieces
- 2 garlic cloves
- 3 cups of long grain white rice
- 2 tbsp. of canola or vegetable oil
- Salt to taste, if needed
- ¼ tsp. of cumin
- 1 tsp. of white vinegar
- 2-3 tbsp. of fresh lime juice

Directions:
1. Blend in a blender water, cilantro, poblano, green onion and garlic until well blend and smooth.
2. Add the rice in a fine mesh colander and place it under cold running water to rinse until the water runs clear.
3. Press the "Sauté" function on your Instant Pot and adjust to more. When hot, add the oil. Add the rinsed rice.
4. Toast the rice for about 3 minutes or until some of the moisture is absorbed and rice appears a little toasted and coated with oil, stirring constantly.
5. Add the water and cilantro mixture, salt, cumin, vinegar and give everything a good stir to combine. Bring the pot to a boil.
6. Secure the lid in place and ensure that the valve is in sealing position. Select Manual High Pressure for 8 minutes.
7. Do a natural pressure release for about 5 minutes, then quick release the remaining pressure. Carefully open the lid and give everything a good stir.
8. Sprinkle lime juice over the cooked rice. Fluff rice with a fork and serve immediately.

VEGETABLES

MASHED CHILI CARROTS

Preparation Time: 5 Mins
Total Time: 25 Mins
Servings: 4

Ingredients:
- 1 ½ pounds Carrots, chopped
- 1 tsp Chili Powder
- 1 tbsp Coconut Cream
- 1 tbsp Coconut Oil
- 1 ½ cups Water

Direction
1. Pour the water into the IP.
2. Place the carrots inside the basket and then lower it into the pot.
3. Put the lid on and seal.
4. Set the Instant Pot to MANUAL.
5. Cook on HIGH for 4 minutes.
6. Release the pressure quickly.
7. Open the lid and transfer the carrots to a food processor.
8. Add the coconut cream, coconut oil, and chili powder.
9. Process until the mixture becomes smooth and creamy.
10. Serve and enjoy!

Nutrition Values:
Calories 45
Total Fats 1g
Carbs: 11g
Protein 1g
Dietary Fiber: 1g

TASTY PEPPER SALAD

Preparation Time: 5 Mins
Total Time: 15 Mins
Servings: 4

Ingredients:
- 2 red capsicums, sliced into strips
- 2 yellow capsicums, sliced into strips
- 1 green capsicum, sliced into strips
- ½ teaspoon olive oil
- 1 red onion
- 2 garlic cloves
- 3 tomatoes, chopped
- basil, chopped
- salt and pepper

Directions :
1. Add oil to your instant pot and sauté onions until tender; add 1 garlic clove, and capsicums and cook until browned.
2. Add the chopped tomatoes, salt and pepper and stir to mix; lock lid and cook on high pressure for 5 minutes and then release pressure naturally.
3. Press the remaining garlic clove and set aside.
4. Remove capsicums into a bowl and add olive oil, garlic and chopped basil; mix well and serve.

Nutrition Values:
Calories 48
Total Fats 1.1g
Carbs: 9.2g
Protein 1.8g
Dietary Fiber: 2.9g

INSTANT POT COCONUT CABBAGE

Preparation Time: 15 Mins
Total Time: 25 Mins
Servings: 7

Ingredients :
- 1 tablespoon coconut oil
- 1 tablespoon olive oil
- ½ cup desiccated unsweetened coconut
- 2 tablespoons lemon juice
- 1 medium carrot, sliced
- 1 medium brown onion, sliced
- 1 medium cabbage, shredded
- 1 tablespoon turmeric powder
- 1 tablespoon mild curry powder
- 1 teaspoon mustard powder
- ½ long red chili, sliced
- 2 large cloves of garlic, diced
- 1 + ½ teaspoons salt
- ⅓ cup water

Directions :
1. Turn your instant pot on sauté mode and add coconut oil; stir in onion and salt and cook for about 4 minutes.
2. Stir in spices, chili and garlic for about 30 seconds.
3. Stir in the remaining ingredients and lock the lid; set on manual high for 5 minutes.
4. When done, natural release the pressure and stir the mixture. Serve with beans or rice.

Nutrition Values:
Calories 231
Total Fats 2.5g
Carbs: 15.9g

Protein 5.9g
Dietary Fiber: 8.5g

INSTANT POT GARLICKY MASHED POTATOES

Preparation Time: 5 Mins
Total Time: 9 Mins
Servings: 4

Ingredients :

- 6 cloves garlic, chopped
- 1 cup Homemade vegetable broth
- 4 Yukon gold potatoes, diced
- 1/2 cup almond milk
- 1/4 cup chopped parsley
- 1/8 teaspoon sea salt

Directions :

1. In your instant pot, mix garlic, broth and potatoes and lock the lid; set to manual for 4 minutes and then release the pressure naturally.
2. Transfer the potato mixture to a large bowl and mash with a potato masher until smooth.
3. Add soy milk to your desired consistency and then stir in parsley and salt. Serve hot!

Nutrition Values:

Calories 243
Total Fats 0.8g
Carbs: 24.7g
Protein 4.5g
Dietary Fiber: 11.2g

INSTANT POT RATATOUILLE

Preparation Time: 15 Mins
Total Time: 35 Mins
Servings: 4

Ingredients :

- 1 egg plant, halved then sliced
- 1 green pepper, cut in strips deseeded
- 1 onion, halved then sliced
- 1 tomatoes, wedged
- 2 small zucchinis, sliced
- 75 ml tomato paste
- 1/8 cup olive oil
- 2tbsp fresh parsley
- 1tsp dried basil
- ½ tsp. oregano
- ½ tsp. freshly ground black pepper
- Salt and red pepper flakes to taste

Directions :

1. Layer the vegetables on your instant pot by starting with onions, eggplant, zucchini, garlic, followed by the peppers and finally the tomatoes.
2. Sprinkle with half the dried herbs, parsley, salt and the pepper flakes.
3. Add half the tomato paste and repeat the layering in the same order.
4. Next, drizzle with the olive oil and lock lid and cook on high pressure for 20 minutes. Release the pressure naturally and serve.

Nutrition Values:

Calories 137
Total Fats 6.9g
Carbs: 19.1g
Protein 3.7g
Dietary Fiber: 7.2g

ARUGULA, ORANGE &KAMUT SALAD

Preparation Time: 10 Mins
Total Time: 40 Mins
Servings: 7

Ingredients :

- 1 cup whole Kamut grains, rinsed
- 1 teaspoon vegetable oil
- 2 cups water
- 1 teaspoon sea salt
- ½ lemon
- ¼ cup chopped walnuts
- 1 tablespoon extra-virgin olive oil
- 2 medium blood oranges, sliced
- 2 cups rocket Arugula

Directions :

1. In a bowl, combine kamut grains, lemon juice and 4 cups of water; soak overnight.
2. Strain the kamut and add to an instant pot along with oil, salt and water; lock the lid and cook on high pressure for 18 minutes.
3. Release the pressure naturally and then transfer to a serving bowl; stir in olive oil, walnuts, orange pieces and arugula.
4. Serve right away.

Nutrition Values:

Calories 63
Total Fats 8.6g
Carbs: 11.7g
Protein 2.8g
Dietary Fiber: 2.1g

SAGE-INFUSED BUTTERNUT SQUASH ZUCCHINI NOODLES

Preparation Time: 10 Mins
Total Time: 25 Mins
Servings: 4

Ingredients :

- 3 large zucchinis, Spiralized or julienned into

- noodles
- 3 cups cubed butternut squash
- 2 cloves garlic, finely chopped
- 1 yellow onion, chopped
- 2 tablespoons olive oil
- 2 cups homemade vegetable broth
- ¼ teaspoon red pepper flakes
- Freshly ground black pepper
- 1 tablespoon fresh sage, finely chopped
- Salt, to taste and smoked salt for garnish

Directions:
1. Add the oil to a pan over medium heat and sauté the sage once it's hot until it turns crisp.
2. Transfer to a small bowl and season lightly with salt then set aside.
3. Add the onion, butternut, garlic, broth, salt and pepper flakes to in instant pot and lock the lid; cook on high pressure for 10 minutes and then release pressure naturally.
4. Meanwhile, steam the zucchini noodles in your microwave or steamer until crisp-tender.
5. Once the butternut mixture is ready, remove from heat and let cool off slightly then transfer to a blender and process until smooth.
6. Combine the zucchini noodles and the butternut puree in the skillet over medium heat and cook until heated through and evenly coated for 2 minutes.
7. Sprinkle with fried sage and smoked salt and serve hot.

Nutrition Values:
Calories 301
Total Fats 28.5g
Carbs: 13.8g
Protein 1.9g
Dietary Fiber: 3.4g

CAULIFLOWER TIKKA MASALA

Preparation Time:3Mins
Cook Time:7Mins
Servings: 4

Ingredients:
- 1 large cauliflower head, chopped into florets
- ½ cup unsweetened coconut cream or unsweetened non-dairy yogurt
- 1 medium beet, peeled, peeled, diced
- ½ cup pumpkin puree
- ½ cup organic low-sodium bone broth
- 2 Tablespoons ghee or non-dairy butter
- 1 medium red onion, finely chopped, 4 garlic cloves, minced
- 1 1-inch fresh ginger, peeled, grated, 1 Tablespoon dried fenugreek leaves
- 1 Tablespoon fresh parsley, finely chopped
- 1 Tablespoon garam masala
- 1 teaspoon smoked or regular paprika
- 1 teaspoon organic ground turmeric
- 1 teaspoon organic chili powder
- Garnish: roasted cashews, finely chopped cilantro

Direction
1. Press "Sauté" function on Instant Pot. Add the ghee.
2. Once melted, add onion. Cook 3 minutes. Add garlic, grated ginger. Cook 2 minutes more. Add fenugreek, paprika, chili powder, turmeric, garam masala, and parsley. Cook 1 minute, stirring frequently.
3. In a blender, combine the beet, pumpkin puree, and bone broth. Blend until slightly chunky. Add to ingredients in the Instant Pot. Stir in the cauliflower.
4. Lock, seal the lid. Press "Manual" button. Cook on HIGH 2 minutes.
5. When done, allow to sit for 1 minute before quick releasing pressure. Remove lid.
6. Stir in cream until well combined. Ladle in bowls. Garnish with roasted cashews, cilantro. Serve.

Nutrition Values:
Calories: 243 , Fat: 8.3g , Carbohydrates: 33.23g, Dietary Fiber: 11.96g, Protein: 13.4g

BARBECUE JACKFRUIT

Preparation Time:5Mins
Cook Time:10Mins
Servings: 4

Ingredients:
- 2 x 8-ounce cans jackfruit, drained, chopped
- 1/2 cup homemade low-sodium vegetable broth
- 1/2 cup ghee or non-dairy butter, melted
- ½ cup vinegar
- Juice from 1 fresh lemon
- 1/2 Tablespoon Worcestershire sauce
- 1/2 teaspoons paprika
- 1/4 teaspoon onion powder
- 1/4 teaspoon garlic powder
- 1/2 teaspoons salt
- 1/4 teaspoon pepper
- Lettuce leaves for serving

Direction
1. Add jackfruit and vegetable broth to Instant

Pot.
2. Lock, seal the lid. Press "Manual" button. Cook on HIGH 5 minutes.
3. When done, naturally release pressure. Remove the lid.
4. Using a colander, drain liquid from jackfruit. Return fruit to Instant Pot. Using a potato masher, smash the fruit slightly.
5. In a bowl, combine melted ghee, vinegar, lemon juice, Worcestershire sauce, paprika, garlic powder, onion powder, salt, and black pepper. Stir well. Pour mixture over the jackfruit.
6. Press "Sauté" function. Warm for 5 minutes. Ladle over lettuce leaves. Serve.

Nutrition Values:
Calories: 488, Fat: 34.8g, Carbohydrates: 45.7g, Dietary Fiber: 3g, Protein: 3.7g

CAULIFLOWER RISOTTO
Preparation Time:10Mins
Cook Time:27Mins
Servings: 4

Ingredients:
- 12 asparagus, remove woodsy stem, diced
- 1 cup organic fresh broccoli florets, 1 cup organic baby carrots
- 1 cup fresh leeks, finely chopped, 2 garlic cloves, minced
- 1 cup fresh baby spinach, ½ bunch chives, thinly sliced
- 1 medium yellow onion, finely chopped
- 1½ cups cauliflower rice
- 4 cups homemade low-sodium vegetable broth
- 2 Tablespoons olive oil
- 1 teaspoon fresh thyme, ½ teaspoon garlic powder, ¼ teaspoon red pepper flakes
- 1 teaspoon fresh lemon zest, 2 Tablespoons fresh lemon juice
- ¼ cup ghee or non-dairy butter
- Pinch of salt, pepper

Direction
1. Line a baking sheet with parchment paper. Place asparagus, broccoli, and carrots in a single layer on the tray. Drizzle olive oil. Season with salt and pepper.
2. Place baking sheet in 400°F oven 15 minutes, until broccoli is tender. Remove, set aside. Once cooled, dice in small pieces.
3. Press "Sauté" function on Instant Pot. Add 1 tablespoon of olive oil.
4. Once hot, add onion. Cook 4 minutes. Add garlic, leeks. Cook 2 minutes. Add cauliflower rice. Sauté 1 minute.
5. Stir in vegetable broth, ghee or non-dairy butter, and fresh thyme.
6. Lock, seal the lid. Press "Manual" button. Cook on HIGH 7 minutes.
7. When done, quick release pressure. Remove the lid.
8. Press "Sauté" function. Stir in asparagus, broccoli, carrots, leeks, spinach, garlic powder, red pepper flakes, lemon zest, and lemon juice. Sauté 1 minute, until spinach wilts. Ladle in bowls. Garnish with chives. Serve.

Nutrition Values:
Calories: 278, Fat: 21.5g, Carbohydrates: 15.3g, Dietary Fiber: 4.3g, Protein: 8.4g

MEXICAN-INSPIRED POSOLE
Preparation Time:20Mins
Cook Time:30Mins
Servings: 4

Ingredients:
- 1/2 large head cauliflower, finely chopped
- 1/2 medium yellow onion, finely chopped
- 4 garlic cloves, minced
- 2 x 10-ounce cans jackfruit
- ½ cup coconut oil or olive oil
- ½ cup New Mexico red chile powder
- 1/2 teaspoon organic ground cumin powder
- 1/2 teaspoon organic Mexican dried oregano
- ¾ cup coconut flour or almond flour
- 3 cups homemade low-sodium vegetable broth
- Pinch of salt, pepper

Direction
1. Press "Sauté" function on Instant Pot. Add coconut oil.
2. Once hot, add onion. Cook 4 minutes. Add garlic. Cook 1 minute.
3. Stir in coconut flour, red chile powder, cumin, oregano, salt, pepper. Cook 3 minutes. Stir in 2 cups of the vegetable broth, jackfruit, and cauliflower florets.
4. Break the jackfruit and cauliflower florets apart using a potato masher. Stir in remaining vegetable broth.
5. Close, seal the lid. Press "Manual" button. Cook on HIGH 10 minutes.
6. When done, naturally release pressure. Remove the lid. Stir ingredients.
7. Ladle into bowls. Serve.

Nutrition Values:
Calories: 314, Fat: 17.4g, Carbohydrates: 39.3g, Dietary

Fiber: 3.7g, Protein: 7.3g

MUSHROOM STIR-FRY

Preparation Time: 4Mins
Cook Time:
30Mins
Servings: 2

Ingredients:
- 4 cups mushrooms, finely sliced
- 2 Tablespoons of olive oil
- 1 teaspoon of cumin seeds
- 1 strand curry leaves
- 3 Tablespoons homemade low-sodium vegetable broth
- ½ teaspoon mustard seeds
- ¼ teaspoon turmeric powder
- Pinch of salt, pepper

Direction
1. Press "Sauté" function on Instant Pot. Add the olive oil.
2. Once hot, add cumin seeds, mustard seeds, curry leaves, turmeric, salt, pepper. Stir. Add the mushrooms and vegetable broth. Turn off "Sauté" function.
3. Close, seal the lid. Press "Steam" function. Cook on HIGH 2 minutes.
4. When done, quick release pressure. Remove the lid.
5. Press "Sauté" function. Simmer until all liquid has evaporated.
6. Ladle in bowls. Garnish with fresh parsley. Serve.

Nutrition Values:
Calories: 150, Fat: 14.4g, Carbohydrates: 4.7g, Dietary Fiber: 1.4g, Protein: 4.4g

MASHED CAULIFLOWER WITH SPINACH

Preparation Time: 5Mins
Cook Time: 31Mins
Servings: 4

Ingredients:
- 1 large head of cauliflower, cut into florets
- 1 Tablespoon flavorless oil
- 1 small yellow onion, finely chopped
- 2 cups organic baby spinach
- 2 garlic cloves, minced
- 2 Tablespoons ghee or non-dairy butter
- ½ cup unsweetened coconut cream or organic heavy cream
- Pinch of salt, pepper
- 1 cup homemade vegetable broth
- 6 sprigs fresh thyme

Direction
1. Press "Sauté" function on Instant Pot. Add the oil.
2. Add onion. Cook 4 minutes. Add garlic. Cook 2 minutes. Stir in thyme.
3. Add 1 cup of water, and trivet to Instant Pot. Place cauliflower on top.
4. Lock, seal the lid. Press "Manual" button. Cook on HIGH 15 minutes.
5. When done, naturally release pressure 10 minutes, then quick release remaining pressure. Remove the lid.
6. Remove trivet. Discard liquid. Return cauliflower to pot.
7. While pot is still hot, add ghee, spinach, salt, black pepper, and cream. Using potato masher, mash ingredients until combined. Season. Transfer to bowl. Serve.

Nutrition Values:
Calories: 111, Fat: 4.3g, Carbohydrates: 9.8g, Dietary Fiber: 4.1g, Protein: 9.83g

PESTO FARFALE

Preparation Time: 5 Mins
Total Time: 10 Mins
Servings: 2

Ingredients:
- 7 ounces pasta Farfale
- 2/3 cup Pesto Sauce
- 3 cups Water
- ½ cup halved Cherry Tomatoes
- 1 tbsp chopped Basil
- 2 tbsp grated Parmesan Cheese

Direction
1. Combine the pasta and water in the IP and close the lid.
2. Cook for 7 minutes on HIGH.
3. DO a quick pressure release.
4. Drain and return to the IP.
5. Stir in the cherry tomatoes and pesto and cook for 1 more minute.
6. Divide between two plates.
7. Top with basil and parmesan.
8. Serve and enjoy!

Nutrition Values:
Calories 395
Total Fats 10g
Carbs: 40g
Protein 8g
Dietary Fiber: 1g

SPINACH AND MUSHROOM RISOTTO

Preparation Time: 5 Mins
Total Time: 25 Mins
Servings: 2

Ingredients:

- ¼ Onion, diced
- 1 cup Spinach
- 2 tbsp Lemon Juice
- 4 ounces Mushrooms, sliced
- ¼ cup dry White Wine
- 1 tbsp Butter
- 2/3 cup Arborio Rice
- 1 tbsp Nutritional Yeast
- 2 ½ cups Vegetable Broth
- 1 tbsp Olive Oil

Direction

1. Heat the oil in the IP on SAUTE.
2. Add the onions and cook for 3 minutes.
3. Stir in the rice, and mushrooms, and cook for 2 minutes.
4. Add broth and wine and stir to combine.
5. Close the lid and set the IP to MANUAL.
6. Cook on HIGH for 6 minutes.
7. Do a quick pressure release.
8. Stir in the butter, spinach, and yeast.
9. Let sit for 2 minutes before serving.
10. Enjoy!

Nutrition Values:

Calories 320
Total Fats 8g
Carbs: 45g
Protein 10g
Dietary Fiber: 6g

STUFFED EGGPLANT

Preparation Time: 5 Mins
Total Time: 50 Mins
Servings: 2

Ingredients:

- 2 Eggplants
- ½ pound Mushrooms, chopped
- ½ cup diced Celery
- 1 tbsp Oil
- ½ Onion, diced
- ¾ cup grated Cheddar Cheese
- 1 tbsp chopped Parsley
- 1 ½ cups Water

Direction

1. Cut the eggplants in half lengthwise and scoop out the flesh. Reserve it.
2. Pour the water into the IP and lower the rack.
3. Place the eggplants on the rack and drizzle with oil.
4. Close the lid and cook on HIGH for 5 minutes.
5. In a bowl, combine the remaining ingredients, including the reserved flesh.
6. Do a quick pressure release and divide the mixture between the eggplants.
7. Return the eggplants to the rack and cook for 10 minutes on HIGH.
8. Release the pressure quickly.
9. Serve and enjoy!

Nutrition Values:

Calories 175
Total Fats 7g
Carbs: 25g
Protein 6g
Dietary Fiber: 3g

VEGGIE PATTIES

Preparation Time: 5 Mins
Total Time: 30 Mins
Servings: 2

Ingredients:

- ½ Zucchini, grated
- 1 Carrot, grated
- 1 cup Broccoli Florets
- 1 cup Sweet Potato cubes
- 2 tbsp Olive Oil
- ½ tsp Turmeric
- 1 ½ cups Cauliflower Florets
- 2/3 cup Veggie Broth

Direction

1. Heat half of the oil in the IP on SAUTE.
2. Add the onions and cook for 3 minutes.
3. Add carrots and cook for another minute.
4. Stir in the potatoes and broth and close the lid.
5. Cook for 6 minutes on HIGH.
6. Do a quick pressure release.
7. Stir in the remaining vegetables.
8. Close the lid and cook for 3 more minutes.
9. Release the pressure quickly and mash the veggies with a potato masher.
10. Let cool until safe to handle and shape into patties.
11. Wipe the pot clean and heat the remaining oil in it.
12. Add the patties and cook on SAUTE until golden.
13. Serve and enjoy!

Nutrition Values:

Calories 220
Total Fats 7g
Carbs: 34g
Protein 4g
Dietary Fiber: 6.5g

LEAFY RISOTTO

Preparation Time: 5 Mins
Total Time: 20 Mins
Servings: 2

Ingredients:
- 2/3 cup Arborio Rice
- ½ cup chopped Spinach
- ½ cup chopped Kale
- ¼ cup grated Parmesan Cheese
- ¼ cup diced Onion
- 1 tsp minced Garlic
- 2 ½ cups Veggie Broth
- 1 tbsp Oil
- 1 tbsp Butter

Direction
1. Heat the oil in the IP on SAUTE.
2. Add the onions and cook for 3 minutes.
3. Add garlic and cook for 1 minute.
4. Stir in the rice and cook for an additional minute.
5. Pour the broth over, stir to combine, and close the lid.
6. Cook on RICE for 6 minutes.
7. Do a quick pressure release.
8. Drain if there is excess liquid.
9. Stir in the butter, parmesan, and greens.
10. Serve after 2 minutes.
11. Enjoy!

Nutrition Values:
Calories 272
Total Fats 11g
Carbs: 140g
Protein 6g
Dietary Fiber: 3g

SPAGHETTI "BOLOGNESE"

Preparation Time: 5 Mins
Total Time: 25 Mins
Servings: 2

Ingredients:
- 2 cups cooked Spaghetti
- 1 tbsp Tomato Paste
- ½ cup Cauliflower Florets
- 1 tbsp Balsamic Vinegar
- 5 ounces Mushrooms
- 14 ounces canned diced Tomatoes
- 1 tsp dried Basil
- ¼ tsp Oregano
- 1 tbsp Agave Nectar
- ¼ cup chopped Eggplant

Direction
1. Place the cauliflower, eggplants, and mushrooms, in your food processor. Pulse until ground.
2. Transfer the mixture to the Instant Pot.
3. Stir in the rest of the ingredients, except the spaghetti.
4. Close the lid and cook on HIGH for 6 minutes.
5. Do a quick pressure release.
6. Stir in the spaghetti. Serve and enjoy!

Nutrition Values:
Calories 360
Total Fats 2.3g
Carbs: 72g
Protein 14g
Dietary Fiber: 8g

BEAN AND RICE BAKE

Preparation Time: 5 Mins
Total Time: 40 Mins
Servings: 2

Ingredients:
- ½ cup Beans, soaked and rinsed
- 2 ½ cups Water
- 1 cup Brown Rice
- 1 tsp Chili Powder
- 3 ounces Tomato Sauce
- 1 Garlic Clove, minced
- 1 tsp Onion Powder
- ¼ tsp Salt

Direction
1. Place all of the ingredients in your IP.
2. Close the lid and set it to POULTRY.
3. Cook for 27 minutes.
4. Do a quick pressure release.
5. Serve and enjoy!

Nutrition Values:
Calories 320
Total Fats 2g
Carbs: 63g
Protein 6g
Dietary Fiber: 9g

BROCCOLI & TOFU IN A TAMARI SAUCE

Preparation Time: 5 Mins
Total Time: 15 Mins
Servings: 2

Ingredients:
- ½ pound Tofu, cubed
- 2 tsp Rice Vinegar
- 1 tbsp Tahini
- 2 tbsp Tamari
- 1 Garlic Clove, minced
- 1/3 cup Veggie Stock
- 1 cup Onion Slices

- 1 tbsp Sriracha
- 2 tsp Sesame Oil
- 1 tbsp Sesame Seeds
- 1 cup Broccoli Florets
- ½ cup diced Sweet Potato

Direction
1. Heat the oil in the IP.
2. Add the sweet potatoes and onions and cook for 3 minutes.
3. Add garlic and cook for a minute.
4. Stir in the tofu, tamari, vinegar, and broth.
5. Close the lid and cook for 2 minutes on HIGH.
6. So a quick pressure release and stir in the broccoli.
7. Cook for another 2 minutes.
8. Release the pressure quickly, again, and stir in the sriracha.
9. Serve and enjoy!

Nutrition Values:
Calories 250
Total Fats 12g
Carbs: 22g
Protein 17g
Dietary Fiber: 2g

CARROT AND SWEET POTATO MEDLEY
Preparation Time: 5 Mins
Total Time: 30 Mins
Servings: 2

Ingredients:
- ½ Onion, chopped
- 1 pound Baby Carrots, halved
- 1 pound Sweet Potatoes, cubed
- 2 tbsp Olive Oil
- ½ tsp Italian Seasoning
- 1 cup Vegetable Broth
- ¼ tsp Garlic Salt

Direction
1. Heat the oil in the IP on SAUTE.
2. Add the onions and cook for about 3-4 minutes.
3. Add the carrots and cook for another 3-4 minutes.
4. Stir in the remaining ingredients.
5. Close the lid and set the IP to MANUAL.
6. Cook for 8 minutes on HIGH.
7. Serve and enjoy!

Nutrition Values:
Calories 413
Total Fats 7g
Carbs: 74g
Protein 7g

Dietary Fiber: 12g

FRUITY WILD RICE CASSEROLE WITH ALMONDS
Preparation Time: 5 Mins
Total Time: 55 Mins
Servings: 2

Ingredients:
- 1/3 cup dried Fruit
- 2 tbsp Apple Juice
- ½ Pear, chopped
- 1 Apple, chopped
- ½ tbsp Maple Syrup
- ¼ cup Slivered Almonds
- ¾ cup Wild Rice
- 2 cups Water
- 1 tsp Oil
- Pinch of Cinnamon

Direction
1. Place the rice and water in the IP and close the lid.
2. Cook on HIGH for 20 minutes.
3. Meanwhile combine the dried fruit and apple juice and let sit for 20 minutes.
4. Drain the fruits and chop them.
5. Do a quick pressure release and stir in the remaining ingredients.
6. Close the lid again and cook for 2 minutes on HIGH.
7. Serve and enjoy!

Nutrition Values:
Calories 410
Total Fats 5g
Carbs: 70g
Protein 9g
Dietary Fiber: 19g

BASIL RISOTTO
Preparation Time: 5 Mins
Total Time: 30 Mins
Servings: 2

Ingredients:
- ¼ Onion, chopped
- 1 cup Rice
- 2 ¼ cup Chicken Broth
- 2 tbsp grated Parmesan Cheese
- 1 tbsp Oil
- A handful of Basil, chopped

Direction
1. Set your Instant Pot to SAUTE and heat the oil in it.
2. Add the onions and cook for 2 minutes.
3. Add the rice and cook for an additional

minute.
4. Pour the broth over, stir to combine, and close the lid.
5. Cook on RICE for 10 minutes.
6. Do a quick pressure release.
7. Drain if there is excess liquid.
8. Stir in the basil and serve topped with parmesan.
9. Enjoy!

Nutrition Values:
Calories 510
Total Fats 7g
Carbs: 80g
Protein 12
Dietary Fiber: 20g

WHEAT BERRIES WITH TOMATOES

Preparation Time: 5 Mins
Total Time: 45 Mins
Servings: 2

Ingredients:
- ¾ cup Wheat Berries
- 1 tbsp Butter
- 8 ounces diced canned Tomatoes
- ½ cup Chicken Broth

Direction
1. Melt the butter in your Instant Pot on SAUTE.
2. Add the wheat berries and cook for about 2 minutes.
3. Stir in the remaining ingredients.
4. Close the lid and set the IP to MANUAL.
5. Cook on HIGH for 25 minutes.
6. Do a natural pressure release.
7. Serve and enjoy!

Nutrition Values:
Calories 140
Total Fats 7g
Carbs: 15 g
Protein 4g
Dietary Fiber: 4g

BLACK BEAN HASH

Preparation Time: 5 Mins
Total Time: 10 Mins
Servings: 2

Ingredients:
- 2 cups cubed Sweet Potatoes
- ½ cup chopped Onions
- 1 tsp Chili Powder
- 1/3 cup Veggie Broth
- 1 cup canned Black Beans, drained
- ¼ cup chopped Scallions
- 1 tbsp Olive Oil

Direction
1. Heat the oil in your IP on SAUTE.
2. Add the onions and cook for 3 minutes.
3. Add the rest of the ingredients.
4. Give it a good stir to combine well.
5. Close the lid and set the IP to MANUAL.
6. Cook for 3 minutes on HIGH.
7. Release the pressure quickly.
8. Serve and enjoy!

Nutrition Values:
Calories 266
Total Fats 9g
Carbs: 28g
Protein 5g
Dietary Fiber: 6g

GREEN BEANS AND BEETS

Preparation time: 10 minutes
Cooking time: 20 minutes
Servings: 4

Ingredients:
- 1 and ½ cups chicken stock
- 4 beets, peeled and cubed
- 1 red onion, sliced
- 1 pound green beans, trimmed and halved
- A pinch of salt and black pepper
- 1 tablespoon dill, chopped
- 1 tablespoon balsamic vinegar

Directions:
1. In your instant pot, combine the beets with the green beans and the rest of the ingredients, put the lid on and cook on High for 20 minutes.
2. Release the pressure naturally for 10 minutes, divide everything between plates and serve.

Nutrition Value: calories 162, fat 3, fiber 1, carbs 4, protein 5

BRUSSELS SPROUTS AND GARLIC

Preparation time: 10 minutes
Cooking time: 20 minutes
Servings: 4

Ingredients:
- 1 pound Brussels sprouts
- 1 cup chicken stock
- 2 green onions, chopped
- 4 garlic cloves, minced
- A pinch of salt and black pepper
- 1 tablespoon dill, chopped

Directions:
1. In your instant pot, mix the sprouts with the stock and the rest of the ingredients, put the lid on and cook on High for 20 minutes.

2. Release the pressure naturally for 10 minutes, divide the mix between plates and serve.

Nutrition Value: calories 142, fat 2, fiber 1, carbs 3, protein 4

BELL PEPPERS AND RICE

Preparation time: 10 minutes
Cooking time: 20 minutes
Servings: 4

Ingredients:
- 1 pound red bell peppers, cut into wedges
- 1 cup white rice, already cooked
- 2 cup veggie stock
- 1 tablespoon chives, chopped
- 1 tablespoon walnuts, chopped

Directions:
1. In your instant pot, mix the bell peppers with the rice and the rest of the ingredients, put the lid on and cook on High for 20 minutes.
2. Release the pressure naturally for 10 minutes, divide the mix between plates and serve.

Nutrition Value: calories 152, fat 2, fiber 2, carbs 4, protein 5

GARLIC PEPPERS MIX

Preparation time: 10 minutes
Cooking time: 15 minutes
Servings: 4

Ingredients:
- 1 pound mixed bell peppers, cut into thick strips
- ½ cup veggie stock
- 3 garlic cloves, minced
- A pinch of cayenne pepper
- A pinch of salt and black pepper
- 1 tablespoon cilantro, chopped

Directions:
1. In your instant pot, combine the bell peppers with the stock and the rest of the ingredients, put the lid on and cook on High for 15 minutes.
2. Release the pressure naturally for 10 minutes, divide the mix between plates and serve.

Nutrition Value: calories 121, fat 2, fiber 2, carbs 4, protein 5

BELL PEPPERS AND PINE NUTS

Preparation time: 5 minutes
Cooking time: 15 minutes
Servings: 4

Ingredients:
- 1 pound mixed bell peppers, cut into wedges
- 1 cup veggie stock
- ¼ cup pine nuts, toasted
- 1 tablespoon olive oil
- 1 tablespoon spring onions, chopped

Directions:
1. In your instant pot, combine the bell peppers with the rest of the ingredients, put the lid on and cook on High for 15 minutes.
2. Release the pressure naturally for 10 minutes, divide the mix between plates and serve.

Nutrition Value: calories 110, fat 2, fiber 2, carbs 4, protein 4

BACON AND MUSTARD BELL PEPPERS

Preparation time: 5 minutes
Cooking time: 15 minutes
Servings: 4

Ingredients:
- 1 pound mixed bell peppers, cut into strips
- A pinch of salt and black pepper
- ½ cup bacon, cooked and chopped
- 1 tablespoon mustard
- 1 cup chicken stock

Directions:
1. In your instant pot, combine the bell peppers with the rest of the ingredients, put the lid on and cook on High for 15 minutes.
2. Release the pressure naturally for 5 minutes, divide the mix between plates and serve.

Nutrition Value: calories 151, fat 2, fiber 3, carbs 5, protein 4

BEETS AND PARMESAN

Preparation time: 10 minutes
Cooking time: 30 minutes
Servings: 4

Ingredients:
- 1 pound beets, peeled and cubed
- Juice of 1 lime
- A pinch of salt and black pepper
- 1 cup chicken stock
- 3 tablespoons parmesan, grated

Directions:
1. In your instant pot, combine the beets with the rest of the ingredients except the parmesan, put the lid on and cook on High for 30 minutes.
2. Release the pressure naturally for 10 minutes, divide the beets between plates, sprinkle the parmesan on top and serve.

Nutrition Value: calories 126, fat 1, fiber 2, carbs 4, protein 4

POTATOES AND CHEDDAR

Preparation time: 10 minutes
Cooking time: 20 minutes
Servings: 4

Ingredients:
- 1 and ½ pounds sweet potatoes, peeled and cut into wedges
- 1 cup cheddar cheese, grated
- 1 and ½ tablespoons tomato sauce
- 1 cup beef stock
- A pinch of salt and black pepper
- 1 tablespoon dill, chopped

Directions:
1. In your instant pot, mix the potatoes with the rest of the ingredients except the cheese, toss, put the lid on and cook on High for 20 minutes.
2. Release the pressure naturally for 10 minutes, divide the mix between plates, sprinkle the cheddar on top and serve.

Nutrition Value: calories 162, fat 8, fiber 2, carbs 4, protein 7

CAULIFLOWER AND COLLARD GREENS

Preparation time: 10 minutes
Cooking time: 12 minutes
Servings: 6

Ingredients:
- 1 pound collard greens, trimmed
- 1 pound cauliflower florets
- 1 cup coconut cream
- 1 tablespoon chili powder
- A pinch of salt and black pepper
- 1 tablespoon chives, chopped

Directions:
1. In your instant pot, combine the cauliflower with the collard greens and the rest of the ingredients except the chives, put the lid on and cook on High for 12 minutes.
2. Release the pressure naturally for 10 minutes, divide the mix between plates, sprinkle the chives on top and serve.

Nutrition Value: calories 122, fat 2, fiber 2, carbs 5, protein 3

BALSAMIC COLLARD GREENS

Preparation time: 10 minutes
Cooking time: 20 minutes
Servings: 4

Ingredients:
- 1 bunch collard greens, trimmed
- ½ cup chicken stock
- 2 tablespoons tomato puree
- A pinch of salt and black pepper
- 1 tablespoon balsamic vinegar

Directions:
1. In your instant pot, mix the collard greens with the stock and the rest of the ingredients, put the lid on and cook on High for 20 minutes.
2. Release the pressure naturally for 10 minutes, divide the mix between plates and serve.

Nutrition Value: calories 130, fat 2, fiber 2, carbs 4, protein 6

COLLARD GREENS AND APPLES MIX

Preparation time: 10 minutes
Cooking time: 20 minutes
Servings: 4

Ingredients:
- 1 sweet onion, chopped
- 3 garlic cloves, minced
- 2 and ½ pounds collard greens, chopped
- A pinch of salt and black pepper
- 1 cup chicken stock
- 1 cup green apple, cored and cubed
- 1 tablespoon cilantro, chopped

Directions:
1. In your instant pot, combine the collard greens with the sweet onion and the rest of the ingredients, put the lid on and cook on High for 20 minutes.
2. Release the pressure naturally for 10 minutes, divide the mix between plates and serve.

Nutrition Value: calories 140, fat 2, fiber 2, carbs 5, protein 7

DILL ENDIVES AND CHIVES

Preparation time: 10 minutes
Cooking time: 12 minutes
Servings: 4

Ingredients:
- 4 endives, trimmed and halved
- A pinch of salt and black pepper
- 1 cup chicken stock
- 1 tablespoon chives, chopped
- 1 tablespoon dill, chopped

Directions:
1. In your instant pot, mix the endives with the rest of the ingredients, put the lid on and cook on High for 12 minutes.
2. Release the pressure naturally for 10 minutes, divide the mix between plates and serve.

Nutrition Value: calories 114, fat 2, fiber 2, carbs 4, protein 4

NUTMEG ENDIVES

Preparation time: 10 minutes
Cooking time: 12 minutes
Servings: 4

Ingredients:
- 4 endives, trimmed
- A pinch of salt and black pepper
- ½ cup coconut milk
- ½ teaspoon nutmeg, ground

Directions:
1. In your instant pot, combine the endives with the rest of the ingredients, put the lid on and cook on High for 12 minutes.
2. Release the pressure naturally for 10 minutes, divide the mix between plates and serve.

Nutrition Value: calories 124, fat 2, fiber 1, carbs 3, protein 4

WINE-GLAZED MUSHROOMS
Servings: 6
Preparation Time: 5 minutes
Cooking Time: 6 minutes

Ingredients
- 2 tablespoons olive oil
- 6 garlic cloves, minced
- 2 lbs. fresh mushrooms, sliced
- 1/3 cup balsamic vinegar
- 1/3 cup white wine
- Salt and black pepper to taste

Directions
1. Add the oil and garlic to the Instant Pot and Select the "Sauté" function to cook for 1 minute.
2. Now add all the remaining ingredients to the cooker.
3. Switch the cooker to the "Manual" function with high pressure and 5 minutes cooking time.
4. After it is done, do a Quick release then remove the lid.
5. Sprinkle some salt and black pepper if desired then serve.

Nutrition Values:
Calories: 91
Carbohydrate: 6.5g
Protein: 5g
Fat: 5.1g
Sugar: 2.8g
Sodium: 38mg

STEAMED ARTICHOKE
Servings: 4
Preparation Time: 5 minutes
Cooking Time: 10 minutes

Ingredients
- 4 artichokes, trimmed
- 2 lemons, one juiced and one sliced
- ½ tablespoon peppercorns, whole
- 1 ½ garlic cloves, chopped
- ½ tablespoons olive oil
- 2 cups water
- Salt and pepper to taste

Directions
1. Pour the water and peppercorns into the insert of the Instant Pot.
2. Place the steamer trivet inside.
3. Arrange the artichokes over the trivet.
4. Secure the lid and select the "Manual" function with low pressure for 5 minutes.
5. After the beep, do a Natural release and remove the lid.
6. Strain the artichokes and return them back to the pot.
7. Add the oil and all the remaining ingredients back into the Instant Pot, and then "Sauté" for 5 minutes while stirring.
8. Serve hot.

Nutrition Values:
Calories: 103
Carbohydrate: 20.5g
Protein: 5.7g
Fat: 2.1g
Sugar: 2.4g
Sodium: 201mg

GREEN BEANS WITH TOMATOES
Servings: 8
Preparation Time: 05 minutes
Cooking Time: 7 minutes

Ingredients
- 2 tablespoons olive oil
- 2 garlic cloves, crushed
- 4 cups fresh tomatoes, diced
- 2 lbs. green beans
- Salt to taste

Directions
1. Add the oil and garlic to the Instant Pot and "Sauté" for 1 minute.
2. Stir in tomatoes and sauté for another 1 minute.
3. Set the steamer trivet in the pot and arrange green beans over it.
4. Secure the lid and select the "Manual" function with high pressure for 5 minutes.
5. After it is done, do a Natural release to release the steam.
6. Remove the lid and the trivet along with green

beans.
7. Add the beans to tomatoes in the pot.
8. Sprinkle salt and stir well. Serve hot.

Nutrition Values:
Calories: 82
Carbohydrate: 11.8g
Protein: 2.9g
Fat: 3.8g
Sugar: 4g
Sodium: 31mg

AVOCADO QUINOA SALAD

Servings: 4
Preparation Time: 5 minutes
Cooking Time: 1 minute

Ingredients
- ½ cup quinoa, rinsed
- ¾ cup water
- ¼ teaspoon salt
- ½ carrot, peeled and shredded
- ½ cup avocados, diced
- ½ cup green onions
- ½ cup cabbage, chopped
- 1 tablespoon lime juice
- 1 tablespoon avocado oil
- 1 tablespoon freshly grated ginger
- A pinch of red pepper flakes

Directions
1. Add the quinoa, salt, and water to the Instant Pot.
2. Secure the lid and select the "Manual" function with high pressure for 1 minute.
3. After the beep, do a quick release and remove the lid.
4. Meanwhile, add the remaining ingredients to a bowl and mix them well.
5. Add the cooked quinoa to the prepared mixture and mix well.
6. Serve as a salad.

Nutrition Values:
Calories: 163
Carbohydrate: 19.3g
Protein: 3.9g
Fat: 8.5g
Sugar: 1.3g
Sodium: 160mg

PEPPER SALAD

Servings: 4
Preparation Time: 5 minutes
Cooking Time: 10 minutes

Ingredients
- 2 red peppers, thinly sliced into strips
- 2 yellow peppers, thinly sliced
- 1 green pepper, thinly sliced
- 2 cups tomato puree
- 1 red onion, thinly sliced into strips
- 2 garlic cloves
- 1 bunch parsley, chopped
- 1 tablespoon olive oil
- Salt and black pepper to taste

Directions
1. Add the oil and all the vegetables to the Instant Pot.
2. Select "Sauté" and stir-fry for 5 minutes with constant stirring.
3. Stir in tomato puree, salt, and pepper.
4. Secure the lid and select the "Manual" function for 5 minutes at high pressure.
5. After the beep, do a quick release and remove the lid.
6. Stir well and serve.

Nutrition Values:
Calories: 132
Carbohydrate: 23.7g
Protein: 4.1g
Fat: 4.2g
Sugar: 9.2g
Sodium: 81mg

ASPARAGUS STICKS

Servings: 3
Preparation Time: 10 minutes
Cooking Time: 03 minutes

Ingredients
- 1 cup water
- 8 oz. thinly sliced Prosciutto*
- 1lb. thick Asparagus sticks
- Salt to taste
- Pepper to taste

Directions
1. Wrap each prosciutto slice over the asparagus sticks.
2. Pour a cup of water into the Instant Pot.
3. Arrange a steamer trivet inside.
4. Place the wrapped asparagus sticks over the trivet.
5. Secure the lid and select "Manual" with high pressure for 3 minutes.
6. After the beep, do a natural release then remove the lid.
7. Transfer the steamed asparagus sticks to the platter.
8. Sprinkle some salt and pepper then serve.

Nutrition Values:
Calories: 164

Carbohydrate: 9.6g
Protein: 17.6g
Fat: 5.7g
Sugar: 3g
Sodium: 1337mg

INSTANT MASHED POTATO

Servings: 4
Preparation Time: 5 minutes
Cooking Time: 18 minutes

Ingredients

- 2 cups water
- 6-8 medium potatoes (peeled)
- 1 teaspoon coarse rock salt
- 2 tablespoons full cream
- Additional salt and pepper to taste

Directions

1. Add the water, potatoes, and salt to the Instant Pot.
2. Secure the lid and select the "Manual" function for 18 minutes with high pressure.
3. After the beep, do a Natural release for 10 minutes and remove the lid.
4. Drain the water from the pot and leave the potatoes inside.
5. Use a potato masher to mash the potatoes in the pot.
6. Stir in cream, pepper, and additional salt. Mix them well.
7. Serve and enjoy.

Nutrition Values:

Calories: 394
Carbohydrate: 62.5g
Protein: 10.3g
Fat: 9.9g
Sugar: 8.5g
Sodium: 216mg

CHICKPEA HUMMUS

Servings: 4
Preparation Time: 5 minutes
Cooking Time: 20 minutes

Ingredients

- ½ cup dry chickpeas, soaked
- 1 bay leaf
- 1 tablespoon olive oil
- 2 garlic cloves
- 3 cups water
- 1 tablespoon tahini
- ½ lemon, juiced
- ¼ teaspoon powdered cumin
- ¼ teaspoon sea salt
- ¼ bunch Parsley, chopped
- ¼ teaspoon paprika

Directions

1. Add 3 cups of water, chickpeas, bay leaf and garlic cloves to the Instant Pot.
2. Secure the lid and select the "Manual" function for 18 minutes with high pressure.
3. After the beep, do a Natural release and remove the lid.
4. Strain and rinse the cooked chickpeas. Discard the bay leaf.
5. Add the oil and all the remaining ingredients to the Instant Pot and "Sauté" for 2 minutes.
6. Return the chickpeas to the pot and use an immerse blender to form a smooth puree.
7. Stir and serve.

Nutrition Values:

Calories: 149
Carbohydrate: 17.4g
Protein: 5.7g
Fat: 7.1g
Sugar: 2.9g
Sodium: 128mg

POTATO & CAULIFLOWER MASH

Servings: 8
Preparation Time: 5 minutes
Cooking Time: 25 minutes

Ingredients

- 3 cups water
- 4 lbs. potatoes (peeled)
- 16 oz. cauliflower florets
- 1 teaspoon coarse rock salt
- 2 tablespoons full cream
- Additional salt and pepper to taste

Directions

1. Add the water, potatoes, cauliflower, and salt to the Instant Pot.
2. Secure the lid and select the "Manual" function for 25 minutes with high pressure.
3. After the beep, do a Natural release in 10 minutes and remove the lid.
4. Drain the water from the pot and leave the potatoes and cauliflower inside.
5. Use a potato masher to mash the cauliflower and potatoes in the pot.
6. Stir in cream, pepper, and the additional salt. Mix them well.
7. Serve and enjoy.

Nutrition Values:

Calories: 204
Carbohydrate: 38.7g
Protein: 6.6g
Fat: 2.1g
Sugar: 6.4g

Sodium: 62mg

GREEN BEANS SALAD

Servings: 4
Preparation Time: 5 minutes
Cooking Time: 7 minutes

Ingredients
- ½ oz. dry porcini mushrooms, soaked
- 1 cup water
- 1 lb. green beans, trimmed
- 1 lb. potatoes, quartered
- ½ teaspoon sea salt, divided
- Black pepper ground to taste

Directions
1. Add the water, potatoes, mushrooms, and salt to the Instant Pot.
2. Place the steamer trivet over the potatoes. Arrange all the green beans in the steamer.
3. Secure the lid and select the "Manual" function for 7 minutes with high pressure.
4. After the beep, do a Natural release for 10 minutes and remove the lid.
5. Transfer the green beans to a platter. Strain the potatoes and mushrooms.
6. Add the potatoes and mushroom to the green beans.
7. Mix gently, sprinkle some pepper and salt on top and serve.

Nutrition Values:
Calories: 127
Carbohydrate: 27.7g
Protein: 4.9g
Fat: 0.3g
Sugar: 2.9g
Sodium: 249mg

TASTY CORN COBS

Servings: 4
Preparation Time: 10 minutes
Cooking Time: 2 minutes

Ingredients
- 4 ears corn
- 2 cups water
- Salt and pepper to taste
- 1 tablespoon lemon juice
- 1 tablespoon melted butter

Directions
1. Add the water and arrange the corn ears vertically in the Instant Pot.
2. Keep the larger end of the corn ears dipped in the water or arrange diagonally.
3. Secure the lid and select the "Manual" function with high pressure for 2 minutes.
4. After the beep, do a Natural release then remove the lid carefully.
5. Strain the corn ears and transfer them to a platter.
6. Drizzle some lemon juice along with melted butter on top.
7. Sprinkle salt and pepper then serve hot.

Nutrition Values:
Calories: 158
Carbohydrate: 29.1g
Protein: 5.1g
Fat: 4.7g
Sugar: 5.1g
Sodium: 48mg

FRESH RED BEETS

Servings: 3
Preparation Time: 5 minutes
Cooking Time: 7 minutes

Ingredients
- 3 red beets, red part only, quartered
- 1 cup water
- Salt and pepper to taste

Directions
1. Pour a cup of water into the insert of the Instant Pot.
2. Place the steamer trivet inside.
3. Arrange the beets over the trivet.
4. Secure the lid and select the "Manual" function with high pressure for 7 minutes.
5. After the beep, do a Natural release and remove the lid.
6. Transfer the beets to the platter, sprinkle some salt and water on top.
7. Serve.

Nutrition Values:
Calories: 44
Carbohydrate: 10g
Protein: 1.7g
Fat: 0.2g
Sugar: 8g
Sodium: 77mg

JUICY QUINOA OLIVES

Servings: 4
Preparation Time: 10 minutes
Cooking Time: 1 minute

Ingredients
- ½ cup quinoa, rinsed
- ¾ cup water
- ¼ teaspoon salt
- ½ carrot, peeled and shredded
- ½ cup green onions
- ¼ cup black olives, sliced
- 1 tablespoon lime juice

- 1 tablespoon olive oil
- 1 tablespoon freshly grated ginger
- A pinch of red pepper flakes

Directions
1. Add the quinoa, salt, and water to the Instant Pot.
2. Secure the lid and select the "Manual" function with high pressure for 1 minute.
3. After the beep, do a quick release and remove the lid.
4. Meanwhile, add the remaining ingredients to a bowl and mix them well.
5. Add the cooked quinoa to the prepared mixture and mix well.
6. Serve as a salad.

Nutrition Values:
Calories: 133
Carbohydrate: 17.8g
Protein: 3.5g
Fat: 5.8g
Sugar: 0.9g
Sodium: 231mg

SOUPS AND STEWS

TOMATO SOUP

Servings: 4
Preparation Time: 6 minutes'
Cooking Time: 13 minutes

Ingredients
- ½ garlic clove, minced
- 1 small onion, chopped
- 2 tablespoons olive oil
- 1 ½ lbs fresh tomatoes, chopped
- 1 teaspoon dried parsley, crushed
- 1 tablespoon tomato sauce
- 1 teaspoon dried basil, crushed
- 1 ¼ cups vegetable broth
- 1 tablespoon sugar
- ½ tablespoon balsamic vinegar
- Freshly ground black pepper, to taste
- Cilantro and fresh cream to garnish

Directions
1. Pour the oil into the inner pan of the instant pot and select the 'sauté" function.
2. Add the garlic and onions to the oil and cook for 3 minutes.
3. Hit 'cancel', then add the tomato sauce, broth, herbs, tomatoes and black pepper.
4. Secure the lid and select the 'Soup' function on your instant pot. Set the timer to cook for 10 minutes.
5. When you hear the beep, 'quick release' the steam and remove the lid.
6. Stir in the vinegar and sugar.
7. Garnish with fresh cream and cilantro, then serve hot.

Nutrition Values:
Calories: 56
Carbohydrate: 12g
Protein: 2.4g
Fat: 0.4g
Sugar: 8.4g
Sodium: 55mg

POTATO AND CORN SOUP

Servings: 4
Preparation Time: 6 minutes
Cooking Time: 12 minutes

Ingredients
- 1 cup fresh corn kernels
- 1 tablespoon unsalted butter, melted
- ½ medium onion, chopped
- 1 celery stalk, chopped
- 1 garlic clove, chopped
- 1 large russet potato, peeled and chopped
- 1 ½ carrots, peeled and chopped
- 1 tablespoon dried parsley, crushed
- 3 cups vegetable broth
- 1½ tablespoon corn starch
- Freshly ground black pepper, to taste
- ¼ cup water

Directions
1. Pour the melted butter into the instant pot and press the 'sauté' key. Add the celery, onion, carrot and garlic to the pot, then cook for 3 minutes.
2. Now add the broth, potatoes, corns, black pepper and parsley to the pot, and secure the lid.
3. Select the 'manual' function, set to high pressure and the timer to 6 minutes.
4. After the beep, 'quick release' the steam and remove the lid.
5. Meanwhile, prepare the corn starch slurry by mixing it with some water.
6. Pour the corn starch slurry into the soup, stirring continuously.
7. Set the cooker to the 'sauté' function and cook for 3 minutes.
8. Serve hot

Nutrition Values:
Calories: 168
Carbohydrate: 30.5g
Protein: 5.1g
Fat: 3.5g
Sugar: 3.9g
Sodium: 282mg

CHICKEN AND KALE SOUP

Servings: 8
Preparation Time: 10 minutes'
Cooking Time: 12 minutes

Ingredients
- 2 cups water
- 6 celery stalks, chopped
- 4 carrots, peeled and chopped
- 2 medium onions, chopped
- 4 bay leaves
- 2 tablespoons olive oil
- ½ teaspoon dried oregano, crushed
- Freshly ground black pepper to taste
- ½ teaspoon dried thyme, crushed

- 8 cups low-sodium chicken broth
- 2 lbs cooked chicken, shredded
- 4 cups fresh kale, trimmed and chopped
- 1 teaspoon Worcestershire sauce

Directions
1. Pour the oil into the instant pot and select the 'sauté' function.
2. Add the carrot, celery and onion to the oil and sauté for 5 minutes.
3. Now stir in the herbs, bay leaves and black pepper and cook for another minute.
4. Pour the water and chicken broth into the pot and secure the lid.
5. Select the 'soup' function on the control panel and cook for 4 minutes.
6. When you hear the beep, 'quick release' the steam, then remove the lid.
7. Stir in the kale and chicken then cook on 'sauté' for 2 minutes.
8. Add the Worcestershire sauce, then serve hot.

Nutrition Values:
Calories: 261
Carbohydrate: 11.2g
Protein: 36.6g
Fat: 7g
Sugar: 3g
Sodium: 198mg

GREEN BEAN SOUP
Servings: 3
Preparation Time: 10 minutes
Cooking Time: 30 minutes

Ingredients
- ½ pound lean ground beef
- ½ tablespoon garlic, minced
- ½ tablespoon olive oil
- ½ medium onion, chopped
- 1 teaspoon dried thyme, crushed
- ½ teaspoon ground cumin
- 1½ cups fresh tomatoes, chopped finely
- ½ pound fresh green beans, trimmed and cut into 1-inch pieces
- 2 cups low-sodium beef broth
- Freshly ground black pepper, to taste
- ⅛ cup Parmesan cheese, freshly grated

Directions
1. Select the 'sauté' function on your instant pot. Pour in the oil, add the beef, and cook for 5 minutes.
2. Add the thyme, cumin and garlic, then cook for 3 minutes.
3. Now stir in the beans, tomatoes and broth and secure the lid.
4. Set the 'manual' function to low pressure and cook for 20 minutes.
5. 'Quick release' the steam and remove the lid.
6. 6.Drizzle some black pepper and Parmesan cheese on top.
7. Serve hot.

Nutrition Values:
Calories: 226
Carbohydrate: 11.5g
Protein: 27.9g
Fat: 7.7g
Sugar: 4.2g
Sodium: 371mg

PORK AND CABBAGE SOUP
Servings: 3
Preparation Time: 10 minutes
Cooking Time: 30 minutes

Ingredients
- ½ tablespoon olive oil
- ½ lb ground pork
- ½ large onion, chopped
- 1 cup carrots, peeled and shredded
- ¼ head cabbage, chopped
- 2 cups chicken broth
- ½ cup coconut aminos*
- ½ teaspoon ground ginger
- Freshly ground black pepper, to taste

Directions
1. Select the 'sauté' function on the instant pot, add the oil and pork to the pot and cook for 5 minutes.
2. Press 'cancel', add the remaining ingredients, and secure the lid.
3. 3 Cook for 25 minutes at high pressure on the 'manual setting.
4. 'Quick release' the steam after the beep, then remove the lid.
5. Serve immediately.

Nutrition Values:
Calories: 179
Carbohydrate: 10.3g
Protein: 22.5g
Fat: 5.1g
Sugar: 4.8g
Sodium: 127mg
(Note: Coconut Aminos* - Coconut-based sauce satisfies, awesome tasting and healthy coconut sugar mixed with mineral-rich sea Salt-Aged to perfection)

CHICKEN AND MUSHROOM STEW
Servings: 3
Preparation Time: 10 minutes
Cooking Time: 15 minutes)

Ingredients
- ½ tablespoon olive oil
- ½ lb fresh cremini mushrooms, stemmed and quartered
- ½ small onion, chopped
- ½ tablespoon tomato paste
- 1½ garlic cloves, minced
- 4 (5-oz) skinless chicken thighs
- ½ cup green olives, pitted and halved
- 1 cup fresh cherry tomatoes
- ¼ cup low-sodium chicken broth
- Freshly ground black pepper to taste
- ¼ cup fresh parsley, chopped

Directions
1. Place the oil, onion and mushrooms into the instant pot and cook on the 'sauté' function for 5 minutes.
2. Stir in the tomato paste, along with the garlic, and cook for another minute.
3. Add the broth, chicken, olives and tomatoes to the pot, then secure the lid.
4. Set the 'manual' function to high pressure for 10 minutes cooking time.
5. After the beep, 'Quick release' the steam and remove the lid.
6. Sprinkle some black pepper and parsley on top.
7. Serve immediately.

Nutrition Values:
Calories: 423
Carbohydrate: 7.8g
Protein: 57.6g
Fat: 16.7g
Sugar: 3.7g
Sodium: 202mg

BEEF AND VEGGIE STEW
Servings: 4
Preparation Time: 10 minutes
Cooking Time: 40 minutes

Ingredients
- 1½ tablespoons olive oil
- 1½ lb chuck roast, trimmed and cubed
- 1 cup homemade tomato sauce
- ½ teaspoon smoked paprika
- 1 cup low-sodium chicken broth
- 1 large onion, cut into bite-sized pieces
- ½ lb carrots, peeled and cut into bite-sized pieces
- ½ lb potatoes, peeled and cut into bite-sized pieces
- ½ garlic clove, minced
- ¼ cup fresh cilantro to garnish, chopped

Directions
1. Put the oil and beef into the instant pot and cook on the 'sauté' function for 5 minutes.
2. Stir in the paprika, broth and tomato sauce, then secure the lid.
3. Cook on 'manual' settings at high pressure for 15 minutes.
4. Once done, 'quick release' the steam pressure, then remove the lid.
5. Add all the vegetables and re-lock the lid. Cook for another 20 minutes at high pressure on 'manual' settings.
6. 'Quick release' the steam, remove the lid and add the cilantro.
7. Serve immediately.

Nutrition Values:
Calories: 320
Carbohydrate: 21.6g
Protein: 26.9g
Fat: 13.7g
Sugar: 7.1g
Sodium: 285mg

MIXED VEGGIE STEW
Servings: 5
Preparation Time: 10 minutes
Cooking Time: 10 minutes)

Ingredients
- 1 tablespoon olive oil
- ½ carrot, peeled and minced
- ½ celery stalk, minced
- ½ small onion, minced
- 1 garlic clove, minced
- ½ teaspoon dried sage, crushed
- ½ teaspoon dried rosemary, crushed
- 4 oz. fresh Portabella mushrooms, sliced
- 4 oz. fresh white mushrooms, sliced
- ¼ cup red wine
- 1 Yukon Gold potato, peeled and chopped
- ¾ cup fresh green beans, trimmed and chopped
- 1 cup tomatoes, chopped
- ½ cup tomato paste
- ½ tablespoon balsamic vinegar
- 1¼ cups water
- 1 tablespoon corn starch
- ⅛ cup water
- Salt and freshly ground black pepper to taste
- 2 oz. frozen peas

Directions
1. Select the 'sauté' function on your instant pot

and pour in the oil. Add the celery, carrot and onion. Cook for 3 minutes.
2. Add the herbs and garlic to the pot and cook for another minute.
3. Now add the mushrooms and sauté for 5 minutes. Stir in the wine and cook for 2 minutes.
4. Add the green beans, potatoes, tomato paste, tomatoes, water and vinegar, and secure the lid.
5. Set to high pressure in the 'manual' function for 15 minutes. When finished, 'quick release' the steam.
6. Combine the corn starch with water in a separate bowl to make a slurry.
7. Remove the lid of the cooker and add the corn starch slurry, the peas, black pepper and salt.
8. Cook for 1 minute on the 'sauté' setting; transfer to a bowl and serve hot.

Nutrition Values:
Calories: 197
Carbohydrate: 36.9g
Protein: 6.6g
Fat: 3.2g
Sugar: 12.6g
Sodium: 224mg

BEEF WITH BEANS CHILI
Servings: 8
Preparation Time: 10 minutes
Cooking Time: 20 minutes

Ingredients
- 1 tablespoon olive oil
- 2 lbs ground beef
- 1 onion, chopped
- 1 green bell pepper, seeded and chopped
- 2 garlic cloves, minced
- 1 teaspoon dried oregano, crushed
- 3 tablespoons red chili powder
- 1 tablespoon ground cumin
- 3½ cups tomatoes, chopped finely
- 1½ cups cooked red kidney beans
- 1½ cups water
- ½ cup sour cream

Directions
1. Place the oil and the beef in the instant pot and cook for 5 minutes on the 'sauté' function.
2. Once cooked, transfer the beef to a plate.
3. Add all the vegetables and stir fry for 5 minutes.
4. Add the beef and all the remaining ingredients, except the sour cream, then secure the lid.
5. Cook on the 'manual' function for 10 minutes at high pressure.
6. Once done, 'Quick release' the steam and then remove the lid.
7. Serve with sour cream topping.

Nutrition Values:
Calories: 769
Carbohydrate: 96.4g
Protein: 67.3g
Fat: 14.6g
Sugar: 13.4g
Sodium: 150mg

THREE BEANS MIX CHILI
Servings: 4
Preparation Time: 5 minutes
Cooking Time: 20 minutes

Ingredients
- 1 tablespoon olive oil
- 1 cup onion, chopped
- ½ green bell pepper, seeded and chopped
- ½ cup carrot, peeled and chopped
- 2 tablespoons celery stalk, chopped
- ½ tablespoon garlic, minced
- ¼ dried kidney beans, rinsed, soaked for 8 hours and drained
- ¼ cup dried pinto beans, rinsed, soaked for 8 hours and drained
- ¼ cup dried black beans, rinsed, soaked for 8 hours and drained
- 1 cup fresh tomatoes, chopped
- 1 cup homemade tomato paste
- 1 teaspoon dried oregano, crushed
- 1 tablespoon mild chili powder
- ½ teaspoon smoked paprika
- ½ teaspoons ground cumin
- ¼ teaspoon ground coriander
- 2 cups low-sodium vegetable broth
- Scallions to garnish, chopped

Directions
1. Select the 'sauté' function on the instant pot, add the oil, bell pepper, celery, onion, carrot and garlic, and cook for 5 minutes.
2. Add the remaining ingredients to the pot then secure the lid.
3. Select the 'manual' function and set to high pressure. Cook for 15 minutes.
4. After the beep, use the 'natural release' function to vent the steam, then remove the lid.

5. Garnish with scallion* and serve.

Nutrition Values:
Calories: 282
Carbohydrate: 50g
Protein: 13g
Fat: 4.7g
Sugar: 12.8g
Sodium: 213mg

(Note: Scallion* - Scallions are vegetables of various Allium onion species. Scallions have a milder taste than most onions.)

FULL MEAL TURKEY SOUP

Servings: 3
Preparation Time: 15 minutes
Cooking Time: 30 minutes)

Ingredients
- ½ tablespoon olive oil
- ½ lb lean ground turkey
- ½ small yellow onion, chopped
- 1 cup carrots, peeled and shredded
- ¼ head cabbage, chopped
- 2 cups homemade chicken broth
- 2 teaspoons low-sodium soy sauce
- ½ teaspoon ground ginger
- Freshly ground black pepper to taste

Directions
1. Add the oil and turkey in the instant pot and select the 'sauté' function to cook for 5 minutes.
2. Select 'cancel', then add the remaining ingredients. Cover and lock the lid.
3. Set the cooker to 'manual' and select high pressure for 25 minutes.
4. After the beep, 'quick release' the steam and then remove the lid.
5. Serve hot.

Nutrition Values:
Calories: 190
Carbohydrate: 9.2g
Protein: 19.5g
Fat: 8.7g
Sugar: 4.9g
Sodium: 798mg

GOURMET MEXICAN BEEF SOUP

Servings: 4
Preparation Time: 15 minutes
Cooking Time: 15 minutes

Ingredients
- ½ teaspoon olive oil
- 1 lb grass-fed, lean ground beef
- 10 oz. canned sugar-free diced tomatoes with green chilies
- 4 oz. cream cheese
- ¼ cup heavy cream
- 2 cups homemade beef broth
- 2 garlic cloves, minced
- 1 tablespoon chili powder
- 1 teaspoon ground cumin
- Salt and freshly ground black pepper to taste
- ¼ cup cheddar cheese, shredded

Directions
1. Pour the oil into the instant pot and Select the 'sauté' function. Stir in the beef and cook for 10 minutes.
2. Add the remaining ingredients, except for the cheese, then secure the lid.
3. Select the 'soup' function and cook for 5 minutes. Once done, vent the steam by using 'natural release'.
4. Remove the lid and serve hot with cheddar cheese on top.

Nutrition Values:
Calories: 390
Carbohydrate: 5.6g
Protein: 29.5g
Fat: 26.5g
Sugar: 2.1g
Sodium: 620mg

BEEF SOUP

Servings: 3
Preparation Time: 15 minutes
Cooking Time: 33 minutes

Ingredients
- ½ tablespoon olive oil
- ½ lb grass-fed, lean ground beef
- ½ small yellow onion, chopped
- ½ tablespoon garlic, minced
- 1 teaspoon dried thyme, crushed
- ½ teaspoon ground cumin
- 1½ cups fresh tomatoes, chopped finely
- ¼ lbs fresh green beans, trimmed and cut into 1-inch pieces
- 2¼ cups homemade beef broth
- Salt and freshly ground black pepper to taste
- ¼ cup Parmesan cheese, freshly grated

Directions
1. Put the oil and beef into the instant pot and select the 'sauté' function. Cook for 5 minutes.
2. Now add the cumin, garlic, thyme and onion, and cook for another 3 minutes.
3. Add the broth, tomatoes and green beans, then secure the lid on the pot.

4. Switch the cooker to the 'manual' function at low pressure and cook for 25 minutes.
5. When it's cooked, 'quick release' the steam, then remove the lid.
6. Sprinkle some salt and black pepper on top, then garnish with Parmesan cheese.
7. Serve hot.

Nutrition Values:
Calories: 227
Carbohydrate: 8.4g
Protein: 22.7g
Fat: 10.8g
Sugar: 3.4g
Sodium: 1449mg

BACON AND VEGGIE SOUP
Servings: 3
Preparation Time: 15 minutes
Cooking Time: 20 minutes

Ingredients
- ½ tablespoon olive oil
- ½ small yellow onion, chopped
- 1 garlic clove, minced
- ½ head cauliflower, chopped roughly
- ½ green bell pepper, seeded and chopped
- Salt, and freshly ground black pepper to taste
- 2 cups homemade chicken broth
- 1 cup Cheddar cheese, shredded
- ½ cup half-and-half cream*
- 3 cooked turkey bacon slices, chopped
- 2 dashes hot pepper sauce

Directions
1. Add the oil with onion and garlic in the instant pot and "Sauté" for 3 minutes
2. Stir in the broth, salt, black pepper, cauliflower and bell pepper then secure the lid.
3. Select the 'soup'" function and cook for 15 minutes.
4. After the beep, 'quick release' the steam then remove the lid.
5. Stir in the remaining ingredients and cook on the 'sauté' function for 5 minutes.
6. Serve hot.

Nutrition Values:
Calories: 293
Carbohydrate: 18.1g
Protein: 18.1g
Fat: 21g
Sugar: 3.3g
Sodium: 814mg

(Note: Half-and-half cream* - Half-and-half, also known as half cream in the United Kingdom, is a simple blend of equal parts whole milk and light cream. It averages 10 to 12% fat, which is more than milk but less than light cream.)

BROCCOLI SOUP
Servings: 3
Preparation Time: 15 minutes
Cooking Time: 13 minutes

Ingredients
- 1 tablespoon olive oil
- 1 medium carrot, peeled and chopped
- ½ small yellow onion, chopped
- 1 tablespoon almond flour
- ½ garlic clove, minced
- 1½ cups homemade vegetable broth
- 2½ cups broccoli florets
- ½ teaspoon dill weed
- ½ teaspoon smoked paprika
- Salt and freshly ground black pepper to taste
- 2 American cheese slices, cut into pieces
- ½ cup Colby Jack cheese, shredded
- ½ cup Pepper Jack cheese, shredded
- ¼ cup Parmesan cheese, shredded
- ½ cup half-and-half cream

Directions
1. Select the 'sauté' function on the instant pot and add the oil, onion and carrot. Cook for 3 minutes.
2. Stir in the garlic and flour, then 'sauté' for another minute.
3. Pour in the broth and cook for one more minute, stirring continuously.
4. Add the broccoli and secure the lid. Cook on 'manual' settings, at high pressure for 8 minutes.
5. After the beep, 'quick release' the steam, then remove the lid.
6. Add the salt, paprika, black pepper, dill weed, cream and all the cheeses, and let it sit for around 2 minutes until the cheeses melt completely.
7. Stir well to combine the ingredients, then serve hot

Nutrition Values:
Calories: 525
Carbohydrate: 59.8g
Protein: 30.1g
Fat: 19.3g
Sugar: 17.3g
Sodium: 827mg

SPICY PARSNIP SOUP
Servings: 2-4
Preparation Time: 15 minutes

Ingredients

- 2 tbsp vegetable oil
- 1 red onion, finely chopped
- 3 parsnips, chopped
- 2 garlic cloves, crushed
- 2 tsp garam masala
- ½ tsp chili powder
- 1 tbsp plain flour
- 4 cups vegetable stock
- 1 whole lemon, juiced
- 1 tsp salt
- ½ tsp black pepper, ground
- Strips of lemon rind, to garnish

Directions

1. Heat oil on Sauté, and stir-fry onion, parsnips and garlic for 5 minutes, or until soft but not changed color. Stir in garam masala and chili powder and cook for 30 seconds. Stir in flour, for another 30 seconds.
2. Pour in the stock, lemon rind and lemon juice, and seal the lid. Cook on Manual/Pressure Cook for 5 minutes on High. Do a quick release, remove a third of the vegetable pieces with a slotted spoon and reserve.
3. Process the remaining soup and vegetables in a food processor for about 1 minute, to a smooth puree. Return to the pot, and stir in the reserved vegetables. Press Keep Warm and heat the soup for 2 minutes until piping hot. Season with salt and pepper, then ladle into bowls. Garnish with strips of lemon, to serve.

MEXICAN-STYLE CHICKEN SOUP

Servings: 2-4
Preparation Time: 35 minutes

Ingredients

1. 4 boneless, skinless chicken thighs
2. 4 cups chicken broth
3. 14 ounces canned whole tomatoes, chopped
4. 2 jalapeno peppers, stemmed, cored, chopped
5. 2 tbsp tomato puree
6. 3 cloves garlic, minced
7. 1 tbsp chili powder
8. 1 tbsp ground cumin
9. ½ tsp dried oregano
10. 1 (14.5-ounce) can black beans, rinsed and drained
11. 2 cups frozen corn kernels, thawed
12. Crushed tortilla chips for garnish
13. ¼ cup cheddar cheese, shredded for garnish
14. Fresh cilantro, chopped for garnish

Directions

1. Add chicken, oregano, garlic, tomato puree, stock, cumin, tomatoes, chili, and jalapeno peppers. Seal the lid and cook on High Pressure for 10 minutes.
2. Once cooking is done, release the pressure quickly. Transfer the chicken to a plate. On Sauté mode; cook corn and black beans. Shred the chicken with a pair of forks, and return to the pot, stirring well.
3. Select Keep Warm and simmer the soup for 5 minutes until heated through. Divide among serving plates; add a topping of cilantro, shredded cheese and crushed tortilla chips.

TRADITIONAL BOLOGNESE SAUCE

Servings: 4-6
Preparation Time: 45 minutes

Ingredients

- 4 slices bacon, chopped
- 1 tbsp olive oil
- 1 onion, minced
- 2 celery stalks, minced
- 1 carrot, chopped
- 1½ pounds ground beef
- 3 tbsp red wine
- 28 ounces canned tomatoes, crushed
- 2 bay leaves
- Salt and pepper to taste
- ½ cup yogurt
- ¼ cup chopped fresh basil

Directions

1. Set on Sauté, and cook bacon until crispy, for 4 to 5 minutes. Mix in celery, butter, carrots, and onion, and continue cooking for about 5 minutes until vegetables are softened.
2. Mix in ¼ teaspoon pepper, ½ teaspoon salt, and beef, and cook for 4 minutes until golden brown. Stir in the wine and allow to soak, approximately 4 more minutes.
3. Add in bay leaves, tomatoes, and remaining pepper and salt. Seal the lid and cook for 15 minutes on High Pressure. Release Pressure naturally, for 10 minutes. Add yogurt and stir. Serve alongside noodles and use basil to garnish.

RAMEN SPICY SOUP WITH COLLARD GREENS

Servings: 2-4
Preparation Time: 20 minutes

Ingredients

- 1 tbsp olive oil
- ½ tsp ground ginger
- 2 tbsp garlic, minced

- 6 cups chicken broth stock
- 2 tbsp soy sauce
- 1 tbsp chili powder
- 1 cup mushrooms, chopped
- 10 ounces ramen noodles
- 1 (1-pound) package fresh collard greens, trimmed
- A bunch of fresh cilantro, chopped to serve
- 1 red chilli, chopped to serve

Directions
1. On Sauté, warm oil, stir in garlic and ginger, and cook for 2 minutes until soft. Add stock, ,ix in chili powder, ramen noodles and soy sauce.
2. Seal the lid and cook on High Pressure for 10 minutes. Release pressure quickly. Stir in collard greens until wilted. Ladle the soup into serving bowls and add red chili and cilantro to serve.

SPICY BORSCHT SOUP

Servings:2-4
Preparation Time: 30 minutes

Ingredients
- 2 tbsp olive oil
- 1 cup leeks, chopped
- 1 tsp garlic, smashed
- 2 beets, peeled and diced
- 1 tbsp cayenne pepper, finely minced
- 1 dried habanero pepper, crushed
- 4 cups beef stock
- 3 cups white cabbage, shredded
- 1 tsp salt
- 2 tsp red wine apple cider vinegar
- ¼ tsp paprika
- Greek yogurt for garnish

Directions
1. Warm oil on Sauté. Stir in garlic and leeks and cook for 5 minutes until soft. Mix in, stock, paprika, salt, peppers, vinegar, beets, white cabbage, cayenne pepper, and crushed red pepper.
2. Seal the lid and cook on High Pressure for 20 minutes. Do a quick release. Place in serving bowls and top with Greek yogurt to serve.

VICHYSSOISE WITH TOFU

Servings:2-4
Preparation Time: 25 minutes

Ingredients
- 3 large leeks
- 3 tbsp butter
- 1 onion, chopped
- 1 lb potatoes, chopped
- 5 cups vegetable stock
- 2 tsp lemon juice
- ¼ tsp nutmeg
- ¼ tsp ground coriander
- 1 bay leaf
- 5 oz silken tofu
- Salt and white pepper
- Freshly snipped chives, to garnish

Directions
1. Remove most of the green parts of the leeks. Slice the white parts very finely. Melt butter on Sauté, and stir-fry leeks and onion for 5 minutes without browning. Add potatoes, stock, juice, nutmeg, coriander and bay leaf. Season to taste with salt and pepper, and seal the lid.
2. Press Manual/Pressure Cook and set the timer to 10 minutes. Cook on High Pressure. Do a quick release and discard the bay leaf. Process the soup in a food processor until smooth. Season to taste, add silken tofu. Serve the soup sprinkled with freshly snipped chives.

HEARTY WINTER VEGETABLE SOUP

Servings:2-4
Preparation Time: 30 minutes

Ingredients
- 2 tbsp olive oil
- 1 onion, chopped
- 2 carrots, peeled and chopped
- 1 cup celery, chopped
- 2 cloves garlic, minced
- 5 cups chicken broth
- 2 turnips, peeled and chopped
- 28 ounces canned tomatoes
- 15 oz canned garbanzo beans, rinsed and drained
- 1 cup frozen green peas
- 2 bay leaves
- 1 sprig fresh sage
- Salt and black pepper to taste
- ¼ cup Parmesan cheese, grated

Directions
1. On Sauté, warm oil, stir in celery, carrots, and onion and cook for 4 minutes until soft. Add in garlic and cook for 30 seconds until crispy. Add vegetable broth, parsnip, garbanzo beans, bay leaves, tomatoes, pepper, salt, peas, and sage. Seal the lid and cook on High Pressure for 12 minutes. Allow natural pressure release,

for about 5 minutes. Serve topped with Parmesan cheese.

LEEK AND POTATO SOUP WITH SOUR CREAM

Servings: 2-4
Preparation Time: 30 minutes

Ingredients
- 2 tbsp butter
- 3 leeks, white part only, chopped
- 2 cloves garlic, minced
- 3 cups vegetable broth
- 3 potatoes, peeled and cubed
- ½ cup sour cream
- 2 tbsp rosemary
- 2 bay leaves
- Salt and black pepper to taste
- 2 tbsp fresh chives, to garnish

Directions
2. Melt butter on Sauté mode. Stir in garlic and leeks and cook for 3 to 4 minutes, until soft. Stir in bay leaves, potatoes, and broth. Seal the lid and cook on High Pressure for 15 minutes. Release pressure quickly. Remove the bay leaves and cobs and discard.
3. Transfer soup to immersion blender and puree soup to obtain a smooth consistency. Season with salt and pepper. Top with diced chives and sour cream.

TWO-BEAN ZUCCHINI SOUP

Servings: 2-4
Preparation Time: 35 minutes

Ingredients
- 1 tbsp olive oil
- 1 onion, chopped
- 2 cloves garlic, minced
- 4 cups vegetable broth
- 1 cup dried chickpeas
- ½ cup pinto beans, soaked overnight
- ½ cup navy beans, soaked overnight
- 3 carrots, chopped
- 1 large celery stalk, chopped
- 1 tsp dried thyme
- 16 oz zucchini noodles
- Sea salt and ground black pepper, to taste

Directions
1. Warm oil on Sauté. Stir in garlic and onion and cook for 5 minutes until golden brown. Mix in pepper, broth, carrots, salt, celery, beans, and thyme.
2. Seal the lid and cook for 15 minutes on High Pressure. Release the pressure naturally for 10 minutes. Mix zucchini noodles into the soup and stir until wilted. Taste and adjust the seasoning.

QUICK CHICKEN RICE SOUP

Servings: 2-4
Preparation Time: 20 minutes

Ingredients
- 1 lb chicken breast, boneless, skinless, cubed
- 1 large carrot, chopped
- 1 onion, chopped
- ¼ cup rice
- 1 potato, finely chopped
- ½ tsp salt
- 1 tsp cayenne pepper
- A handful of parsley, finely chopped
- 3 tbsp olive oil
- 4 cups chicken broth

Directions
1. Add all ingredients, except parsley, to the pot, and seal the lid. Cook on Soup/Broth for 15 minutes on High. Do a quick pressure release. Stir in fresh parsley and serve.

TOMATO & RICE SOUP

Servings: 2-4
Preparation Time: 25 minutes

Ingredients
- 1 cup tomato puree
- ¼ cup rice
- ¼ tsp salt
- 2 tbsp olive oil
- 4 cups vegetable broth

Directions
1. Add all ingredients to the pot and seal the lid. Set the steam release handle and cook on Soup/Broth mode for 30 minutes on High Pressure. Release the pressure naturally, for about 10 minutes.

BUTTERNUT SQUASH CURRY

Servings: 2-4
Preparation Time: 30 minutes

Ingredients
- 1½ pounds butternut squash, chopped
- 4 cups chicken stock
- ½ cup buttermilk
- 4 spring onions, chopped into lengths
- 2 tbsp curry powder
- 1½ tsp ground turmeric
- 1½ tsp ground cumin
- ¼ tsp cayenne pepper

- 2 bay leaves
- Salt and black pepper, to taste
- A bunch of cilantro leaves, chopped

Directions
1. In the pot, stir in squash, buttermilk, curry, turmeric, spring onions, stock, cumin, and cayenne. Season with pepper and salt. Add bay leaves to the liquid and ensure they are submerged.
2. Seal the lid, press Soup/Broth and cook for 10 minutes on High. Naturally release the pressure for 10 minutes. Discard bay leaves. Transfer the soup to a blender and process until smooth.
3. Use a fine-mesh strainer to strain the soup. Divide into plates and garnish with cilantro before serving.

CREAMY QUINOA AND MUSHROOM PILAF
Servings:2-4
Preparation Time: 20 minutes

Ingredients
- 4 cups vegetable broth
- 1 carrot, peeled and chopped
- 1 stalk celery, diced
- 2 cups quinoa, rinsed
- 1 cup mushrooms, sliced
- 1 onion, chopped
- 2 garlic cloves, smashed
- 1 tsp salt
- ½ tsp dried thyme
- 3 tbsp butter
- ½ cup heavy cream

Directions
1. Melt the butter on Sauté. Add onion, garlic, celery, and carrot, and cook for 8 minutes until tender. Mix in broth, thyme, quinoa, mushrooms, and salt.
2. Seal the lid and cook on High Pressure for 10 minutes. Release pressure quickly. Stir in heavy cream. Cook for 2 minutes to obtain a creamy consistency. Serve warm.

FAVORITE CHICKEN SOUP
Servings:2-4
Preparation Time: 40 minutes

Ingredients
- 1 lb chicken breast, boneless, skinless, chopped
- 1 onion, chopped
- 1 carrot, chopped
- 2 small potatoes, peeled, chopped
- 1 tsp cayenne pepper
- 2 egg yolks
- 1 tsp salt
- 3 tbsp lemon juice
- 3 tbsp olive oil
- 4 cups water

Directions
1. Add all ingredients to the pot, and seal the lid. Set the steam release handle and cook on Soup/Broth mode for 20 minutes on High. Release the pressure naturally, for 10 minutes, open the lid and serve.

SPICY PORK SOUP
Servings:2-4
Preparation Time: 65 minutes

Ingredients
- o   lb pork ribs
- 1 large leek, chopped into bite-sized pieces
- 1 onion, chopped
- 1 cup celery root, diced
- ½ cup parsley, chopped
- 4 cups beef broth
- 1 tsp salt
- ¼ tsp chili flakes
- 2 bay leaves
- A handful of fresh basil, torn
- 3 tbsp oil

Directions
1. Heat oil on Sauté. Add the ribs in batches and brown on all sides, for 5-6 minutes. Add the remaining ingredients. Seal the lid and cook on Meat/Stew mode on High for 30 minutes. Do a quick release.

SNACKS AND APPETIZERS

ITALIAN MUSSELS APPETIZER

Preparation time: 10 minutes
Cooking time: 5 minutes
Servings: 3

Ingredients:
- 28 ounces canned tomatoes, no-salt-added and crushed
- ½ cup white onion, chopped
- 2 jalapeno peppers, chopped
- ¼ cup low-sodium veggie stock
- ¼ cup olive oil
- ¼ cup balsamic vinegar
- 2 pounds mussels, cleaned and scrubbed
- 2 tablespoons red pepper flakes
- 2 garlic cloves, minced
- ½ cup basil, chopped

Directions:
1. Set your instant pot on Sauté mode, add tomatoes, onion, jalapenos, stock, oil, vinegar, garlic and pepper flakes, stir and bring to a boil.
2. Add mussels, stir, cover and cook on Low for 5 minutes.
3. Discard unopened mussels, add basil, stir, divide into bowls and serve as an appetizer.
4. Enjoy!

Nutrition Value: calories 200, fat 4, fiber 7, carbs 18, protein 7

SPICY ITALIAN MUSSELS

Preparation time: 10 minutes
Cooking time: 8 minutes
Servings: 4

Ingredients:
- 2 pounds mussels, scrubbed
- 2 tablespoons olive oil
- 1 yellow onion, chopped
- 1 teaspoon red pepper flakes
- ½ teaspoon hot paprika
- 14 ounces tomatoes, chopped
- 2 teaspoons garlic, minced
- ½ cup low-sodium chicken stock
- 2 teaspoons oregano, dried

Directions:
1. Set your instant pot on Sauté mode, add oil, heat it up, add onions, stir and cook for 3 minutes.
2. Add pepper flakes, paprika, garlic, stock, oregano, tomatoes and mussels, stir, cover, cook on Low for 5 minutes, divide into bowls and serve as an appetizer.
3. Enjoy!

Nutrition Value: calories 200, fat 4, fiber 7, carbs 18, protein 5

SEAFOOD PLATTER

Preparation time: 10 minutes
Cooking time: 18 minutes
Servings: 4

Ingredients:
- 12 shell clams
- 12 mussels
- 1 and ½ pounds shrimp, peeled and deveined
- 1 cup low-fat butter
- 2 yellow onions, chopped
- 3 garlic cloves, minced
- ½ cup parsley, chopped
- 20 ounces canned tomatoes, chopped
- 1 tablespoon basil, dried
- Black pepper to the taste

Directions:
1. Set your instant pot on Sauté mode, add butter, melt it, add onion and garlic, stir and cook for 2 minutes.
2. Add tomatoes, parsley, basil, bay leaves and pepper, stir, cover and cook on High for 10 minutes.
3. Set the pot to Sauté mode again, add clams, shrimp and mussels, cover, cook on Low for 6 minutes.
4. Divide into bowls and serve as an appetizer.
5. Enjoy!

Nutrition Value: calories 271, fat 4, fiber 7, carbs 19, protein 16

SPANISH CLAMS APPETIZER

Preparation time: 10 minutes
Cooking time: 14 minutes
Servings: 4

Ingredients:
- 30 clams
- 2 chorizo links, low-sodium and sliced
- 1 pound baby red potatoes
- 1 yellow onion, chopped
- 10 ounces low-sodium veggie stock
- 2 tablespoons parsley, chopped
- 1 teaspoon olive oil

- Lemon wedges for serving

Directions:
1. Set your instant pot on Sauté mode, add oil, heat it up, add chorizo and onions, stir and cook for 4 minutes.
2. Add clams, potatoes and stock, stir, cover and cook on High for 10 minutes.
3. Add parsley, stir, divide into bowls and serve with lemon wedges on the side as an appetizer.
4. Enjoy!

Nutrition Value: calories 261, fat 3, fiber 7, carbs 29, protein 6

CHEESY CLAMS

Preparation time: 10 minutes
Cooking time: 5 minutes
Servings: 4

Ingredients:
- 24 clams, shucked
- 3 garlic cloves, minced
- 4 tablespoons olive oil
- ¼ cup parsley, chopped
- ¼ cup fat-free cheddar cheese, grated
- 1 teaspoon oregano, dried
- 1 cup whole wheat breadcrumbs
- 2 cups water
- Lemon wedges

Directions:
1. In a bowl, mix breadcrumbs with cheese, oregano, parsley, oil and garlic, stir and stuff clams with this mix.
2. Add the water to your instant pot, add steamer basket, add clams, cover, cook on High for 5 minutes, arrange them on a platter and serve as an appetizer.
3. Enjoy!

Nutrition Value: calories 200, fat 6, fiber 7, carbs 18, protein 6

ARTICHOKES DIP

Preparation time: 10 minutes
Cooking time: 8 minutes
Servings: 6

Ingredients:
- 14 ounces canned artichoke hearts, no-salt-added
- 8 ounces fat-free cream cheese
- 16 ounces fat-free cheddar cheese, grated
- 10 ounces spinach
- ½ cup low-sodium chicken stock
- ½ cup coconut cream
- 3 garlic cloves, minced
- 1 teaspoon onion powder

Directions:
1. In your instant pot, mix artichokes with stock, garlic, spinach, cream cheese, coconut cream and onion powder, stir, cover and cook on High for 8 minutes.
2. Add cheddar, blend using an immersion blender, divide into bowls and serve.
3. Enjoy!

Nutrition Value: calories 300, fat 8, fiber 15, carbs 19, protein 7

ARTICHOKE APPETIZER

Preparation time: 10 minutes
Cooking time: 22 minutes
Servings: 2

Ingredients:
- 2 artichokes, washed and halved
- 1 bay leaf
- 1 cup water
- 2 garlic cloves, chopped
- 1 lemon, halved
- For the dressing:
- ¼ cup extra virgin olive oil
- 2 tablespoons lemon juice
- 3 garlic cloves

Directions:
1. Add water to the instant pot, add lemon halves, 2 garlic cloves and bay leaf, add steamer basket, add artichokes inside, cover, cook on High for 20 minutes and divide artichokes between plates.
2. In a bowl, mix 3 garlic cloves with the oil and the lemon juice and whisk really well.
3. Arrange artichokes on a platter, drizzle the dressing all over and serve.
4. Enjoy!

Nutrition Value: calories 261, fat 3, fiber 6, carbs 18, protein 5

WRAPPED ASPARAGUS

Preparation time: 5 minutes
Cooking time: 4 minutes
Servings: 4

Ingredients:
- 1 pound asparagus, trimmed
- 8 ounces prosciutto slices, low-sodium
- 2 cups water

Directions:
1. Add the water to your instant pot, add steamer basket, wrap asparagus spears in prosciutto slices, put them in the basket, cover, cook on High for 4 minutes, arrange

the asparagus canes on a platter and serve as an appetizer.
2. Enjoy!

Nutrition Value: calories 121, fat 3, fiber 8, carbs 9, protein 6

ITALIAN SWEET POTATO AND LENTILS DIP

Preparation time: 10 minutes
Cooking time: 20 minutes
Servings: 8

Ingredients:
- 56 ounces canned tomatoes, no-salt-added and crushed
- 3 garlic cloves, minced
- ½ cup red lentils, rinsed
- 1 cup sweet potato, chopped
- Black pepper to the taste
- 1 and ½ cups low-sodium veggie stock

Directions:
1. Set your instant pot on Sauté mode, add lentils, sweet potatoes, pepper, garlic, stock and tomatoes, stir, cover the pot and cook on High for 20 minutes.
2. Puree everything using an immersion blender, divide into bowls and serve.
3. Enjoy!

Nutrition Value: calories 152, fat 4, fiber 7, carbs 16, protein 6

APPLE DIP

Preparation time: 10 minutes
Cooking time: 8 minutes
Servings: 4

Ingredients:
- 8 apples, cored and chopped
- 1 teaspoon cinnamon powder
- ½ cup apple juice
- Directions:
- Put apples in your instant pot, add the juice, cover the pot and cook on High for 8 minutes.
- Add cinnamon, blend using an immersion blender, divide into bowls and serve.
- Enjoy!

Nutrition Value: calories 181, fat 3, fiber 7, carbs 19, protein 6

ORANGE CRANBERRY DIP

Preparation time: 10 minutes
Cooking time: 15 minutes
Servings: 4

Ingredients:
- 2 and ½ teaspoons orange zest, grated
- 12 ounces cranberries
- ¼ cup orange juice
- 2 tablespoons maple syrup

Directions:
1. In your instant pot, mix orange juice with maple syrup, orange zest and cranberries, stir, cover and cook on High for 15 minutes.
2. Stir well, divide into bowls and serve as a party dip.
3. Enjoy!

Nutrition Value: calories 201, fat 4, fiber 5, carbs 11, protein 5

GINGER AND ONIONS DIP

Preparation time: 5 minutes
Cooking time: 7 minutes.
Servings: 4

Ingredients:
- 1 cup low-sodium veggie stock
- Black pepper to the taste
- 1 tablespoon olive oil
- 4 spring onions, chopped
- 1-inch ginger piece, chopped
- Zest of 1 orange, grated
- Juice of 1 orange

Directions:
1. In your instant pot, mix stock with pepper, olive oil, onions, ginger, orange juice and zest, stir well, cover, cook on High for 7 minutes, blend using an immersion blender, divide into bowls and serve.
2. Enjoy!

Nutrition Value: calories 270, fat 4, fiber 6, carbs 15, protein 5

ZUCCHINI DIP

Preparation time: 10 minutes
Cooking time: 10 minutes
Servings: 4

Ingredients:
- 1 yellow onion, chopped
- 1 tablespoon olive oil
- 1 and ½ pounds zucchini, chopped
- ½ cup low-sodium veggie stock
- 1 bunch basil, chopped
- 2 garlic cloves, minced

Directions:
1. Set your instant pot on Sauté mode, add oil, heat it up, add onion, stir and cook 4 minutes.
2. Add zucchini, stock, basil and garlic, stir, cover, cook on High for 7 minutes, blend everything using an immersion blender, divide into bowls and serve.

3. Enjoy!

Nutrition Value: calories 200, fat 2, fiber 3, carbs 11, protein 4

GARLIC MUSHROOM DIP

Preparation time: 10 minutes
Cooking time: 30 minutes
Servings: 6

Ingredients:
- 1 yellow onion, chopped
- ¼ cup olive oil
- Black pepper to the taste
- 1 tablespoon thyme, chopped
- 3 garlic cloves, minced
- 1 and ¼ cup low-sodium chicken stock
- 30 ounces white mushrooms, chopped
- 1-ounce fat-free cheddar cheese, grated
- ½ cup coconut cream
- 1 tablespoons parsley, chopped

Directions:
1. Set your instant pot on Sauté mode, add oil, heat it up, add onion, stir and cook for 5 minutes.
2. Add garlic, thyme, stock and mushrooms, stir, cover and cook on High for 25 minutes.
3. Add cream, cheese and parsley, stir, divide into bowls and serve as a dip.
4. Enjoy!

Nutrition Value: calories 200, fat 3, fiber 7, carbs 18, protein 5

CAULIFLOWER HUMMUS

Preparation time: 10 minutes
Cooking time: 10 minutes
Servings: 6

Ingredients:
- 2 tablespoons low-fat butter
- 8 garlic cloves, minced
- ½ cup low-sodium veggie stock
- 6 cups cauliflower florets
- Black pepper to the taste
- 3 tablespoons fat-free milk

Directions:
1. Set your instant pot on Sauté mode, add butter, melt it, add garlic, stock and cauliflower to the pot, heat up, cover and cook on High for 10 minutes.
2. Transfer cauliflower, garlic and 2 tablespoons stock to your blender, add pepper and milk, pulse well, divide into bowls and serve.
3. Enjoy!

Nutrition Value: calories 181, fat 3, fiber 7, carbs 15, protein 6

TURKEY MEATBALLS

Preparation time: 10 minutes
Cooking time: 40 minutes
Servings: 8

Ingredients:
- 1 pound turkey meat, ground
- 1 yellow onion, minced
- ¼ cup fat-free cheddar cheese, grated
- 4 garlic cloves, minced
- ¼ cup parsley, chopped
- Black pepper to the taste
- 1 teaspoon oregano, dried
- 1 egg, whisked
- ¼ cup almond milk
- 2 teaspoons coconut aminos
- 12 cremini mushrooms, chopped
- 1 cup low-sodium chicken stock
- 2 tablespoons olive oil

Directions:
1. In a bowl, mix turkey meat with the cheese, black pepper, onion, garlic, parsley, oregano, egg, milk and aminos, stir and shape 16 meatballs.
2. Set your instant pot on sauté mode, add the oil, heat it up, add meatballs, brown them for 1 minutes on each side and transfer them to a plate.
3. Add stock and cremini mushrooms, cover and cook on High for 10 minutes.
4. Return the meatballs, cover the pot and cook on High for 6 minutes.
5. Arrange the meatballs on a platter, drizzle some of the mushrooms sauce all over and serve as an appetizer.
6. Enjoy!

Nutrition Value: calories 271, fat 4, fiber 6, carbs 18, protein 17

CHICKEN MEATBALLS

Preparation time: 10 minutes
Cooking time: 10 minutes
Servings: 8

Ingredients:
- 1 and ½ pounds chicken meat, ground
- 2 tablespoons parsley, chopped
- 1 egg
- 2 garlic cloves, minced
- Black pepper to the taste
- 1 cup low-sodium stock
- ½ teaspoon nutmeg, ground
- 2 tablespoons whole wheat flour

- ½ teaspoon sweet paprika
- 2 tablespoons olive oil
- 2 carrots, chopped
- ¾ cup fresh peas

Directions:
1. In a bowl, combine the meat with the egg, pepper, parsley, paprika, garlic, nutmeg and 1 tablespoons stock, stir and shape medium meatballs out of this mix.
2. Set your instant pot on Sauté mode, add oil, heat it up, add meatballs and brown them on all sides.
3. Add carrots, peas and stock, cover the pot, cook on High for 6 minutes, arrange meatballs on a platter and serve them.
4. Enjoy!

Nutrition Value: calories 288, fat 8, fiber 8, carbs 19, protein 7

PORK MEATBALLS APPETIZER

Preparation time: 10 minutes
Cooking time: 10 minutes
Servings: 6

Ingredients:
- 1 yellow onion, chopped
- 1/3 cup fat-free cheddar, grated
- ½ teaspoon oregano, dried
- Black pepper to the taste
- ½ cup almond milk
- 1 pound pork meat, ground
- 1 tablespoon olive oil
- 1 egg, whisked
- 1 carrot, chopped
- ½ celery stalk, chopped
- 2 and ¾ cups tomato puree, no-salt-added
- 1 cup water

Directions:
1. In a bowl, combine the meat with the cheese, onion, oregano, pepper, milk and egg, stir and shape medium meatballs.
2. Set your instant pot on Sauté mode, add oil, heat it up, add celery, carrot, tomato puree, water and the meatballs, cover and cook on High for 10 minutes.
3. Divide the meatballs and the sauce into bowls and serve as an appetizer.
4. Enjoy!

Nutrition Value: calories 200, fat 3, fiber 6, carbs 16, protein 6

CHICKPEAS SPREAD

Preparation time: 10 minutes
Cooking time: 25 minutes
Servings: 4

Ingredients:
- 3 teaspoons olive oil
- 1 cup chickpeas
- 3 cups low-sodium chicken stock
- 1 yellow onion, chopped
- 2 teaspoons cumin, ground
- ¼ teaspoon garlic powder
- ¼ teaspoon red pepper flakes
- Black pepper to the taste

Directions:
1. Set your instant pot on Sauté mode, add the oil, heat it up, add onions, stir and cook for 4 minutes.
2. Add cumin, garlic powder, pepper flakes, pepper, chickpeas and stock, stir, cover, cook on High for 20 minutes, transfer to your blender, pulse well, divide into bowls and serve.
3. Enjoy!

Nutrition Value: calories 200, fat 4, fiber 8, carbs 10, protein 8

APRICOT DIP

Preparation time: 10 minutes
Cooking time: 20 minutes
Servings: 6

Ingredients:
- 5 ounces apricots, dried and halved
- 2 cups water
- ½ teaspoon vanilla extract

Directions:
1. In your instant pot, combine the apricots with the water and vanilla, stir, cover, cook on Low for 20 minutes, transfer to a blender, pulse, divide into bowls and serve as a party dip with some fruit chips on the side.
2. Enjoy!

Nutrition Value: calories 152, fat 3, fiber 1, carbs 7, protein 6

WHOLE WHEAT SALAD

Preparation time: 10 minutes
Cooking time: 10 minutes
Servings: 4

Ingredients:
- ½ cup cracked whole wheat
- 1 and ½ cups water
- 2 tomatoes, chopped
- 3 teaspoons olive oil
- 1 carrot, grated
- 5 cauliflower florets, chopped

- Salt and black pepper to the taste
- ¼ teaspoon mustard seeds
- 1 teaspoon ginger, grated
- 2 garlic cloves, minced
- 1 yellow onion, chopped

Directions:
1. Set your instant pot on Sauté mode, add the oil, heat up, add mustard seeds, onion, garlic, ginger, carrot, cauliflower and tomatoes, stir and cook for 4 minutes.
2. Add wheat, pepper and water, stir, cover and cook on High for 5 minutes.
3. Divide the mix into bowls and serve as an appetizer.
4. Enjoy!

Nutrition Value: calories 162, fat 4, fiber 4, carbs 10, protein 5

ASIAN SPROUTS SALAD

Preparation time: 10 minutes
Cooking time: 8 minutes
Servings: 4

Ingredients:
- 2 pounds Brussels sprouts, trimmed
- 1 teaspoon red pepper flakes
- ¼ cup coconut aminos
- 2 teaspoons garlic powder
- 1 tablespoon smoked paprika
- 2 tablespoons sesame oil
- 1 tablespoon balsamic vinegar
- A pinch of black pepper

Directions:
1. Set your instant pot on sauté mode, add oil, heat up, add sprouts, pepper flakes, aminos, garlic powder, paprika, vinegar and pepper, toss, cover, cook on High for 8 minutes, divide into bowls and serve as an appetizer.
2. Enjoy!

Nutrition Value: calories 265, fat 7, fiber 3, carbs 10, protein 5

OKRA SALAD

Preparation time: 10 minutes
Cooking time: 15 minutes
Servings: 6

Ingredients:
- 1 pound okra, trimmed
- 6 scallions, chopped
- Back pepper to the taste
- 2 tablespoons olive oil
- 6 tomatoes, chopped
- 2 tablespoons low-sodium veggie stock

Directions:
1. Set your instant pot on Sauté mode, add oil, heat up, add scallions, stir and cook for 5 minutes.
2. Add okra, pepper, stock and tomatoes, stir, cover, cook on High for 10 minutes, divide into bowls and serve as an appetizer.
3. Enjoy!

Nutrition Value: calories 201, fat 3, fiber 3, carbs 11, protein 5

LEEK STICKS

Preparation time: 10 minutes
Cooking time: 8 minutes
Servings: 4

Ingredients:
- 4 leeks, washed, roots and ends cut off and cut into sticks
- Black pepper to the taste
- 1 teaspoons sweet paprika
- 1 teaspoon cumin, ground
- 1/3 cup low-sodium chicken stock
- 1 tablespoon olive oil

Directions:
1. Put leeks in your instant pot, add stock, oil, cumin, paprika and black pepper, cover and cook on High for 5 minutes.
2. Set the pot on sauté mode, cook leeks for 3 minutes more, arrange them on a platter and serve as a snack.
3. Enjoy!

Nutrition Value: calories 123, fat 3, fiber 4, carbs 8, protein 4

BALSAMIC CABBAGE APPETIZER SALAD

Preparation time: 5 minutes
Cooking time: 5 minutes
Servings: 4

Ingredients:
- 2 cups red cabbage, shredded
- 2 tablespoons water
- 1 tablespoon olive oil
- 1 tablespoon homemade mayonnaise
- Black pepper to the taste
- 2 teaspoons balsamic vinegar

Directions:
1. Put cabbage in your instant pot, add the water, cover, cook on High for 5 minutes, drain, transfer to a bowl, add oil, mayo, black pepper and vinegar, toss well, divide into small cups and serve as an appetizer.
2. Enjoy!

Nutrition Value: calories 200, fat 1, fiber 5,

carbs 16, protein 4

BELL PEPPER DIP

Preparation time: 10 minutes
Cooking time: 15 minutes
Servings: 10

Ingredients:
- 2 cups low-sodium veggie stock
- 10 red bell peppers, deseeded and roughly chopped
- A pinch of black pepper
- 3 tablespoons olive oil
- ½ cup lemon juice
- 2 garlic cloves, roasted and chopped
- 1 cup sesame seeds, toasted

Directions:
1. Put the bell peppers and the stock in your instant pot, add a pinch of black pepper, cover and cook on High for 15 minutes.
2. Transfer the bell peppers to your blender, add the oil, lemon juice and garlic and pulse really well.
3. Add 1 tablespoon of cooking liquid, pulse really well again, divide into bowls, sprinkle sesame seeds on top and serve as a snack.
4. Enjoy!

Nutrition Value: calories 200, fat 6, fiber 8, carbs 14, protein 7

CHICKEN APPETIZER SALAD

Preparation time: 10 minutes
Cooking time: 10 minutes
Servings: 2

Ingredients:
- 1 avocado, pitted, peeled and sliced
- 2 tablespoons fat-free yogurt
- 2 tablespoons mayonnaise
- 1 cup low-sodium chicken stock
- Black pepper to the taste
- 1 chicken breast, skinless and boneless and cubed

Directions:
1. In your instant pot, mix chicken with stock and pepper, cover, cook on High for 10 minutes, transfer to a bowl, add mayo, avocado and yogurt, toss well, divide between appetizer plates and serve.
2. Enjoy!

Nutrition Value: calories 304, fat 16, fiber 4, carbs 17, protein 8

SPINACH PUFFS

Preparation time: 10 minutes
Cooking time: 20 minutes
Servings: 12

Ingredients:
- ½ cup almond flour
- 2 and ½ cups fat-free mozzarella, shredded
- 2 eggs
- 1 and ½ cups water
- 4 ounces fat-free cream cheese
- 6 ounces spinach, torn
- 1 teaspoon avocado oil

Directions:
1. Set your instant pot on sauté mode, add the oil, heat it up, add spinach, stir and sauté for 2 minutes.
2. Add cream cheese, cover and cook on High for 2 minutes.
3. Meanwhile, in a bowl, mix the flour with mozzarella and eggs and stir until you obtain a dough.
4. Flatten dough with a rolling pin, cut into 12 rectangles, place them all on a working surface, divide spinach mix on each, roll and seal edges.
5. Add water to your instant pot, add steamer basket, add spinach puffs inside, cover, cook on High for 15 minutes, arrange them on a platter and serve as an appetizer.
6. Enjoy!

Nutrition Value: calories 260, fat 15, fiber 4, carbs 17, protein 14

BASIL ZUCCHINI AND CAPERS DIP

Preparation time: 10 minutes
Cooking time: 10 minutes
Servings: 4

Ingredients:
- 1 shallot, chopped
- 1 and ½ pounds zucchinis, chopped
- 1 tablespoon olive oil
- 2 garlic cloves, minced
- A pinch of salt and black pepper
- 1 tablespoon capers, drained and chopped
- ¼ cup veggie stock
- 1 bunch basil, chopped

Directions:
1. Set your instant pot on Sauté mode, add the oil, heat it up, add the shallot and the garlic, stir and sauté for 2 minutes.
2. Add the zucchinis and the rest of the ingredients, put the lid on and cook on High for 8 minutes.
3. Release the pressure naturally for 10 minutes, blend everything using an immersion blender,

divide into bowls and serve.

Nutrition Value: calories 75, fat 2.5, fiber 0.1, carbs 0.6, protein 1.2

LIME SPINACH AND LEEKS DIP

Preparation time: 10 minutes
Cooking time: 20 minutes
Servings: 4

Ingredients:
- 1 shallot, chopped
- 2 tablespoons avocado oil
- 2 leeks, chopped
- 2 garlic cloves, minced
- 4 cups spinach, torn
- ¼ cup veggie stock
- ¼ cup lime juice
- 1 bunch basil, chopped
- A pinch of salt and black pepper

Directions:
1. Set your instant pot on Sauté mode, add the oil, heat it up, add the shallot, leeks and garlic and sauté for 5 minutes.
2. Add the rest of the ingredients, put the lid on and cook on High for 15 minutes.
3. Release the pressure naturally for 10 minutes, blend the mix using an immersion blender, transfer to bowls and serve as a snack.

Nutrition Value: calories 56, fat 1.8, fiber 0.5, carbs 1.6, protein 1.7

CHILI TOMATO AND ZUCCHINI DIP

Preparation time: 10 minutes
Cooking time: 15 minutes
Servings: 4

Ingredients:
- 2 cups tomatoes, cubed
- 2 cups zucchinis, cubed
- 1 tablespoon hot paprika
- 2 red chilies, chopped
- ¼ cup veggie stock
- 1 tablespoon basil, chopped
- A pinch of salt and black pepper
- 2 scallions, chopped
- 1 tablespoon olive oil

Directions:
1. Set the instant pot on Sauté mode, add the oil, heat it up, add the chilies and the scallions and sauté for 2 minutes.
2. Add the tomatoes and the rest of the ingredients except the basil, put the lid on and cook on High for 12 minutes.
3. Release the pressure naturally for 10 minutes, blend the mix with an immersion blender, divide into bowls, sprinkle the basil on top and serve.

Nutrition Value: calories 58, fat 3.5, fiber 1.9, carbs 2.3, protein 1.6

PARMESAN MUSHROOM SPREAD

Preparation time: 10 minutes
Cooking time: 20 minutes
Servings: 4

Ingredients:
- 1 shallot chopped
- 2 tablespoons olive oil
- 1 tablespoon rosemary, chopped
- A pinch of salt and black pepper
- 3 garlic cloves, minced
- 1 cup chicken stock
- 2 pounds white mushrooms, sliced
- ½ cup parmesan, grated
- ½ cup coconut cream
- 1 tablespoons parsley, chopped

Directions:
1. Set your instant pot on Sauté mode, add the oil, heat it up, add the shallot and garlic and sauté for 2 minutes.
2. Add the mushrooms and sauté for 5 minutes.
3. Add the rest of the ingredients, put the lid on and cook on High for 15 minutes.
4. Release the pressure naturally, divide the mix into bowls and serve as a party spread.

Nutrition Value: calories 187, fat 12.4, fiber 2.1, carbs 4.5, protein 8.2

BROCCOLI DIP

Preparation time: 10 minutes
Cooking time: 15 minutes
Servings: 6

Ingredients:
- 2 tablespoons avocado oil
- 8 garlic cloves, minced
- 2 cups veggie stock
- 6 cups broccoli florets
- 1 cup Greek yogurt
- 1 tablespoon dill, chopped
- A pinch of salt and black pepper
- ½ cup coconut cream

Directions:
1. Set your instant pot on Sauté mode, add the oil, heat it up, add the garlic and cook for 2 minutes.
2. Add the rest of the ingredients except the dill and the yogurt, put the lid on and cook on

High for 13 minutes.
3. Release the pressure naturally for 10 minutes, add the yogurt, blend the mix with an immersion blender, divide into bowls, sprinkle the dill on top and serve.

Nutrition Value: calories 136, fat 8.6, fiber 4.8, carbs 5.6, protein 5.1

GINGER CAULIFLOWER SPREAD

Preparation time: 10 minutes
Cooking time: 15 minutes
Servings: 4

Ingredients:
- 1 shallot, chopped
- 1 tablespoon avocado oil
- 2 tablespoons ginger, minced
- 1 pound cauliflower florets
- ¼ cup chicken stock
- 2 red hot chilies, chopped
- 1 and ¼ tablespoon balsamic vinegar

Directions:
1. Set your instant pot on Sauté mode, add the oil, heat it up, add the ginger and the shallot and sauté for 2 minutes.
2. Add the rest of the ingredients, put the lid on and cook on High for 13 minutes.
3. Release the pressure naturally for 10 minutes, blend the mix a bit with an immersion blender, divide into bowls and serve as a party spread.

Nutrition Value: calories 45, fat 2.5, fiber 1.3, carbs 2 , protein 2.6

RADISH SALSA

Preparation time: 10 minutes
Cooking time: 15 minutes
Servings: 4

Ingredients:
- 2 cups red radishes, sliced
- 1 shallot, chopped
- 2 spring onions, chopped
- 2 tomatoes, cubed
- 1 avocado, peeled and cubed
- 1 tablespoon olive oil
- ¼ cup chicken stock
- A pinch of salt and black pepper
- 1 tablespoon oregano, chopped
- 1 tablespoon chives, chopped

Directions:
1. In your instant pot, combine the radishes with the stock, oregano, salt and pepper, put the lid on and cook on Low for 15 minutes.
2. Release the pressure naturally for 10 minutes, transfer the radishes to a bowl, add the rest of the ingredients, toss, divide into small cups and serve as an appetizer.

Nutrition Value: calories 160, fat 13.7, fiber 5.5, carbs 10.1, protein 2.2

MUSTARD GREENS DIP

Preparation time: 5 minutes
Cooking time: 14 minutes
Servings: 4

Ingredients:
- 6 ounces mustard greens, chopped
- 1 tablespoon olive oil
- 1 tablespoon basil, chopped
- 1 garlic clove, minced
- ¼ cup veggie stock
- 1 tablespoon balsamic vinegar
- 2 tablespoon coconut cream
- A pinch of salt and black pepper

Directions:
1. Set your instant pot on Sauté mode, add the oil, heat it up, add the garlic and cook for 1 minute
2. Add the rest of the ingredients, put the lid on and cook on High for 13 minutes.
3. Release the pressure fast for 5 minutes, blend the mix with an immersion blender, divide into bowls and serve.

Nutrition Value: calories 60, fat 5.4, fiber 1.6, carbs 2.8, protein 1.4

SPINACH AND ARTICHOKES SPREAD

Preparation time: 10 minutes
Cooking time: 15 minutes
Servings: 6

Ingredients:
- 14 ounces canned artichoke hearts, drained
- 8 ounces mozzarella cheese, shredded
- 1 pound spinach, torn
- 1 teaspoon garlic powder
- ½ cup chicken stock
- ½ cup coconut cream
- A pinch of salt and black pepper

Directions:
1. In your instant pot, mix the artichokes with the rest of the ingredients, put the lid on and cook on High for 15 minutes.
2. Release the pressure naturally for 10 minutes, blend the mix using an immersion blender, stir well, transfer to a bowl and serve as a snack.

Nutrition Value: calories 204, fat 11.5, fiber 3.1, carbs 4.2, protein 5.9

ARTICHOKES AND SALMON BOWLS

Preparation time: 5 minutes
Cooking time: 8 minutes
Servings: 4

Ingredients:

- 1 cup canned artichoke hearts, drained
- 1 pound smoked salmon, skinless, boneless and cubed
- 1 tablespoon olive oil
- A pinch of salt and black pepper
- 1 cup cherry tomatoes, cubed
- ¼ cup coconut cream
- 1 tablespoon chives, chopped

Directions:

1. In your instant pot, mix the artichoke hearts with the salmon and the rest of the ingredients, toss, put the lid on and cook on High for 8 minutes.
2. Release the pressure fast for 5 minutes, divide the mix into small bowls and serve as an appetizer.

Nutrition Value: calories 206, fat 12.4, fiber 0.9, carbs 2.6, protein 21.5

SALMON AND COD CAKES

Preparation time: 10 minutes
Cooking time: 10 minutes
Servings: 4

Ingredients:

- 1 tablespoon olive oil
- 1 egg, whisked
- 1 cup tomato passata
- 4 tablespoons almond flour
- ½ pound cod fillets, boneless and chopped
- 1 pound salmon meat, minced
- 1 tablespoon parsley, chopped
- 2 tablespoons lime zest
- A pinch of salt and black pepper

Directions:

1. In a bowl, combine the cod and salmon meat with the rest of the ingredients except the oil and tomato passata, stir and shape medium cakes out of this mix.
2. Set your instant pot on sauté mode, add the oil, heat it up, add the patties and cook them for 2 minutes on each side.
3. Add the tomato passata, put the lid on and cook on High for 8 minutes.
4. Release the pressure naturally for 10 minutes, arrange the cakes on a platter and serve as an appetizer.

Nutrition Value: calories 62, fat 4.7, fiber 1.3, carbs 3.9, protein 2.3

GREEN BEANS AND COD SALAD

Preparation time: 10 minutes
Cooking time: 15 minutes
Servings: 4

Ingredients:

- 1 pound cod fillets, skinless, boneless and cubed
- 2 tablespoons parsley, chopped
- 2 teaspoons lime juice
- 2 cups green beans, trimmed and halved
- A pinch of salt and black pepper
- 1 cup coconut cream
- 1 tablespoon oregano, chopped
- 1 tablespoon chives, chopped

Directions:

1. In your instant pot, combine the cod with the green beans and the rest of the ingredients except the oregano and chives, put the lid on and cook on High for 15 minutes.
2. Release the pressure naturally for 10 minutes, divide the mix into small bowls, sprinkle the oregano and the chives on top and serve as an appetizer.

Nutrition Value: calories 160, fat 14.5, fiber 3.8, carbs 8.1, protein 2.6

SHRIMP AND LEEKS PLATTER

Preparation time: 5 minutes
Cooking time: 5 minutes
Servings: 6

Ingredients:

- 2 pounds shrimp, peeled and deveined
- 2 leeks, sliced
- 1 tablespoon sweet paprika
- 1 tablespoon olive oil
- 1 tablespoon chives, chopped
- ½ cup veggie stock
- 2 garlic cloves, minced

Directions:

1. Set instant pot on Sauté mode, add the oil, heat it up, add the leeks and garlic and sauté for 1 minute.
2. Add the rest of the ingredients except the chives, put the lid on and cook on High for 4 minutes.
3. Release the pressure fast for 5 minutes, arrange the shrimp and leeks on a platter and serve as an appetizer.

Nutrition Value: calories 224, fat 5.1, fiber 1, carbs 3.9, protein 35.1

BALSAMIC MUSSELS BOWLS

Preparation time: 10 minutes
Cooking time: 10 minutes
Servings: 4

Ingredients:
- 2 cups tomato passata
- 2 pounds mussels, scrubbed
- 2 chili peppers, chopped
- ¼ cup veggie stock
- 1 tablespoon olive oil
- ¼ cup balsamic vinegar
- 2 garlic cloves, minced
- A pinch of salt and black pepper
- ½ cup oregano, chopped

Directions:
1. Set your instant pot on Sauté mode, add oil heat it up, add the chili peppers and the garlic and cook for 2 minutes.
2. Add the rest of the ingredients, put the lid on and cook on High for 8 minutes.
3. Release the pressure naturally for 10 minutes, divide the mix into bowls and serve as an appetizer.

Nutrition Value: calories 306, fat 9.8, fiber 4.8, carbs 6.5, protein 20.5

TOMATO AND ZUCCHINI SALSA

Preparation time: 10 minutes
Cooking time: 10 minutes
Servings: 4

Ingredients:
- 1 pound tomatoes, cubed
- 2 zucchinis, cubed
- 2 tablespoons olive oil
- ¼ cup chicken stock
- ½ teaspoon red pepper flakes
- 2 teaspoons garlic, minced
- 2 teaspoons ginger, chopped
- 1 tablespoon cilantro, chopped
- 2 teaspoons oregano, dried

Directions:
1. Set your instant pot on Sauté mode, add the oil, heat it up, add the pepper flakes, garlic and ginger and sauté for 2 minutes.
2. Add the rest of the ingredients, put the lid on and cook on High for 8 minutes.
3. Release the pressure naturally for 10 minutes, divide the salsa into bowls and serve cold.

Nutrition Value: calories 105, fat 7.6, fiber 3, carbs 6.7, protein 2.5

SWEET SHRIMP BOWLS

Preparation time: 5 minutes
Cooking time: 5 minutes
Servings: 6

Ingredients:
- 2 pounds shrimp, peeled and deveined
- 2 scallions, chopped
- 1 cup veggie stock
- 1 tablespoon olive oil
- 2 garlic cloves, minced
- 1 avocado, peeled, pitted and cubed
- 1 tablespoon sweet paprika

Directions:
1. Set your instant pot on Sauté mode, add the oil, heat it up, add the scallions and the ginger, stir and cook for 1 minute.
2. Add the rest of the ingredients, put the lid on and cook on High for 4 minutes.
3. Release the pressure fast for 5 minutes, divide the mix into bowls and serve as an appetizer.

Nutrition Value: calories 274, fat 11.6, fiber 2.8, carbs 6.5, protein 35.4

PARSLEY CLAMS PLATTER

Preparation time: 10 minutes
Cooking time: 12 minutes
Servings: 4

Ingredients:
- 20 clams, scrubbed
- 2 spring onions, chopped
- 1 and ½ cups veggie stock
- 2 tablespoons parsley, chopped
- 2 teaspoons lime zest, grated
- 1 tablespoon lime juice

Directions:
1. In your instant pot, combine the clams with the stock and the rest of the ingredients, put the lid on and cook on High for 12 minutes.
2. Release the pressure naturally for 10 minutes, arrange the clams on a platter and serve.

Nutrition Value: calories 224, fat 4.5, fiber 1.2, carbs 2.7, protein 1.3

ZUCCHINIS AND WALNUTS SALSA

Preparation time: 10 minutes
Cooking time: 12 minutes
Servings: 4

Ingredients:
- 4 zucchinis, sliced
- ½ cup veggie stock
- 3 garlic cloves, minced
- 1 tablespoon ghee, melted
- 1 cup walnuts, chopped

- ¼ cup parsley, chopped
- ¼ cup parmesan cheese, grated
- 1 teaspoon oregano, dried
- 1 teaspoon balsamic vinegar

Directions:
1. In your instant pot, combine the zucchinis with the stock and the rest of the ingredients except the parmesan, put the lid on and cook on High for 12 minutes.
2. Release the pressure naturally for 10 minutes, divide the mix into bowls, sprinkle the parmesan on top and serve as an appetizer.

Nutrition Value: calories 259, fat 22.1, fiber 4.6, carbs 5.9, protein 10.2

SHRIMP AND BEEF BOWLS

Preparation time: 10 minutes
Cooking time: 10 minutes
Servings: 4

Ingredients:
- 1 and ½ pounds shrimp, peeled and deveined
- ½ pound beef, cut into strips
- 1 tablespoon Italian seasoning
- 1 cup chicken stock
- A pinch of salt and black pepper
- 1 tablespoon olive oil
- 1 tablespoon sweet paprika
- 1 tablespoon cilantro, chopped
- 1 teaspoon red pepper flakes, crushed

Directions:
1. Set the instant pot on Sauté mode, add the oil, heat it up, add the beef and brown for 2 minutes.
2. Add the rest of the ingredients, put the lid on and cook on High for 8 minutes.
3. Release the pressure naturally fro 10 minutes, divide the mix into bowls and serve as an appetizer.

Nutrition Value: calories 155, fat 8.5, fiber 0.8, carbs 1.8, protein 17.7

COCONUT SHRIMP PLATTER

Preparation time: 10 minutes
Cooking time: 4 minutes
Servings: 4

Ingredients:
- 2 pounds shrimp, peeled and deveined
- 2 tablespoons coconut aminos
- 3 tablespoons balsamic vinegar
- ¾ cup veggie stock
- 1 tablespoon chives, chopped
- 1 tablespoon basil, chopped
- 1 tablespoon chervil, chopped

Directions:
1. In your instant pot, combine the shrimp with the aminos and the rest of the ingredients, put the lid on and cook on High for 5 minutes.
2. Release the pressure naturally for 10 minutes, arrange the shrimp on a platter and serve.

Nutrition Value: calories 273, fat 3.9, fiber 0.1, carbs 3.8, protein 17.8

MARINATED SHRIMP

Preparation time: 10 minutes
Cooking time: 6 minutes
Servings: 4

Ingredients:
- 1 and ½ pounds shrimp, peeled and deveined
- ¼ cup chicken stock
- 1 tablespoon avocado oil
- Juice of ½ lemon
- 4 garlic cloves, minced
- 2 thyme springs, chopped
- 1 tablespoon rosemary, chopped
- Salt and black pepper to the taste

Directions:
1. In your instant pot, combine the shrimp with the stock and the rest of the ingredients, put the lid on and cook on High for 6 minutes.
2. Release the pressure naturally for 10 minutes, arrange the shrimp on a platter and serve as an appetizer.

Nutrition Value: calories 282, fat 4.5, fiber 0.6, carbs 2.3, protein 30.4

EGGPLANT AND SPINACH DIP

Preparation time: 10 minutes
Cooking time: 15 minutes
Servings: 4

Ingredients:
- 2 eggplants, cubed
- 1 cup baby spinach
- ¼ cup veggie stock
- ¼ cup coconut cream
- A pinch of salt and black pepper
- 2 garlic cloves, minced
- 1 tablespoon lemon juice

Directions:
1. In your instant pot, combine the eggplants with the spinach and the rest of the ingredients, put the lid on and cook on High for 15 minutes.
2. Release the pressure naturally for 10 minutes, blend the mix with an immersion blender, divide into bowls and serve as a party dip.

Nutrition Value: calories 108, fat 4.1, fiber 2.6, carbs 3.7, protein 3.5

BALSAMIC ENDIVES

Preparation time: 10 minutes
Cooking time: 12 minutes
Servings: 4

Ingredients:
- 4 endives, trimmed and halved lengthwise
- A pinch of salt and black pepper
- 2 tablespoons lime juice
- ¼ cup olive oil
- 2 teaspoons balsamic vinegar
- 1 teaspoon thyme, dried
- 2 cups water

Directions:
1. Put the water in the instant pot, add steamer basket, add the endives inside, put the lid on and cook on High for 12 minutes.
2. Release the pressure naturally for 10 minutes, transfer the endives to a bowl, add the rest of the ingredients, toss gently, arrange everything on a platter and serve.

Nutrition Value: calories 109, fat 12.6, fiber 0.1, carbs 0.2, protein 1

ITALIAN ASPARAGUS

Preparation time: 4 minutes
Cooking time: 4 minutes
Servings: 4

Ingredients:
- 1 cup water
- 1 pound asparagus, trimmed
- ½ tablespoon Italian seasoning
- A pinch of salt and black pepper
- 1 tablespoon cilantro, chopped
- 1 tablespoon lemon juice
- 1 teaspoon olive oil

Directions:
Put the water in your instant pot, add steamer basket, add the asparagus, put the lid on and cook on High for 4 minutes.
Release the pressure fast for 4 minutes, transfer the asparagus to a bowl, add the rest of the ingredients, toss, arrange everything on a platter and serve.
Nutrition Value: calories 39, fat 2.1, fiber 1.1, carbs 1.3, protein 2.5

FENNEL AND LEEKS PLATTER

Preparation time: 5 minutes
Cooking time: 8 minutes
Servings: 4
Ingredients:
- 4 leeks, roughly sliced
- 2 fennel bulbs, halved
- 1 tablespoon smoked paprika
- 1 teaspoon chili sauce
- A pinch of salt and black pepper
- 1 tablespoon ghee, melted
- ½ cup chicken stock

Directions:
1. In your instant pot, combine the leeks with the fennel, salt, pepper and the stock, put the lid on and cook on High for 8 minutes.
2. Release the pressure fast for 5 minutes, arrange the leeks and fennel on a platter, sprinkle the paprika on top, drizzle the chili sauce and the ghee and serve as an appetizer.

Nutrition Value: calories 124, fat 4, fiber 2.1, carbs 3.3, protein 3.2

NUTMEG ENDIVES

Preparation time: 10 minutes
Cooking time: 10 minutes
Servings: 4

Ingredients:
- 4 endives, trimmed and halved
- 1 cup water
- Salt and black pepper to the taste
- 2 tablespoons olive oil
- 1 teaspoon nutmeg, ground
- 1 tablespoon chives, chopped

Directions:
1. Add the water to your instant pot, add steamer basket, add the endives inside, put the lid on and cook on High for 10 minutes.
2. Release the pressure naturally for 10 minutes, arrange the endives on a platter, drizzle the oil, season with salt, pepper and nutmeg, sprinkle the chives at the end and serve as an appetizer.

Nutrition Value: calories 63, fat 7.2, fiber 0.1, carbs 0.3, protein 0.1

DESSERTS

COCONUT CAKE
Preparation Time: 5 Mins
Total Time: 55 Mins
Servings: 2
Ingredients:
- 1 Egg, yolk and white separated
- ½ cup Coconut Flour
- 1 tbsp melted Coconut Oil
- ¼ tsp Coconut Extract
- ¾ cup warm Coconut Milk
- ¼ cup Coconut Sugar
- 1 cup Water

Direction
1. Beat the white until soft form peaks.
2. Bea tin the sugar and yolk.
3. Add the coconut oil and extract and stir to combine.
4. Fold in the coconut flour.
5. Line or grease a small baking dish an pour the batter into it.
6. Pour the water into the IP and lower the trivet.
7. Place the dish on the trivet.
8. Cook for 40 minutes on HIGH.
9. Do a quick pressure release.
10. Serve and enjoy!

Nutrition Values:
Calories 350
Total Fats 14g
Carbs: 47g
Protein 7g
Dietary Fiber: 7g

YOGURT VANILLA LIGHTER CHEESECAKE
Preparation Time: 5 Mins
Total Time: 6 hours and 60 Mins
Servings: 2
Ingredients:
- 1 small Egg
- ½ cup Yogurt
- ¼ tsp Vanilla
- 2 tbsp melted Butter
- ½ cup Graham Cracker Crumbs
- 2 ounces Cream Cheese, softened
- 1 tbsp Sugar
- 1 cup Water

Direction
1. Pour the water into the Instant Pot and lower the trivet.
2. Combine the butter and crackers and press the mixture into the bottom of a greased small baking dish.
3. Bea the yogurt, vanilla, sugar, and cream cheese.
4. Beat in the egg.
5. Pour over the crust.
6. Place the baking dish on the trivet and close the id.
7. Cook on HIGH for 20 minutes.
8. Do a quick pressure release.
9. Let cool to room temperature then place it in the fridge for 5-6 hours.
10. Serve and enjoy!

Nutrition Values:
Calories 280
Total Fats 9g
Carbs: 26g
Protein 6g
Dietary Fiber: 1g

MOLTEN LAVA CAKE
Preparation Time: 5 Mins
Total Time: 20 Mins
Servings: 2
Ingredients:
- 1 tbsp Butter, melted
- 3 tbsp Almond Flour
- ½ cup chopped Dark Chocolate
- 1 cup Water
- 1 Egg, beaten
- ¼ tsp Vanilla
- ¼ cup Coconut Sugar

Direction
1. Pour the water into the Instant Pot. Lower the trivet.
2. Combine all of the remaining ingredients in a bowl.
3. Grease two ramekins and divide the batter among them.
4. Place them on the trivet and close the lid.
5. Cook for 9 minutes on HIGH.
6. Do a quick pressure release.
7. Serve and enjoy!

Nutrition Values:
Calories 414
Total Fats 23g
Carbs: 48g
Protein 8g
Dietary Fiber: 2.6g

STUFFED PEACHES
Preparation Time: 5 Mins
Total Time: 35 Mins
Servings: 2
Ingredients:
- 2 Peaches
- 2 tbsp Butter
- ¼ tsp Almond Extract
- Pinch of Cinnamon
- 2 tbsp Cassava Flour
- 2 tbsp Maple Syrup
- 2 tsp chopped Almonds
- 1 ½ cups Water

Direction
1. Pour the water into the Instant Pot. Lower the rack.
2. Slice the tops off the peaches and discard the pits.
3. Combine the rest of the ingredients in a bowl.
4. Stuff the peaches with the mixture.
5. Place them on the rack and close the lid.
6. Cook for 3 minutes on HIGH.
7. Do a quick pressure release.
8. Serve and enjoy!

Nutrition Values:
Calories 145
Total Fats 5g
Carbs: 25g
Protein 1.5g
Dietary Fiber: 1g

BLUEBERRY JAM
Preparation Time: 5 Mins
Total Time: 30 Mins
Servings: 2
Ingredients:
- ¼ cup Honey
- ½ cup Blueberries

Direction
1. Combine the honey and blueberries in the IP.
2. Set it to KEEP WARM and let it sit until the honey turns liquid.
3. When the honey becomes liquid, set the IP to SAUTE and bring it to a boil.
4. Cover, press CANCEL, and set to MANUAL.
5. Cook on HIGH for 2 minutes.
6. Do a natural pressure release.
7. Serve and enjoy!

Nutrition Values:
Calories 180
Total Fats 0g
Carbs: 40g
Protein 1g
Dietary Fiber: 1g

VANILLA RICE PUDDING
Preparation Time: 5 Mins
Total Time: 30 Mins
Servings: 2
Ingredients:
- 1/3 cup Basmati Rice
- ½ tsp Vanilla Extract
- ¼ cup Heavy Cream
- 2/3 cup Milk
- 1 ½ tbsp Maple Syrup
- Pinch of Salt

Direction
1. Combine everything in the Instant Pot, except the cream.
2. Close the lid and set the IP to PORRIDGE.
3. Cook for 17 minutes.
4. Do a natural pressure release.
5. Stir in the heavy cream.
6. Serve and enjoy!

Nutrition Values:
Calories 240
Total Fats 7g
Carbs: 38g
Protein 5g
Dietary Fiber: 7g

PRESSURE COOKED BROWNIES
Preparation Time: 5 Mins
Total Time: 45 Mins
Servings: 2
Ingredients:
- 1 tbsp Honey
- 2 cups Water
- ½ cup Sugar
- 1 Egg
- 2 tbsp Cocoa Powder
- Pinch of Salt
- ¼ cup melted Butter
- 2/3 cup Flour
- 1/3 cup Baking Powder

Direction
1. Pour the water into the Instant Pot. Lower the trivet.
2. Whisk the wet ingredients in one bowl.
3. Stir together the dry ones in another.
4. Combine the two mixtures gently.
5. Grease a baking dish with some cooking spray.
6. Pour the batter into it.
7. Place the dish on the trivet and close the lid.
8. Cook on HIGH for 25 minutes.

9. Do a quick pressure release.
10. Serve and enjoy!

Nutrition Values:
Calories 525
Total Fats 25g
Carbs: 75g
Protein 8g
Dietary Fiber: 3g

ALMOND TAPIOCA PUDDING

Preparation Time: 5 Mins
Total Time: 30 Mins
Servings: 2

Ingredients:
- 2/3 cup Almond Milk
- ¼ cup Tapioca Pearls
- 2 tbsp Sugar
- ½ tsp Almond Extract
- ½ cup Water
- Pinch of Cinnamon

Direction
1. Pour the water into the Instant Pot. Lower the trivet.
2. Take a heat –proof bowl and place all of the ingredients into it.
3. Stir well to combine.
4. Cover with a foil and place the bowl on the trivet.
5. Close the lid and set the IP to MANUAL.
6. Cook on HIGH for 7-8 minutes.
7. Do a natural pressure release.
8. Serve and enjoy!

Nutrition Values:
Calories 190
Total Fats 2.5g
Carbs: 39g
Protein 2.5g
Dietary Fiber: 5.2g

BLONDIES WITH PEANUT BUTTER

Preparation Time: 5 Mins
Total Time: 55 Mins
Servings: 2

Ingredients:
- 1 ½ cups Water
- ¼ cup Brown Sugar
- 2 tbsp White Sugar
- 1/3 cup Oats
- 1/3 cup Flour
- 1 Egg
- 2 tbsp Peanut Butter
- 3 tbsp Butter, softened
- Pinch of Salt

Direction
1. Pour the water into the Instant Pot. Lower the trivet.
2. Grease a baking dish with cooking spray and set aside.
3. Cream together the sugars, egg, butter, peanut butter, and salt, in a mixing bowl.
4. Fold in the dry ingredients.
5. Pour the batter into the greased pan.
6. Place the pan on the trivet and close the lid.
7. Cook on POULTRY for 26 minutes.
8. Wait 10 minutes before doing a quick pressure release.
9. Let it cool for 15 minutes before inverting onto a plate and slicing.
10. Serve and enjoy!

Nutrition Values:
Calories 550
Total Fats 18g
Carbs: 61g
Protein 8g
Dietary Fiber: 1.5g

GINGERY APPLESAUCE

Preparation Time: 5 Mins
Total Time: 15 Mins
Servings: 2

Ingredients:
- 1 ½ pounds Apples, chopped
- 1 ½ tbsp Crystalized Ginger
- ½ cup Water

Direction
1. Pour the water into the Instant Pot.
2. Add the apples and ginger and stir to combine.
3. Close the lid and set the IP to MANUAL.
4. Cook on HIGH for 4 minutes.
5. Wait 10 minutes and then release the pressure naturally.
6. Mashed with a potato masher.
7. Serve and enjoy!

Nutrition Values:
Calories 260
Total Fats 1g
Carbs: 66g
Protein 5g
Dietary Fiber: 5g

PEACH CRUMB

Preparation Time: 5 Mins
Total Time: 55 Mins
Servings: 2

Ingredients:
- ¼ cup Breadcrumbs

- 2 small Peaches, sliced
- 2 tbsp Lemon Juice
- ¼ tsp Lemon Zest
- ¼ cup melted Butter
- ¼ tsp ground Ginger
- Pinch of Cinnamon
- 2 tbsp Sugar
- 1 ½ cups Water

Direction
1. Pour the water into the Instant Pot. Lower the trivet.
2. Grease a baking dish with cooking spray and arrange the peach slices in it.
3. Combine the remaining ingredients in a bowl and spread over the peaches.
4. Place the dish on the trivet and close the lid.
5. Cook on HIGH for 20 minutes.
6. Do a natural pressure release.
7. Serve and enjoy!

Nutrition Values:
Calories 505
Total Fats 25g
Carbs: 70g
Protein 2.5g
Dietary Fiber: 4g

PEAR RICOTTA CAKE

Preparation Time: 5 Mins
Total Time: 30 Mins
Servings: 2

Ingredients:
- 2 tbsp Sugar
- 1 Egg
- 1 Pear, diced
- ½ cup Ricotta
- ½ cup Flour
- ½ tsp Baking Soda
- ½ tsp Vanilla
- 1 ½ tbsp Oil
- 1 tbsp Lemon Juice
- 1 tsp Baking Powder
- 2 cups Water

Direction
1. Pour the water into the Instant Pot. Lower the trivet.
2. Whisk together all of the ingredients in a large bowl.
3. Stir well to avoid leaving any lumos.
4. Grease a baking dish that fits inside the IP, with some cooking spray.
5. Pour the batter into the dish and then place it on the trivet.
6. Close the lid of the IP and set it to MANUAL.
7. Cook on HIGH for 15 minutes.
8. Release the pressure quickly.
9. Serve and enjoy!

Nutrition Values:
Calories 452
Total Fats 20g
Carbs: 60g
Protein 13g
Dietary Fiber: 4g

LEMON AND BLACKBERRY COMPOTE

Preparation Time: 5 Mins
Total Time: 135 Mins
Servings: 2

Ingredients:
- Juice of ½ Lemon
- Pinch of Lemon Zest
- 1 cup Frozen Blackberries
- 5 tbsp Sugar
- 1 tbsp Cornstarch
- 1 tbsp Water

Direction
1. Combine the lemon juice, sugar, zest, and blackberries, in your IP.
2. Close the lid and set the IP to MANUAL.
3. Cook for 3 minutes on HIGH.
4. Do a natural pressure release.
5. Whisk together the water and cornstarch and stir the mixture into the compote.
6. Cook on SAUTE until slightly thickened.
7. Place in the fridge for 1 ½ - 2 hours.
8. Serve and enjoy!

Nutrition Values:
Calories 220
Total Fats 0g
Carbs: 60g
Protein 1g
Dietary Fiber: 4g

POACHED GINGERY ORANGE PEARS

Preparation Time: 5 Mins
Total Time: 20 Mins
Servings: 2

Ingredients:
- 2 Pears
- 1 cup Orange Juice
- 1 tsp minced Ginger
- Pinch of Nutmeg
- Pinch of Cinnamon
- 2 tbsp Sugar

Direction
1. Pour the juice into the IP.

2. Stir in the sugar, ginger, cinnamon, and nutmeg.
3. Peel the pears and cut in half.
4. Place the inside the IP.
5. Close the lid and cook for 7 minutes on HIGH.
6. Do a natural pressure release.
7. Serve drizzled with the sauce.
8. Enjoy!

Nutrition Values:
Calories 170
Total Fats 1g
Carbs: 43g
Protein 1g
Dietary Fiber: 5g

CARAMEL FLAN

Preparation Time: 5 Mins
Total Time: 30 Mins
Servings: 2

Ingredients:
- 1 Egg
- 4 ounces Condensed Milk
- ½ cup Coconut Milk
- ½ tsp Vanilla Extract
- 1 ½ cups plus 3 tbsp Water
- 5 tbsp Sugar

1. **Direction**
2. Combine the sugar and water in the IP on SAUTE.
3. Cook until caramelized.
4. Divide the caramelized sugar immediately otherwise it will harden between 2 greased ramekins.
5. Bea the remaining ingredients in a bowl and then pour on top of the caramel.
6. Cover with aluminum foil.
7. Pour the water into the Instant Pot. Lower the trivet.
8. Place the ramekins on the trivet and close the lid.
9. Cook on HIGH for 5 minutes.
10. Do a natural pressure release.
11. Allow to cool before inverting onto a plate.
12. Serve and enjoy!

Nutrition Values:
Calories 108
Total Fats 3g
Carbs: 16g
Protein 3g
Dietary Fiber: 0g

STRAWBERRY CREAM

Preparation Time: 5 Mins
Total Time: 4 hours and 20 Mins
Servings: 2

Ingredients:
- 1 cup Strawberry Halves
- 1 cup Coconut Milk

Direction
1. Combine the ingredients in your IP.
2. Close the lid and set the IP to MANUAL.
3. Cook on HIGH for 2 minutes.
4. Do a quick pressure release.
5. Let the mixture cool completely.
6. Blend with a hand blender and divide between two glasses.
7. Refrigerate for 4 hours.
8. Serve and enjoy!

Nutrition Values:
Calories 63
Total Fats 3g
Carbs: 9g
Protein 1g
Dietary Fiber: 2g

BERRY COMPOTE

Preparation Time: 5 Mins
Total Time: 2 hours and 30 Mins
Servings: 4

Ingredients:
- 2 tbsp Arrowroot
- 1 cup Raspberries
- 1 cup halved Strawberries
- 1 cup Blackberries
- 1 cup Blueberries
- Juice of 1 Orange
- ½ cup Water

Direction
1. Place the berries, water, and orange juice, in the Instant Pot.
2. Close the lid and set the IP to MANUAL.
3. Cook on HIGH for 3 minutes.
4. Do a quick pressure release.
5. Whisk in the arrowroot and set the IP to SAUTE.
6. Cook until thickened.
7. Let cool completely and transfer to an airtight container.
8. Refrigerate for 2 hours before serving.
9. Enjoy!

Nutrition Values:
Calories 95
Total Fats 0.5g
Carbs: 23g
Protein 1g
Dietary Fiber: 6.7g

CREAMY COCONUT PEACH DESSERT

Preparation Time: 5 Mins
Total Time: 2 hours and 20 Mins
Servings: 4

Ingredients:
- 3 Peaches, peeled and chopped
- ½ cup shredded Coconut
- ½ cup Coconut Milk
- Pinch of Cinnamon

Direction
- Combine all of the ingredients in the IP.
- Close the lid and set the IP to MANUAL.
- Cook on HIGH for about 4 minutes.
- Do a quick pressure release.
- Mash with a fork and let cool.
- Divide between 4 bowls, cover, and refrigerate for 2 hours.
- Serve and enjoy!

Nutrition Values:
Calories 50
Total Fats 1g
Carbs: 9g
Protein 0.5g
Dietary Fiber: 1.5g

BANANA AND ALMOND BUTTER BARS

Preparation Time: 5 Mins
Total Time: 20 Mins
Servings: 2

Ingredients:
- ½ cup Almond Butter
- 3 Bananas
- 2 tbsp 100% Cocoa Powder
- 1 ½ cups Water

Direction
1. In a bowl, mash together the bananas and almond butter.
2. Stir in the cocoa powder.
3. Grease a baking dish and pour the banana mixture into it.
4. Pour the water into the IP and lower the rack.
5. Place the baking dish on the rack and close the lid.
6. Set the IP to MANUAL and cook on HIGH for 15 minutes.
7. Do a quick pressure release.
8. Remove the baking dish from the IP.
9. Let cool and cut into bars.
10. Serve and enjoy!

Nutrition Values:
Calories 141
Total Fats 10g
Carbs: 14g
Protein 3g
Dietary Fiber: 2g

FRUITY SAUCE WITH APPLES

Preparation Time: 5 Mins
Total Time: 15 Mins
Servings: 2

Ingredients:
- 2 Apples, peeled and cubed
- 1 cup mixed Berries
- 1 cup Pineapple chunks
- ¼ cup Fresh Orange Juice
- 2/3 cup Water
- ¼ cup chopped Almonds
- 1 tbsp Coconut Oil

Direction
1. Combine all of the ingredients, except the almonds, in the Instant Pot.
2. Close the lid and set the IP to MANUAL.
3. Cook for 5 minutes on HIGH.
4. Release the pressure quickly.
5. Open the lid and blend the mixture with a hand blender.
6. Stir in the almonds.
7. Serve and enjoy!

Nutrition Values:
Calories 120
Total Fats 4g
Carbs: 15g

WINE-GLAZED APPLES

Servings: 4
Preparation Time: 5 minutes'
Cooking Time: 10 minutes

Ingredients
- 4 apples, cored
- ¾ cup red wine
- 1/3 cup demerara sugar
- ¼ cup raisins
- ¾ teaspoon ground cinnamon
- Cooking oil for topping

Directions
1. Add all the ingredients to the Instant Pot.
2. Secure the lid. Cook on 'Manual' function for 10 minutes at high pressure.
3. After the beep, do a 'Quick release' and remove the lid.
4. Top the apples with some cooking oil and serve.

Nutrition Values:
Calories: 227
Carbohydrate: 51.4g

Protein: 0.9g
Fat: 0.5g
Sugar: 40.6g
Sodium: 9mg

BROWN FUDGE CAKE

Servings: 3
Preparation Time: 6 minutes
Cooking Time: 06 minutes

Ingredients

- ¼ cup milk
- 2 tablespoons extra-virgin olive oil
- 1 egg
- ¼ cup unbleached all-purpose flour
- ¼ cup brown sugar
- 1 tablespoon cocoa powder
- ½ teaspoon baking powder
- 2 teaspoons fresh orange zest, grated finely
- 1 cup water
- Powdered sugar, as required
- 3 ramekins

Directions

1. Add all the ingredients to a large bowl except the powdered sugar.
2. Whisk all the ingredients well to prepare a smooth mixture.
3. Grease the three ramekins and pour the prepared mixture into the ramekins.
4. Pour a cup of water into the Instant Pot. Place the steamer trivet inside.
5. Arrange the ramekins over the trivet.
6. Secure the lid and cook on manual for 6 minutes at high pressure.
7. After the beep, do a quick release and remove the lid.
8. Let the ramekins cool. Sprinkle powdered sugar on top of each cake.
9. Serve.

Nutrition Values:

Calories: 166
Carbohydrate: 21.2g
Protein: 3g
Fat: 8.7g
Sugar: 13.9g
Sodium: 24mg

CHOCOLATE CHEESECAKE

Servings: 3
Preparation Time: 10 minutes'
Cooking Time: 18 minutes

Ingredients

- ¼ cup Swerve brown sugar (Sweetener)
- 3/4 tablespoon cocoa powder
- 2 eggs
- 8 oz. cream cheese softened
- 1 tablespoon powdered peanut butter
- ½ teaspoon pure vanilla extract
- 3 ramekins, greased
- Water as needed

Directions

1. Blend the eggs and cream cheese in a blender to form a smooth mixture.
2. Add the brown sugar, peanut butter and vanilla extract to the egg mixture and blend.
3. Transfer the mixture to a greased ramekin.
4. Pour the water into the Instant Pot and place the trivet inside.
5. Arrange the ramekins over the trivet.
6. Secure the lid and cook on manual function for 18 minutes at high pressure.
7. After the beep, do a quick release and remove the lid.
8. Let the ramekins cool and top it with cocoa powder. Refrigerate the cake for 8 hours.
9. Serve.

Nutrition Values:

Calories:223
Carbohydrate: 17.8g
Protein: 6.5g
Fat: 21.2g
Sugar: 15.4g
Sodium: 195mg

MAPLE-GLAZED FLAN

Servings: 4
Preparation Time: 10 minutes
Cooking Time: 09 minutes

Ingredients

- 2 large eggs
- ½ cup milk
- ½ can sweeten condensed milk
- ¼ cup water
- ½ teaspoon vanilla extract
- A pinch of salt
- ¼ cup maple syrup
- ¼ cup cherries for topping

Directions

1. Beat the eggs in a large bowl and stir in the remaining ingredients except for the maple syrup and cherry
2. Glaze a ramekin with maple syrup and transfer the vanilla mixture in it.
3. Pour a cup of water into the Instant Pot and place the trivet inside.
4. Arrange the ramekin over the trivet.
5. Secure the lid and cook on 'manual' function

for 9 minutes at high pressure.
6. After the beep, do a 'quick release' and remove the lid.
7. Let the ramekin cool and refrigerate the flan for 3 hours.
8. Top with additional maple glaze and cherries then serve.

Nutrition Values:
Calories: 227
Carbohydrate: 35.8g
Protein: 7.2g
Fat: 6.5g
Sugar: 34.2g
Sodium: 139mg

ALMOND CHEESECAKE

Servings: 3
Preparation Time: 10 minutes
Cooking Time: 18 minutes

Ingredients
- ¼ cup powdered brown sugar
- ¼ cup almonds, thinly sliced
- 2 eggs
- 8 oz. cream cheese softened
- 1 tablespoon powdered peanut butter
- ½ teaspoon pure vanilla extract
- 3 ramekins, greased
- 1 cup water

Directions
1. Blend the eggs and cream cheese in a blender to form a smooth mixture.
2. Add the brown sugar, peanut butter and vanilla extract to the egg mixture and blend.
3. Transfer the mixture to a greased ramekin.
4. Pour water into the Instant Pot and place the trivet inside.
5. Arrange the ramekins over the trivet.
6. Secure the lid and cook on manual function for 18 minutes at high pressure.
7. After the beep, do a quick release and remove the lid.
8. Let the ramekins cool and top it with almonds. Refrigerate the cake for 8 hours.
9. Serve.

Nutrition Values:
Calories: 248
Carbohydrate: 11g
Protein: 7.6g
Fat: 24g
Sugar: 8g
Sodium: 195mg

CRÈME BRÛLÉE

Servings: 4
Preparation Time: 10 minutes
Cooking Time: 13 minutes

Ingredients
- 4 ramekins
- 5 egg yolks
- 2 cups heavy cream
- 1 tablespoon vanilla extract
- ½ cup sugar
- 1 cup water
- ¼ cup superfine sugar

Directions
1. Beat the egg yolks, cream, vanilla extract and sugar in a large bowl.
2. Divide the mixture into 4 ramekins.
3. Pour a cup of water into the Instant Pot and place the trivet inside.
4. Arrange the ramekins over the trivet.
5. Secure the lid and cook on manual function for 13 minutes at high pressure.
6. After the beep, do a quick release and remove the lid.
7. Let the ramekin cool and refrigerate for 4 hours.
8. Sprinkle superfine sugar on top and serve.

Nutrition Values:
Calories: 377
Carbohydrate: 27.8g
Protein: 4.6g
Fat: 27.8g
Sugar: 25.6g
Sodium: 33mg

NUTMEG APPLE CRISP

Servings: 4
Preparation Time: 10 minutes
Cooking Time: 07 minutes

Ingredients
- 4 medium apples, peeled, cored and diced
- 1 teaspoon ground cinnamon
- ¼ teaspoon ground nutmeg
- 2 tablespoons pure maple syrup or honey
- 1 cup water

For topping:
- 2/3 cup old-fashioned rolled oats
- 1/3 cup flour
- ¼ cup brown sugar
- ¼ cup unsalted butter, melted
- ¼ tablespoon nutmeg
- ½ tablespoon cinnamon
- A pinch of salt

Directions
1. Combine the diced apples, nutmeg, maple

syrup, and cinnamon in a bowl, toss until well coated.
2. Transfer this mixture to ramekins.
3. Add the topping ingredients in the same bowl and mix them well, cover the apples completely with the mixture.
4. Add a cup of water into the pot and add trivet and stack the ramekins on the trivet.
5. Secure the lid and set the valve in the sealing position. Cook on 'manual' function for 7 minutes. Once it beeps, do a 'quick release' and remove the lid.
6. Let it cool and serve.

Nutrition Values:
Calories: 383
Carbohydrate: 67.8g
Protein: 3.7g
Fat: 13.2g
Sugar: 41g
Sodium: 128mg

CHOCOLATE CRÈME BRÛLÉE

Servings: 4
Preparation Time: 10 minutes
Cooking Time: 13 minutes

Ingredients
- 4 ramekins
- 5 egg yolks
- 2 cups heavy cream
- 1 tablespoon vanilla extract
- ½ tablespoon cocoa powder
- ½ cup sugar
- 1 cup water
- ¼ cup superfine sugar
- ½ tablespoon grated chocolate

Directions
1. Beat the egg yolks, cream, cocoa powder, vanilla extract and sugar in a large bowl.
2. Divide the mixture into 4 ramekins.
3. Pour a cup of water into the Instant Pot and place the trivet inside.
4. Arrange the ramekins over the trivet.
5. Secure the lid and cook on manual function for 13 minutes at high pressure.
6. After the beep, do a quick release and remove the lid.
7. Let the ramekin cool and refrigerate for 4 hours.
8. Sprinkle superfine sugar and grated chocolate on top and serve.

Nutrition Values:
Calories: 386
Carbohydrate: 29g
Protein: 4.8g
Fat: 28.3g
Sugar: 26.3g
Sodium: 34mg

BLUEBERRY CHEESECAKE

Servings: 6
Preparation Time: 10 minutes
Cooking Time: 35 minutes

Ingredients
- 8 oz. cream cheese
- 8 oz. ricotta cheese
- ½ cup sugar
- 2 eggs
- ¼ cup sour cream
- 1 tablespoon vanilla extract
- 10 butter cookies, crushed
- 1 cup water
- 2 tablespoons unsalted butter, melted
- 2 tablespoons powdered sugar
- ¼ cup fresh blueberries, pitted

Directions
1. Blend the eggs, ricotta, sugar and cream cheese in a blender.
2. Stir in vanilla extract and sour cream.
3. Mix the crushed cookies with butter.
4. Layer a 7-inch springform pan with the cookies and cream cheese mixture.
5. Pour the water into the Instant Pot and place the trivet inside.
6. Arrange the pan over the trivet.
7. Secure the lid and cook on manual function for 35 minutes at high pressure.
8. After the beep, do a quick release and remove the lid.
9. Let it cool and top it with powdered sugar and blueberries. Refrigerate the cake for 12 hours.
10. 1Serve.

Nutrition Values:
Calories: 471
Carbohydrate: 29.4g
Protein: 9g
Fat: 35.5g
Sugar: 19.1g
Sodium: 368mg

TAPIOCA PUDDING

Servings: 4
Preparation Time: 05 minutes
Cooking Time: 09 minutes

Ingredients
- 1½ cups water
- ½ cup small pearl tapioca

- ½ cup sugar
- A pinch of salt
- ½ cup milk
- 2 egg yolks
- ½ teaspoon vanilla extract
- ¼ cup fresh raspberries

Directions
1. Add the water and tapioca to the Instant Pot and mix them well.
2. Secure the lid and cook on manual for 6 minutes at high pressure.
3. Do a quick release and remove the lid.
4. Whisk the egg, sugar, salt and milk in a bowl using a beater then add this mix to the pot.
5. Cook on sauté for 3 minutes and stir in the vanilla extract.
6. Let it chill in the refrigerator for 30 minutes.
7. Top with raspberries and then serve.

Nutrition Values:
Calories: 295
Carbohydrate: 63.7g
Protein: 3.3g
Fat: 3.9g
Sugar: 35.8g
Sodium: 88mg

CHERRY CHEESECAKE
Servings: 6
Preparation Time: 10 minutes
Cooking Time: 35 minutes

Ingredients
- 8 oz. cream cheese
- 8 oz. ricotta cheese
- ¼ cup sugar
- 2 eggs
- ¼ cup sour cream
- 1 tablespoon vanilla extract
- 10 Oreo cookies, crushed
- 1 cup water
- 2 tablespoons unsalted butter, melted
- 2 tablespoons powdered sugar
- ¼ cup fresh cherries, pitted

Directions
1. Blend the eggs, ricotta, sugar and cream cheese in a blender.
2. Stir in vanilla extract and sour cream.
3. Mix the crushed Oreos with butter.
4. Layer a 7-inch springform pan with the cookies and cream cheese mixture.
5. Pour the water into the Instant Pot and place the trivet inside.
6. Arrange the pan over the trivet.
7. Secure the lid and cook on manual function for 35 minutes at high pressure.
8. After the beep, do a quick release and remove the lid.
9. Let it cool and top it with powdered sugar and cherries. Refrigerate the cake for 12 hours.
10. 1Serve.

Nutrition Values:
Calories: 366
Carbohydrate: 21.5g
Protein: 10.3g
Fat: 26.7g
Sugar: 12.3g
Sodium: 293mg

LAVENDER CRÈME BRÛLÉE
Servings: 4
Preparation Time: 10 minutes
Cooking Time: 13 minutes

Ingredients
- 4 ramekins
- 5 egg yolks
- 2 cups heavy cream
- 1 tablespoon vanilla extract
- ½ cup sugar
- 1 cup water
- ¼ cup superfine sugar
- ½ tablespoon lavender buds

Directions
1. Beat the egg yolks, cream, vanilla extract and sugar in a large bowl.
2. Divide the mixture into 4 ramekins.
3. Pour a cup of water into the Instant Pot and place the trivet inside.
4. Arrange the ramekins over the trivet.
5. Secure the lid and cook on manual function for 13 minutes at high pressure.
6. After the beep, do a quick release and remove the lid.
7. Let the ramekin cool and refrigerate for 4 hours.
8. Sprinkle superfine sugar and lavender buds on top and serve.

Nutrition Values:
Calories: 377
Carbohydrate: 27.8g
Protein: 4.6g
Fat: 27.8g
Sugar: 25.6g
Sodium: 33mg

PUMPKIN BUNDT CAKE
Servings: 3
Preparation Time: 15 minutes

Cooking Time: 35 minutes

Ingredients

- 6 tablespoons whole wheat flour
- 6 tablespoons unbleached all-purpose flour
- ¼ teaspoon salt
- ½ teaspoon baking soda
- ¼ teaspoon baking powder
- ¼ teaspoon pumpkin pie spice
- 6 tablespoons sugar
- ½ medium banana mashed
- 1 tablespoon canola oil
- ¼ cup Greek yoghurt
- ¼ (15 oz. can pumpkin puree
- ½ egg
- ¼ teaspoon pure vanilla extract
- ¼ cup chocolate chips
- 3 mini Bundt pans (tools)

Directions

1. Combine all the dry ingredients in a bowl and keep them aside.
2. Mix the banana, sugar, oil, yoghurt, egg, vanilla and pureed pumpkin with the electric mixer.
3. Add all the dry ingredients to the egg mixture and beat until smooth.
4. Fold in chocolate chips and divide the mixture into 3 mini Bundt pans.
5. Pour a cup of water into the Instant Pot and place the trivet inside.
6. Arrange the Bundt pans over the trivet.
7. Secure the lid and cook on manual function for 35 minutes at high pressure.
8. After the beep, do a natural release and remove the lid.
9. Let the Bundt cool then remove the cake.
10. 1Garnish with fresh cream and serve.

Nutrition Values:
Calories: 356
Carbohydrate: 59.7g
Protein: 6.7g
Fat: 10.5g
Sugar: 36.1g
Sodium: 453mg

CINNAMON APPLESAUCE

Servings: 3
Preparation Time: 10 minutes
Cooking Time: 08 minutes

Ingredients

- 6 large apples, peeled, cored and roughly chopped
- 1 cup water
- 1-2 drops cinnamon essential oil
- 1 tablespoon lemon juice
- 1 teaspoon organic cinnamon

Directions

1. Add all the ingredients to the Instant Pot.
2. Secure the lid and cook on manual for 8 minutes at high pressure.
3. After the beep, do a quick release and remove the lid.
4. Let it cool then blend the mixture using an immerse blender.
5. Stir in more cinnamon if needed and serve. You can store in the fridge for up to 10 days.

Nutrition Values:
Calories: 321
Carbohydrate: 62.2g
Protein: 1.2g
Fat: 10.1g
Sugar: 46.4g
Sodium: 6mg

APPLE BREAD PUDDING

Servings: 8
Preparation Time: 15 minutes
Cooking Time: 20 minutes

Ingredients

- 3 apples peeled, cored, and cubed
- 8 thick slices of bread, cubed, toasted
- 1 cup brown sugar
- 2 eggs
- 1 tablespoon vanilla extract
- 1 tablespoon cinnamon
- 3 cups milk
- 2/3 tablespoon cornstarch
- A pinch of salt
- Vanilla Sauce:
- Melt together: 2 tablespoon sugar, 2 tbs brown sugar, ¼ cup milk, 2 tbs butter, ½tbs vanilla

Directions

1. Butter a ½ quart glass dish that can in your instant pot. Add cubed bread.
2. Mix the milk, eggs, cinnamon, vanilla extract, and the salt.
3. Pour over bread, let sit for 10 to 20 minute. Mix the cornstarch and sugar. Stir apples into the mixture. Sprinkle over bread cubes.
4. Can cover with foil if mixture looks full.
5. Pour a cup of water into the Instant Pot and place the trivet inside.
6. Arrange the pan over the trivet. Secure the lid.
7. Cook on manual function for 20 minutes at high pressure.

8. After the beep, do a natural release and remove the lid. If desired, put under the broiler to crisp up the top.
9. Melt the ingredients for vanilla sauce on medium heat on the stove.
10. 1Drizzle the sauce over bread pudding and serve.

Nutrition Values:
Calories: 554
Carbohydrate: 95.4g
Protein: 5.1g
Fat: 18.5g
Sugar: 67g
Sodium: 234mg

ORANGE CHEESECAKE

Servings: 3
Preparation Time: 10 minutes
Cooking Time: 8 minutes

Ingredients
- 3 half pint mason jars
- 8 oz. cream cheese
- ¼ cup sugar
- ½ teaspoon flour
- ¼ teaspoon vanilla
- 2 tablespoons sour cream
- ½ tablespoon orange Juice
- zest of ¼ orange
- 1 ½ eggs
- ½ jar Greek yoghurt
- 3 raspberries
- 1 cup water

Directions
1. Beat the cream cheese, flour and sugar in a large bowl.
2. Add the sour cream, orange juice, zest, vanilla and eggs. Beat again.
3. Layer each Mason jar with the cheese batter and drop of yoghurt on top.
4. Pour a cup of water into the Instant Pot and place the trivet inside.
5. Cover the jars with aluminium foil and arrange them over the trivet.
6. Secure the lid and cook on manual for 8 minutes at high pressure.
7. After the beep, do a quick release and remove the lid.
8. Let the cakes cool then garnish with yoghurt and raspberries.
9. Serve.

Nutrition Values:
Calories: 382
Carbohydrate: 23.3g
Protein: 9.6g
Fat: 28.8g
Sugar: 19.3g
Sodium: 241mg

BANANA CHOCOLATE CHIP CAKE

Servings: 10
Preparation Time: 10 minutes
Cooking Time: 45 minutes

Ingredients
- 1 cup whole wheat flour
- A pinch of salt
- ½ teaspoon baking soda
- 6 tablespoons sugar
- 2 medium bananas mashed
- ½ tablespoon nutmeg
- 1/3 cups unsalted butter, melted
- 1/2 cup Greek yoghurt
- 1 tablespoon cinnamon
- 1 egg
- ½ cup white chocolate chips
- ¼ cups semi-sweet chocolate chips
- 1 teaspoon pure vanilla extract

Directions
1. Combine all the ingredients in a bowl and set aside.
2. Butter a 7-inch Bundt pan, pour batter in evenly.
3. Add 1 cup of water into the pot, place the Bundt pan into the instant pot. Cook on high pressure for 45 minutes.
4. Once done, do a 'natural' release.
5. Remove to a wire rack to cool for 10-15 minutes, then remove from the pan.
6. Serve or store for later use. You can store for up to 1 week.

Nutrition Values:
Calories: 332
Carbohydrate: 63.2g
Protein: 7.7g
Fat: 6.5g
Sugar: 35.4g
Sodium: 427mg

LEMON CHEESECAKE

Servings: 3
Preparation Time: 5 minutes
Cooking Time: 08 minutes

Ingredients
- 3 half pint mason jars
- 8 oz. cream cheese
- ¼ cup sugar
- ½ teaspoon flour

- ¼ teaspoon vanilla
- 2 tablespoons sour cream
- ½ tablespoon lemon juice
- zest of half lemon
- 1 ½ eggs
- ½ jar lemon curd
- 3 raspberries
- 1 cup water

Directions
1. Beat the cream cheese, flour and sugar in a large bowl.
2. Add the sour cream, lemon juice, zest, vanilla and eggs. Beat again.
3. Layer each Mason jar with the cheese batter and lemon curd on top.
4. Pour a cup of water into the Instant Pot and place the trivet inside.
5. Cover the jars with aluminium foil and arrange them over the trivet.
6. Secure the lid and cook on 'manual' function for 8 minutes at high pressure.
7. After the beep, do a quick release and remove the lid.
8. Let the cakes cool then garnish with lemon curd and raspberries.
9. Serve.

Nutrition Values:
Calories: 385
Carbohydrate: 23.6g
Protein: 8.9g
Fat: 28.5g
Sugar: 19.3g
Sodium: 237mg

RUM CHEESECAKE
Preparation Time 30 Minutes
Servings: 10
Ingredients:
- 2 cups almond flour
- 3 cups Mascarpone
- 1/4 cup coconut cream
- 4 large eggs; separated
- 1 cup plain Greek yogurt
- 2-3 drops stevia
- 2 tablespoon almond butter
- 1/4 cup cocoa powder; unsweetened.
- 1/4 cup swerve
- 3 teaspoon baking powder
- 1/2 teaspoon cinnamon powder
- 2 teaspoon rum extract

Directions:
1. Plug in the instant pot and position a trivet. Pour in one cup of water in the stainless steel insert and set aside
2. Beat egg whites and swerve with a hand mixer until light foam appears. Add egg yolks, coconut cream, almond butter, baking powder, and cocoa powder, beating constantly
3. Finally, add almond flour and continue to beat until completely combined.
4. Pour the mixture into lightly greased cake pan and cook for 15 minutes on the *Manual* mode.
5. When done; perform a quick pressure release and open the lid. Remove the cake from the pan and cool for a while
6. Now combine Mascarpone and Greek yogurt. Add rum extract, cinnamon powder, and stevia. Using a hand mixer, mix well until completely combined.
7. Pour the mixture over the crust and refrigerate for a couple of hours before slicing

Nutrition Value: Calories: 247; Total Fats: 18.1g; Net Carbs: 5.6g; Protein: 15.6g; Fiber: 1.7g

VANILLA CHOCOLATE BROWNIES
Preparation Time 40 Minutes
Servings: 8
Ingredients:
For the chocolate layer:
3/4 cup almond flour
1/4 cup coconut flour
5 eggs
3 tablespoon coconut cream
1/4 cup cocoa powder; unsweetened.
1 teaspoon baking powder
4 tablespoon granulated stevia
- 1/2 cup cream cheese

For the vanilla layer:
- 2 tablespoon granulated stevia
- 1/4 cup whipping cream
- 3 tablespoon shredded coconut
- 1/4 cup plain Greek yogurt
- 2 tablespoon butter
- 1 large egg
- 1 teaspoon vanilla extract
- 1 cup almond flour

Directions:
1. In a medium-sized bowl, combine together all the chocolate layer ingredients and beat well with a paddle attachment on medium-high speed, Set aside.
2. In a separate bowl, combine the remaining vanilla ingredients and beat until smooth.

3. Line a small cake pan with some parchment paper and dust with some cocoa powder. Add the chocolate layer and flatten the surface with a kitchen spatula
4. Pour in the vanilla mixture and shake the pan a couple of times
5. Loosely cover with aluminum foil and set aside
6. Plug in the instant pot and set the trivet at the bottom of the inner pot. Pour in one cup of water and add the cake pan.
7. Seal the lid and set the steam release handle to the *Sealing* position. Press the *Manual* button and cook for 25 minutes on high pressure.
8. When done, perform a quick pressure release and open the lid. Remove the cake pan from the pot and cool for a while
9. Slice into 8 brownies and serve.

Nutrition Value: Calories: 218; Total Fats: 17.7g; Net Carbs: 4.3g; Protein: 8.7g; Fiber: 3.8g

KETO COCONUT BARS

Preparation Time 25 Minutes
Servings: 6

Ingredients:
- 2 cups shredded coconut
- 1 tablespoon chia seeds
- 1 tablespoon sesame seeds
- 1/4 cup flaxseed meal
- 1/2 cup coconut oil
- 1/4 cup almonds; finely chopped.
- 2 tablespoon almond butter
- 3 large eggs
- 2 tablespoon granulated stevia
- 1 teaspoon vanilla extract
- 1/4 teaspoon salt

Directions:
1. Combine the ingredients in a large bowl and mix until a lightly sticky mixture forms. Optionally, add some more stevia and set aside.
2. Line a small baking pan with some parchment paper and lightly grease with some coconut oil. Add the mixture and press well with the palms of your hands to flatten the surface as evenly as possible
3. Loosely cover with aluminum foil and set aside.
4. Plug in the instant pot and set the trivet at the bottom of the inner pot. Pour in two cups of water and place the baking pan.
5. Seal the lid and set the steam release handle to the *Sealing* position. Cook for 15 minutes on the *Manual* mode.
6. When done; perform a quick pressure release and open the lid. Remove the pan and cool to a room temperature before slicing into bars
7. Refrigerate for one hour before serving

Nutrition Value: Calories: 376; Total Fats: 36.8g; Net Carbs: 2.9g; Protein: 7.2g; Fiber: 4.9g

KETO PECAN BROWNIES

Preparation Time 45 Minutes
Servings: 6

Ingredients:
- 4 tablespoon butter
- 1/4 cup pecans; finely chopped
- 1/2 cup almond flour
- 1/3 cup cocoa powder; unsweetened.
- 2 large eggs
- 1/3 cup swerve
- 4 tablespoon dark chocolate chips; sugar-free
- 2 tablespoon plain Greek yogurt
- 2 teaspoon baking powder
- 1/2 teaspoon cinnamon powder
- 1 teaspoon vanilla extract

Directions:
1. Line a small cake pan with some parchment paper and lightly coat with some cooking spray. Set asde
2. Plug in the instant pot and position a trivet at the bottom of the stainless steel insert. Pour in two cups of water and set aside.
3. In a large mixing bowl, combine together butter, eggs, and swerve. With a paddle attachment on, beat well for 2-3 minutes on medium-high speed
4. Gradually add almond flour and baking powder, beating constantly.
5. Finally, add the remaining ingredients and beat until completely incorporated. Transfer the dough to a clean work surface and shape approximately bite-size balls. Transfer half of the balls to the prepared cake pan and gently flatten each with the palm of your hand.
6. Loosely cover the pan with some aluminum foil and place in the pot. Seal the lid and set the steam release handle to the *Sealing* position. Press the *Manual* button and set the timer for 15 minutes on high pressure
7. When done; perform a quick pressure release and open the lid. Remove the pan from the pot and transfer cookies to a wire rack to cool

8. Repeat the process with the remaining dough

Nutrition Value: Calories: 202; Total Fats: 19.5g; Net Carbs: 2.8g; Protein: 5.1g; Fiber: 3g

CHOCO CINNAMON CAKE

Preparation Time 45 Minutes
Servings: 8
Ingredients:
1 cup coconut flour
1/2 cup granulated stevia
4 tablespoon almond butter
1/2 cup cream cheese
1/2 cup almonds; minced
1 tablespoon unsweetened cocoa powder
2 large eggs
1/4 teaspoon apple pie spice
1/4 teaspoon cinnamon; ground.
1/4 teaspoon salt

Directions:
1. Combine coconut flour, almonds, granulated stevia, salt, cinnamon, and apple pie spice in a large mixing bowl. Using a spatula, mix until combined.
2. Gradually, add eggs, butter, and cream cheese. Beat with a hand mixer until well incorporated.
3. Plug in your instant pot and pour 1 cup of water in the stainless steel insert. Set the trivet on the bottom.
4. Line a fitting springform pan with some parchment paper and grease the walls with some cooking spray. Pour in the mixture and cover the top with some aluminum foil.
5. Set the pan on top of the trivet and close the lid. Adjust the steam release handle and press the *Manual* button. Set the timer for 35 minutes on *High* pressure.
6. When you hear the cooker's end signal, perform a quick pressure release and open the pot. Using oven mitts, remove the pan to a wire rack and let it cool completely.
7. Sprinkle with cocoa and enjoy!

Nutrition Value: Calories: 285; Total Fats: 20.5g; Net Carbs: 7.9g; Protein: 10.4g; Fiber: 10.4g

KETO MOCHA BROWNIES

Preparation Time 45 Minutes
Servings: 6
Ingredients:
For the base:
- 6 eggs; separated
- 2 teaspoon baking powder
- 1 ½ cup swerve
- 3 tablespoon butter; unsalted
- 1 ½ cups of almond flour
- 1/4 teaspoon salt

For the topping:
- 1 ½ cup swerve or stevia crystal
- 2 butter sticks; unsalted
- 1/4 cup black coffee; unsweetened.
- 5 egg yolks

Directions:
1. Place egg whites in a large mixing bowl and beat on medium speed until light and fluffy. Add swerve, almond glour, melted butter, baking powder, and salt. Beat well on medium-high speed until completely incporporated.
2. Line a small cake pan with some parchment paper and add the batter. Tightly wrap with aluminum foil and set aside.
3. Plug in the instant pot and position a trivet at the bottom of the inner pot. Pour in some water and add the cake pan.
4. Securely seal the lid and set the steam release handle to the *Sealing* position. Press the *Manual* button and set the timer for 15 minutes on high pressure
5. When done, perform a quick pressure release and open the lid. Remove the pan from the pot and set aside to cool.
6. Now place a steam basket in the stainless steel insert and pour in some more water, Set aside
7. In a large mixing bowl, combine together the filling ingredients. With a whisking attachment on, beat well on medium-high speed for 2-3 minutes
8. Pour the mixture into an oven-safe bowl and wrap with aluminum foil. Place the bowl in the steam basket and seal the lid
9. Set the steam release handle and cook for 4 minutes on the *Manual* mode
10. When you hear the cooker's end signal, perform a quick pressure release and open the lid. Remove the bowl from the pot and chill for a while.
11. Pour the mixture over the crust and cool to a room temperature. Refrigerate for at least an hour before serving

Nutrition Value: Calories: 236; Total Fats: 21.1g; Net Carbs: 2.3g; Protein: 9.4g; Fiber: 0.8g

CHOCOLATE CUPCAKES

Preparation Time 20 Minutes
Servings: 6
Ingredients:

- 1 ½ cups of almond flour
- 1/4 cup cream cheese
- 1/4 cup swerve
- 2 tablespoon cocoa powder; unsweetened.
- 1 cup shredded coconut
- 2 large eggs
- 3 tablespoon butter
- 2 teaspoon baking powder
- 1/4 cup blueberries
- 3 tablespoon plain Greek yogurt
- 1 teaspoon vanilla extract

Directions:
1. In a large mixing bowl, combine together eggs and butter. Beat well on high speed until light and fluffy mixture. Then add swerve, cream cheese, and Greek yogurt. Continue to mix until smooth.
2. Finally, add almond flour, shredded coconut, and baking powder. Mix well again and fold in blueberries.
3. Divide the mixture between 6 silicone cups and set aside
4. Plug in the instant pot and position a trivet at the bottom of the inner pot. Pour in 1 cup of water and carefully place cups on the trivet
5. Seal the lid and set the steam release handle to the *Sealing* position. Set the timer for 10 minutes on the *Manual* mode
6. Perform a quick pressure release and open the lid. Remove the cups from the pot and cool to a room temperature

Nutrition Value: Calories: 212; Total Fats: 18.9g; Net Carbs: 4.2g; Protein: 6g; Fiber: 2.7g

COCONUT COHOCO BROWNIES
Preparation Time 1 hour 40 Minutes
Servings: 6

Ingredients:
- 1/2 cup shredded coconut
- 1 cup cream cheese
- 4 tablespoon raw cocoa; unsweetened.
- 1/2 cup almond flour
- 4 tablespoon coconut oil
- 2 tablespoon swerve
- 2 teaspoon baking powder
- 1/2 teaspoon cinnamon; ground.
- 1 teaspoon vanilla extract

Directions:
1. In a large mixing bowl, combine shredded coconut, almond flour, swerve, baking powder, and cocoa. Stir well until combined
2. Now; add cream cheese and coconut oil. Using a hand mixer, beat until all well incorporated. Add vanilla extract and cinnamon and beat again for a minute, Set aside.
3. Pour 1 cup of water in the stainless steel insert of your instant pot. Position a trivet on the bottom. Line a fitting springform pan with a parchment paper and pour in the prepared mixture. Gently spread with a spatula and flatten the surface.
4. Set the pan on top a trivet and close the lid. Adjust the steam release handle and press the *Manual* button. Set the timer for 30 minutes and cook on *High* pressure.
5. When done; perform a quick release of the pressure by moving the valve to the *Venting* position.
6. Open the pot and let it chill to a room temperature. Cut into brownies and serve immediately
7. Refrigerate up to 3 days

Nutrition Value: Calories: 260; Total Fats: 26.4g; Net Carbs: 3.3g; Protein: 4.3g; Fiber: 2g

RASPBERRY MUFFINS WITH CHOCOLATE TOPPING
Preparation Time 45 Minutes
Servings: 6

Ingredients:
- 1 cup fresh raspberries
- 1/4 cup coconut butter; melted
- 1 cup almond flour
- 1/4 cup granulated stevia
- 2 large eggs
- 1 teaspoon vanilla extract
- 1/4 cup whole milk
- 1 teaspoon baking powder
- 1/4 teaspoon salt
- For the topping:
- 1/4 teaspoon cinnamon; ground.
- 1/4 cup dark chocolate chips; melted
- 1/4 cup butter

Directions:
1. In a large mixing bowl, combine almond flour, stevia, baking powder, and salt. Mix until combined and set aside.
2. In a separate bowl, combine eggs, milk, and vanilla extract. Beat with a hand mixer until fluffy
3. Now; add the wet ingredients to the bowl with dry ingredients. Mix until you get a thick batter. Add raspberries and stir with a spatula.
4. Pour the mixture in silicone muffin molds and

set aside

5. Plug in the instant pot and pour 1 cup of water in the stainless steel insert. Set the trivet on the bottom and place molds on top
6. Close the lid and adjust the steam release handle. Press the *Manual* button and set the timer for 30 minutes. Cook on *High* pressure.
7. Meanwhile, combine all topping ingredients in a mixing bowl. Beat with a mixer until all well combined and creamy, Set aside.
8. When you hear the cooker's end signal, perform a quick pressure release and open the pot
9. Carefully transfer the muffins to a wire rack and let it cool completely.
10. Using a pipping bag, swirl the mixture over each muffin. Refrigerate for 15 minutes before serving

Nutrition Value: Calories: 193; Total Fats: 14.7g; Net Carbs: 4.2g; Protein: 7.1g; Fiber: 4.4g

MATCHA CHEESECAKE

Preparation Time 70 Minutes
Servings: 6

Ingredients:
- 16-ounce cream cheese; room temperature.
- 2 tablespoons heavy whipping cream
- 1/2 cup Swerve confectioners
- 2 teaspoon coconut flour
- 1/2 teaspoon vanilla extract
- 1 tablespoon matcha powder
- 2 large eggs; at room temperature.
- 1/2 cup sour cream
- 2 teaspoon Swerve confectioners
- 1 ½ cups water
- Sugar-free maple syrup

Directions:
1. Mix first six ingredients in a bowl. Add in the eggs one at a time
2. Pour the cheesecake batter into a well-greased springform pan that fits inside your Instant Pot.
3. Pour 1 ½ cups water into the bottom of your Instant Pot
4. Place the steam tray inside with the handles facing up. Put the cheesecake on top of the tray. Lock the lid and make sure the valve is sealed.
5. Pressure cook on high for 35 minutes, then allow a 20-minute natural pressure release
6. Mix the sour cream and Swerve confectioners together. Distribute evenly over the top of the cheesecake
7. Allow the cheesecake to fully cool then store in the fridge for 3 hours before serving. Making this the day ahead is best
8. Drizzle with sugar-free maple syrup, Serve

Nutrition Value: Calories: 350; Total Carbs: 6.64 g; Net Carbs: 5.8 g; Fat: 33 g; Protein: 8.4g

KETO MINT CAKE

Preparation Time 60 Minutes
Servings: 8

Ingredients:
For the layers:
- 1 cup almond flour
- 1 teaspoon vanilla extract
- 1 cup coconut flour
- 5 large eggs
- 1 tablespoon stevia powder
- 1/4 cup whole milk
- 3 tablespoon butter
- 1/2 teaspoon salt

For the filling:
- 2 teaspoon stevia powder
- 1/4 cup butter
- 1 teaspoon mint extract
- 1/2 cup cream cheese

Directions:
1. In a large mixing bowl, combine almond flour, coconut flour, stevia powder, and salt. Mix until combined and set aside.
2. In a separate bowl, combine eggs, butter, milk, and vanilla extract. Using a hand mixer, beat until fluffy and then gradually add to dry ingredients. Mix until all well incorporated, Set aside
3. In another bowl, combine all filling ingredients. With a paddle attachment on, beat until well combined and set aside.
4. Pour 1 cup of water in the stainless steel of your instant pot. Line a fitting springform pan with some parchment paper. Set the trivet on the bottom of the pot and place the pan on top. Pour half of the layer mixture in the pan and close the lid. Adjust the steam release handle and press the *Manual* button. Set the timer for 20 minutes and cook on *High* pressure
5. When you hear the cooker's end signal, perform a quick pressure release and open the pot. Transfer the layer to a wire rack to cool. Repeat the process with the remaining

mixture.
6. When the second layer is done, spread the filling over and top with the remaining layer. Close the lid of your pot and adjust the steam release handle. Press the *Manual* button and set the timer for 5 minutes on *High* pressure
7. When done; perform a quick pressure release and open the pot
8. Chill to a room temperature before serving and optionally, garnish with some fresh mint

Nutrition Value: Calories: 398; Total Fats: 33.8g; Net Carbs: 6.6g; Protein: 10.5g; Fiber: 7.5g

LEMON CAKE

Preparation Time 45 Minutes
Servings: 8

Ingredients:
For the cake:
- 3 cups almond flour
- 3 teaspoon baking powder
- 1/4 cup butter; softened
- 2 teaspoon lemon extract
- 5 large eggs
- 3 tablespoon stevia powder
- 1/4 cup coconut milk; full-fat
- 1 tablespoon coconut cream
- 1/4 teaspoon salt

For the syrup:
- 1 tablespoon lemon juice; freshly squeeze
- 1/4 cup granulated stevia
- 1/4 cup raspberries
- 1/4 cup blueberries

Directions:
1. In a large mixing bowl, combine together almond flour, stevia powder, baking powder, and salt.
2. Mix well and add eggs, one at the time, beating constantly.
3. Now add coconut milk, coconut cream, butter, and lemon extract. Using a paddle attachment beat for 3 minutes on medium speed.
4. Grease a small cake pan with some oil and line with parchment paper. Pour the mixture in it and tightly wrap with aluminum foil
5. Plug in the instant pot and set the trivet at the bottom of the inner pot. Place the cake pan on top and pour in one cup of water
6. Seal the lid and set the steam release handle to the *Sealing* position. Press the *Manual* button and cook for 25 minutes.
7. When done; perform a quick pressure release and open the lid. Carefully remove the pan and set aside
8. Now press the *Saute* button. Add berries and pour in one cup of water and granulated stevia. Gently simmer for 5-6 minutes, stirring constantly.
9. Finally, add agar powder and give it a good stir. Cook until the mixture thickens.
10. Pour the syrup over chilled cake and refrigerate for 2 hours before serving

Nutrition Value: Calories: 186; Total Fats: 16g; Net Carbs: 3.8g; Protein: 6.4g; Fiber: 1.3g

SWEET POTATO & CINNAMON PATTIES

Preparation Time 30 Minutes
Servings: 4

- **Ingredients:**
- 1 small sweet potato; cubed
- 1/2 cup Mascarpone
- 1/2 cup almond flour
- 1 tablespoon psyllium husk powder
- 3 tablespoon granulated stevia
- 1/4 cup flaxseed meal
- 3 tablespoon coconut oil; softened
- 1/2 teaspoon cinnamon powder
- 1 teaspoon vanilla extract

Directions:
1. Plug in the instant pot and add potatoes. Pour in enough water to cover and seal the lid. Set the steam release handle and cook for 3 minutes on the *Manual* mode.
2. When done, perform a quick pressure release and open the lid.
3. Remove potatoes from the pot and drain. Cool for a while and transfer to a food processor along with the remaining ingredients. Process until smooth
4. Now press the *Saute* button and grease the inner pot with some oil. Add about 1/4 cup of the potato mixture and cook for 3-4 minutes on one side
5. Gently turn over and continue to cook for another 2 minutes
6. Repeat the process with the remaining mixture
7. Optionally, sprinkle with some granulated stevia before serving

Nutrition Value: Calories: 213; Total Fats: 18.1g; Net Carbs: 4g; Protein: 5.8g; Fiber: 2.8g

CHOCOLATE CHIP PUDDING

Preparation Time 10 Minutes
Servings: 4

Ingredients:

- 1 cup unsweetened almond milk
- 1 tablespoon agar powder
- 1 ¼ cup whipping cream
- 2 tablespoon chocolate chips; sugar-free
- 1/2 cup coconut cream
- 1/4 cup swerve
- 1/4 cup almonds; finely chopped
- 2 tablespoon cocoa powder; unsweetened.
- 1 teaspoon vanilla extract

Directions:
1. Plug in the instant pot and pour in the milk. Press the *Saute* button and heat up. Add swerve, cocoa powder, coconut cream, and vanilla extract
2. Bring it to a boil, stirring constantly, and then add agar powder. Continue to cook for 1-2 minutes.
3. Press the *Cancel'* button and stir in finely chopped almonds.
4. Transfer the mixture to a large mixing bowl and pour in the whipping cream. Beat well on high speed for 2-3 minutes
5. Finally, divide the mixture between serving bowls and cool completely before serving

Nutrition Value: Calories: 257; Total Fats: 24.5g; Net Carbs: 6.5g; Protein: 3.9g; Fiber: 2.9g

CHOCO ORANGE MUFFINS
Preparation Time 45 Minutes
Servings: 5

Ingredients:
- 1/2 cup almond flour
- 5 large eggs
- 1 tablespoon flaxseed meal
- 1/4 cup almonds; roughly chopped
- 1 tablespoon chia seeds
- 1/2 cup whole milk
- 1 tablespoon butter
- 1 tablespoon dark chocolate chips
- 1/2 teaspoon baking powder
- 1/4 teaspoon bicarbonate of soda
- 1/4 teaspoon cinnamon; ground
- 1 teaspoon orange extract
- 2 teaspoon stevia powder

Directions:
1. In a large mixing bowl, combine almond flour, almonds, chia seeds, flaxseed meal, baking powder, and bicarbonate of soda. Mix until well combined
2. Add eggs, butter, milk, orange extract, stevia, and cinnamon. With a paddle attachment on, beat with a hand mixer for 2-3 minutes, or until well incorporated
3. Divide the mixture evenly between greased silicone muffin molds. Tuck in the chocolate chips and set aside
4. Plug in the instant pot and set the trivet on the bottom. Place the molds on top and close the lid. Adjust the steam release handle and press the *Manual* button. Set the timer for 30 minutes and cook on *High* pressure.
5. When done, perform a quick pressure release and open the pot. Transfer the molds to a wire rack and let it cool to a room temperature.

Nutrition Value: Calories: 246; Total Fats: 18.3g; Net Carbs: 4.9g; Protein: 11.8g; Fiber: 4.2g

KETO GLUTEN-FREE COCONUT ALMOND CAKE
Preparation Time 70 Minutes
Servings: 8

Ingredients:
Dry Ingredients
- 1 cup almond flour
- 1/3 cup Truvia baking blend
- 1/2 cup unsweetened coconut; shredded.
- 1 teaspoon baking powder
- 1 teaspoon apple pie spice

Wet ingredients
- 2 eggs; lightly whisked
- 1/4 cup butter; melted
- 1/2 cup heavy whipping cream

Directions:
1. Mix all dry ingredients in a large bowl
2. Pour in wet ingredients one by one, mixing well with each addition.
3. Pour into a springform loaf pan and cover the pan with foil.
4. Pour 2 cups of water into your Instant Pot liner, and place a trivet on top
5. Set your Instant Pot to high pressure for 40 minutes. When time is up, let pressure release naturally for 10 minutes, and release remaining pressure
6. Carefully take out the pan and let it chill for 15-20 minutes. Unclasp the sides and remove the cake and serve

Nutrition Value: Calories: 252 ; Total Carbs: 6 g; Net Carbs: 2.5 g; Fat: 24 g; Protein: 5g

CHOCO VANILLA PUDDING
Preparation Time 10 Minutes
Servings: 3

Ingredients:
- 1 cup cream cheese
- 5 large eggs whites
- 5 large egg yolks
- 1 teaspoon erythritol
- 1/4 cup coconut oil
- 3 teaspoon raw cocoa powder
- 1/2 teaspoon glucomannan powder
- 1/4 teaspoon nutmeg; ground.
- 1 teaspoon vanilla extract
- 1/2 teaspoon lemon zest; freshly grated

Directions:
1. Plug in the instant pot and place cream cheese in the stainless steel insert. Press the *Saute* button gently stir with a wooden spatula
2. Stir in the egg yolks, cocoa, erythritol, coconut oil, and glucomannan powder. Cook for 2-3 minutes, or until all well incorporated. Turn off the pot.
3. In a large bowl, combine egg whites, vanilla extract, and ground nutmeg. With a hand mixer, beat until foamy
4. Spoon the egg whites into the pot and give it a good stir.
5. Pour the mixture into a serving bowl while still hot. Set aside to cool completely
6. Refrigerate for 1 hour and optionally, sprinkle with some raw cocoa before serving

Nutrition Value: Calories: 554; Total Fats: 53.1g; Net Carbs: 4.2g; Protein: 16.7g; Fiber: 0.6g

KETO ORANGE NUT COOKIES

Preparation Time 35 Minutes
Servings: 8

Ingredients:
- 2 cups almond flour
- 1/2 cup almonds; finely chopped
- 4 eggs
- 1/4 cup coconut butter; melted
- 2 teaspoon baking powder
- 2 tablespoon sesame seeds
- 3 tablespoon swerve
- 1/4 cup Mascarpone
- 1 teaspoon orange extract
- 1/4 teaspoon salt

Directions:
1. In a large mixing bowl, combine together almond flour, melted coconut butter, eggs, swerve, Mascarpone, almonds, sesame seeds, orange extract, and salt.
2. With a dough hook attachment, beat well on high speed until completely incorporated
3. Dust a clean work surface with some almond flour and knead the dough until smooth
4. Shape bite-sized cookies and flatten each with the palm of your hand. Transfer to a small baking pan lined with some parchment paper
5. Plug in the instant pot and position a trivet. Pour in one cup of water and place the pan on top.
6. Seal the lid and set the steam release handle to the *Sealing* position. Press the *Manual* button and set the timer for 20 minutes on high pressure.
7. When done; perform a quick pressure release and open the lid. Cool for a while before serving

Nutrition Value: Calories: 228; Total Fats: 19.6g; Net Carbs: 3.5g; Protein: 7.8g; Fiber: 4.3g

FAVORITES

FAMILY-STYLE CANAPÉS
Preparation Time: 10 minutes
Servings 8
Nutrition Values: 112 Calories; 5.8g Fat; 1.2g Total Carbs; 12.8g Protein; 0.7g Sugars
Ingredients
- 1 pound tuna fillets
- 1/4 cup mayonnaise, preferably homemade
- 1/2 teaspoon dried dill
- 1/2 teaspoon sea salt
- 1/4 teaspoon ground black pepper, or more to taste
- 2 cucumbers, sliced

Directions
1. Prepare your Instant Pot by adding 1 ½ cups of water and steamer basket to the inner pot.
2. Place the tuna fillets in your steamer basket.
3. Secure the lid. Choose "Manual" mode and High pressure; cook for 4 minutes. Once cooking is complete, use a quick pressure release; carefully remove the lid. Flake the fish with a fork.
4. Add the mayonnaise, dill, salt, and black pepper. Divide the mixture among cucumber slices and place on a serving platter. Enjoy!

YUMMY EGG SALAD "SANDWICH"
Preparation Time: 25 minutes
Servings 4
Nutrition Values: 406 Calories; 37g Fat; 5.3g Total Carbs; 11.6g Protein; 2.2g Sugars
Ingredients
- 6 eggs
- 1/2 cup tablespoons mayonnaise
- 1 teaspoon Dijon mustard
- 1/2 cup cream cheese
- 1 cup baby spinach
- Salt and ground black pepper, to taste
- 2 red bell peppers, sliced into halves
- 2 green bell pepper, sliced into halves

Directions
1. Place 1 cup of water and a steamer basket in your Instant Pot. Next, place the eggs in the steamer basket.
2. Secure the lid. Choose "Manual" mode and Low pressure; cook for 5 minutes. Once cooking is complete, use a quick pressure release; carefully remove the lid.
3. Allow the eggs to cool for 15 minutes. Chop the eggs and combine them with mayonnaise, Dijon mustard, cheese, and baby spinach.
4. Season with salt and pepper. Divide the mixture between four bell pepper "sandwiches". Serve well chilled and enjoy!

BEEF TACO WRAPS
Preparation Time: 15 minutes
Servings 4
Nutrition Values: 219 Calories; 12.5g Fat; 2.7g Total Carbs; 24.1g Protein; 1.2g Sugars
Ingredients
- 1 tablespoon olive oil
- 1/2 red onion, chopped
- 1 pound ground chuck
- 1 bell pepper, seeded and sliced
- 1 teaspoon taco seasoning
- 1 cup beef stock
- Salt and ground black pepper, to taste

Directions
1. Press the "Sauté" button to heat up the Instant Pot. Now, heat the oil and sauté the onion until tender and translucent.
2. Then, add ground chuck and cook an additional 2 minutes or until no longer pink.
3. Then, add bell pepper, taco seasoning, stock, salt, and black pepper.
4. Secure the lid. Choose "Manual" mode and High pressure; cook for 5 minutes. Once cooking is complete, use a natural pressure release; carefully remove the lid.
5. To assemble taco wraps, place a few lettuce leaves on each serving plate. Divide the meat mixture between lettuce leaves. Add toppings of choice and serve. Bon appétit!

HOLIDAY FISH SANDWICHES
Preparation Time: 30 minutes
Servings 3
Nutrition Values: 280 Calories; 19.5g Fat; 4.1g Total Carbs; 22.3g Protein; 2.1g Sugars
Ingredients
- 1/4 cup fresh lemon juice
- 1 cup water
- 3 cod fillets
- 2 tablespoons butter, softened
- 1/2 teaspoon salt
- 1/4 teaspoon ground black pepper
- 1/4 teaspoon paprika

- 1/4 teaspoon dried dill weed
- 1 teaspoon Dijon mustard
- 8 lettuce leaves
- 1 cucumber, thinly sliced

Oopsies:
- 2 eggs, separated yolks and whites
- 1/4 teaspoon sea salt
- 3 ounces cream cheese
- 1/4 teaspoon baking powder

Directions
1. Place 1/4 cup of fresh lemon juice and water in the bottom of your Instant Pot. Add a steamer basket.
2. Rub the cod fillets with softened butter. Season with salt, black pepper, paprika, and dill. Place the fillets in the steamer basket.
3. Secure the lid. Choose "Manual" mode and Low pressure; cook for 3 minutes. Once cooking is complete, use a quick pressure release; carefully remove the lid.
4. To make your oopsies, beat the egg whites together with salt until very firm peaks form.
5. In another bowl, thoroughly combine the egg yolks with cream cheese. Now, add the baking powder and stir well.
6. Next, fold the egg white mixture into the egg yolk mixture. Divide the mixture into 6 oopsies and transfer them to a silicon sheet.
7. Bake in the preheated oven at 290 degrees F for about 23 minutes. Serve fish fillets between 2 oopsies, garnished with mustard, lettuce and cucumber. Enjoy!

KETO MUFFINS

Preparation Time: 10 minutes
Servings 6
Nutrition Values: 189 Calories; 13.4g Fat; 4.3g Total Carbs; 12.5g Protein; 2.8g Sugars
Ingredients
- 6 eggs
- 1/4 cup almond milk, unsweetened
- 1/2 teaspoon salt
- A pinch of ground allspice
- 1/2 teaspoon Mexican oregano
- 1/4 cup green onions, chopped
- 1 tomato, chopped
- 1 ½ cups bell peppers, chopped
- 1 jalapeño pepper, seeded and minced
- 1/2 cup Cotija cheese, crumbled

Directions
1. Prepare your Instant Pot by adding 1 ½ cups of water to the inner pot.
2. Spritz six ovenproof custard cups with a nonstick cooking spray.
3. In a mixing dish, thoroughly combine the eggs, milk, salt, allspice, and Mexican oregano; mix to combine well.
4. Add green onions, tomato, bell peppers, and jalapeño pepper to the custard cups. Pour the egg mixture over them. Top with cheese.
5. Lower 3 custard cups onto a metal trivet; then, place the second trivet on top. Lower the remaining 3 cups onto it.
6. Secure the lid. Choose "Manual" mode and High pressure; cook for 7 minutes. Once cooking is complete, use a quick pressure release; carefully remove the lid. Serve at room temperature.

BACON BISCUITS WITH CHEESE

Preparation Time: 20 minutes
Servings 6
Nutrition Values: 271 Calories; 23.8g Fat; 1.8g Total Carbs; 12.2g Protein; 1.2g Sugars
Ingredients
- 1 cup almond flour
- 1 teaspoon baking powder
- 1/2 teaspoon salt
- 1/4 teaspoon dried oregano
- 1/2 teaspoon dried basil
- 3 teaspoons butter, melted
- 3 eggs, whisked
- 1/2 cup double cream
- 6 ounces Colby cheese, grated
- 4 slices bacon, chopped

Directions
1. Start by adding 1 ½ cups of water and a metal rack to the Instant Pot. Line a cake pan with a piece of parchment paper.
2. Mix almond flour, baking powder, salt, oregano and basil until well combined.
3. Mix in the melted butter, eggs, and double cream; fold in the cheese and bacon; mix until everything is well incorporated.
4. Now, grab your dough, smoothen a little bit and roll it to 1/2-inch thickness. Then, cut down the cookies with a cookie cutter.
5. Arrange the cookies on the prepared cake pan and lower it onto the rack in your Instant Pot.
6. Secure the lid. Choose "Manual" mode and Low pressure; cook for 15 minutes. Once cooking is complete, use a natural pressure release; carefully remove the lid. Bon appétit!

SPECIAL CHICKEN LIVER MOUSSE

Preparation Time: 10 minutes

Servings 8
Nutrition Values: 143 Calories; 10.1g Fat; 2.2g Total Carbs; 10.4g Protein; 1.2g Sugars
Ingredients
- 1 pound chicken livers
- 1 Spanish onion, chopped
- 1/2 cup chicken stock
- 1/2 cup white wine
- 1 tablespoon olive oil
- 1 cup heavy cream
- 1/2 teaspoon dried basil
- 1/2 teaspoon dried oregano
- 1 sprig rosemary
- 1/4 teaspoon ground black pepper
- A pinch of salt
- A pinch of ground cloves

Directions
1. Simply mix all ingredients in your Instant Pot
2. Secure the lid. Choose "Manual" mode and High pressure; cook for 3 minutes. Once cooking is complete, use a quick pressure release; carefully remove the lid.
3. Afterwards, purée the mixture with an immersion blender until smooth and uniform. Serve with veggie sticks. Bon appétit!

CHICKEN LEGS WITH SPICY MAYO SAUCE

Preparation Time: 25 minutes
Servings 4
Nutrition Values: 484 Calories; 42.6g Fat; 2.4g Total Carbs; 22.3g Protein; 0.5g Sugars
Ingredients
- 4 chicken legs, bone-in, skinless
- 2 garlic cloves, peeled and halved
- 1/2 teaspoon coarse sea salt
- 1/4 teaspoon ground black pepper, or more to taste
- 1/2 teaspoon red pepper flakes, crushed
- 1 tablespoon olive oil
- 1/4 cup chicken broth

Dipping Sauce:
- 3/4 cup mayonnaise
- 2 tablespoons stone ground mustard
- 1 teaspoon fresh lemon juice
- 1/2 teaspoon Sriracha

Topping:
1/4 cup fresh cilantro, roughly chopped

Directions
1. Rub the chicken legs with garlic halves; then, season with salt, black pepper, and red pepper flakes. Press the "Sauté" button.
2. Once hot, heat the oil and sauté chicken legs for 4 to 5 minutes, turning once during cooking time. Add a splash of chicken broth to deglaze the bottom of the pan.
3. Secure the lid. Choose "Manual" mode and High pressure; cook for 14 minutes. Once cooking is complete, use a natural pressure release; carefully remove the lid.
4. Meanwhile, mix all ingredients for the dipping sauce; place in the refrigerator until ready to serve.
5. Garnish chicken legs with cilantro. Serve with the piquant mayo sauce on the side. Bon appétit!

HERBES DE PROVENCE CHICKEN DRUMETTES

Preparation Time: 15 minutes
Servings 6
Nutrition Values: 346 Calories; 18.3g Fat; 2.7g Total Carbs; 40.5g Protein; 0.9g Sugars
Ingredients
- 2 tablespoons olive oil
- 2 ½ pounds chicken drumettes, trimmed of fat
- 1 tomato, chopped
- 2 garlic cloves, sliced
- 1 tablespoon Herbes de Provence
- Sea salt, to taste
- 1/3 teaspoon ground black pepper
- 1/2 teaspoon paprika
- 1 cup water
- 2/3 cup mayonnaise
- 2 tablespoons Dijon mustard
- 1/2 lemon, cut into slices

Directions
1. Press the "Sauté" button. Heat the oil and brown chicken drumettes for 2 to 3 minutes on each side.
2. Add tomato, garlic, Herbes de Provence, salt, black pepper, paprika, and water.
3. Secure the lid. Choose "Manual" mode and High pressure; cook for 10 minutes. Once cooking is complete, use a natural pressure release; carefully remove the lid.
4. Serve with mayonnaise, mustard, and lemon slices. Bon appétit!

AROMATIC CHICKEN CHOWDER

Preparation Time: 20 minutes
Servings 5
Nutrition Values: 238 Calories; 17g Fat; 5.4g Total Carbs; 16.4g Protein; 2.6g Sugars

Ingredients
- 2 tablespoons grapeseed oil
- 2 banana shallots, chopped
- 4 cloves garlic, minced
- 1 cup Cremini mushrooms, sliced
- 2 bell peppers, seeded and sliced
- 1 serrano pepper, seeded and sliced
- 2 ripe tomatoes, pureed
- 1 teaspoon porcini powder
- 2 tablespoons dry white wine
- Sea salt and ground black pepper, to your liking
- 1 teaspoon dried basil
- 1/2 teaspoon dried dill weed
- 5 cups broth, preferably homemade
- 4 chicken wings

Directions
1. Press the "Sauté" button and heat the oil. Once hot, sauté the shallots until just tender and aromatic.
2. Add the garlic, mushrooms, and peppers; cook an additional 3 minutes or until softened.
3. Now, stir in tomatoes, porcini powder, white wine, salt, and black pepper. Add the remaining ingredients and stir to combine.
4. Secure the lid. Choose "Manual" mode and High pressure; cook for 18 minutes. Once cooking is complete, use a quick pressure release.
5. Make sure to release any remaining steam and carefully remove the lid. Remove the chicken wings from the Instant Pot. Discard the bones and chop the meat.
6. Add the chicken meat back to the Instant Pot. Ladle into individual bowls and serve warm. Bon appétit!

CHICKEN TACOS
Preparation Time: 30 minutes
Servings 6
Nutrition Values: 443 Calories; 17.3g Fat; 4.6g Total Carbs; 63.7g Protein; 1.7g Sugars
Ingredients
Low Carb Tortillas:
- 2 ounces pork rinds, crushed into a powder
- A pinch of baking soda
- A pinch of salt
- 2 ounces ricotta cheese
- 3 eggs
- 1/4 cup water
- Nonstick cooking spray

Chicken:
- 1 ½ pounds chicken legs, skinless
- 4 cloves garlic, pressed or chopped
- 1/2 cup scallions, chopped
- 1 teaspoon dried basil
- 1/2 teaspoon dried thyme
- 1/2 teaspoon dried rosemary
- 1 teaspoon dried oregano
- Sea salt, to your liking
- 1/3 teaspoon ground black pepper
- 1/4 cup freshly squeezed lemon juice
- 1 cup water
- 1/4 cup dry white wine
- 1/2 cup salsa, preferably homemade

Directions
1. To make low carb tortillas, add pork rinds, baking soda, and salt to your food processor; pulse a few times.
2. Now, fold in the cheese and eggs; mix until well combined. Add the water and process until smooth and uniform.
3. Spritz a pancake pan with a nonstick cooking spray. Preheat the pancake pan over moderate heat.
4. Now, pour the batter into the pan and prepare like you would a tortilla. Reserve keeping the tortillas warm.
5. Then, press the "Sauté" button and cook chicken legs for 2 to 4 minutes per side; reserve. Add the garlic and scallions and cook until aromatic.
6. Add the remaining ingredients, except for salsa. Return the chicken legs back to the Instant Pot.
7. Secure the lid. Choose the "Poultry" setting and cook for 15 minutes. Once cooking is complete, use a quick pressure release; carefully remove the lid.
8. Shred the chicken with two forks and discard the bones; serve with prepared tortillas and salsa. Enjoy!

TRADITIONAL CHICKEN STEW
Preparation Time: 25 minutes
Servings 6
Nutrition Values: 453 Calories; 22.6g Fat; 5.9g Total Carbs; 53.6g Protein; 2.6g Sugars
Ingredients
- 2 slices bacon
- 6 chicken legs, skinless and boneless
- 3 cups water
- 2 chicken bouillon cubes
- 1 leek, chopped

- 1 carrot, trimmed and chopped
- 4 garlic cloves, minced
- 1/2 teaspoon dried thyme
- 1/2 teaspoon dried basil
- 1 teaspoon Hungarian paprika
- 1 bay leaf
- 1 cup double cream
- 1/2 teaspoon ground black pepper

Directions
1. Press the "Sauté" button to heat up your Instant Pot. Now, cook the bacon, crumbling it with a spatula; cook until the bacon is crisp and reserve.
2. Now, add the chicken legs and cook until browned on all sides.
3. Add the water, bouillon cubes, leeks, carrot, garlic, thyme, basil, paprika, and bay leaf; stir to combine.
4. Secure the lid. Choose the "Poultry" setting and cook for 15 minutes at High pressure. Once cooking is complete, use a natural pressure release; carefully remove the lid.
5. Fold in the cream and allow it to cook in the residual heat, stirring continuously. Ladle into individual bowls, sprinkle each serving with freshly grated black pepper and serve warm. Bon appétit!

CHICKEN TERIYAKI

Preparation Time: 15 minutes
Servings 6

Nutrition Values: 326 Calories; 13.2g Fat; 3.1g Total Carbs; 45.6g Protein; 0.7g Sugars

Ingredients
- 1/3 cup coconut aminos
- 1/4 cup rice wine vinegar
- 3 tablespoons Mirin
- 8 drops liquid stevia
- 1 tablespoon cornstarch
- 1/3 cup water
- 2 tablespoons olive oil
- 2 pounds chicken legs, boneless and skinless
- 1 teaspoon garlic powder
- 1 teaspoon ginger powder
- Sea salt and black pepper, to taste
- 1/2 teaspoon sweet paprika
- 2/3 cup chicken stock

Directions
1. Press the "Sauté" button to heat up your Instant Pot. Now, add the coconut aminos, vinegar, Mirin, liquid stevia, and cornstarch; whisk to combine well.
2. Now, pour in water and cook, bringing to a boil; cook until the liquid is thickened; reserve teriyaki sauce.
3. Wipe down the Instant Pot with a damp cloth; then, heat olive oil and cook the chicken until browned. Add garlic powder and ginger powder.
4. Season with salt, black pepper, and paprika.
5. Add chicken stock and 2/3 of teriyaki sauce; stir to combine. Secure the lid. Choose the "Manual" setting and cook for 10 minutes.
6. Once cooking is complete, use a natural pressure release; carefully remove the lid. Serve with the remaining 1/3 of teriyaki sauce and enjoy!

SIMPLE CHICKEN CARNITAS

Preparation Time: 20 minutes
Servings 8

Nutrition Values: 294 Calories; 15.4g Fat; 2.8g Total Carbs; 35.2g Protein; 1.3g Sugars

Ingredients
- 3 pounds whole chicken, cut into pieces
- 3 cloves garlic, pressed
- 1 guajillo chili, minced
- 1 tablespoon avocado oil
- 1/3 cup roasted vegetable broth
- Sea salt, to taste
- 1/2 teaspoon ground bay leaf
- 1/3 teaspoon cayenne pepper
- 1/2 teaspoon paprika
- 1/3 teaspoon black pepper
- 1 cup crème fraiche, to serve
- 2 heaping tablespoons fresh coriander, chopped

Directions
1. Place all of the above ingredients, except for crème fraiche and fresh coriander, in the Instant Pot.
2. Secure the lid. Choose the "Poultry" setting and cook for 15 minutes. Once cooking is complete, use a quick pressure release; carefully remove the lid.
3. Shred the chicken with two forks and discard the bones. Add a dollop of crème fraiche to each serving and garnish with fresh coriander. Enjoy!

THE BEST TURKEY LEGS

Preparation Time: 40 minutes
Servings 6

Nutrition Values: 339 Calories; 19.3g Fat; 1.3g Total Carbs; 37.7g Protein; 0.4g Sugars

Ingredients
- 3 tablespoons sesame oil
- 2 pounds turkey legs
- Sea salt and ground black pepper, to your liking
- A bunch of scallions, roughly chopped
- 1 ½ cups turkey broth

Directions
1. Press the "Sauté" button and heat the sesame oil. Now, brown turkey legs on all sides; season with salt and black pepper.
2. Add the scallions and broth.
3. Secure the lid. Choose the "Manual" setting and cook for 35 minutes. Once cooking is complete, use a natural pressure release; carefully remove the lid.
4. You can thicken the cooking liquid on the "Sauté" setting if desired. Serve warm.

OLD-FASHIONED PAPRIKASH

Preparation Time: 25 minutes
Servings 6
Nutrition Values: 402 Calories; 31.7g Fat; 6.1g Total Carbs; 21g Protein; 2.4g Sugars

Ingredients
- 1 tablespoon lard, at room temperature
- 1 ½ pounds chicken thighs
- 1/2 cup tomato puree
- 1 ½ cups water
- 1 yellow onion, chopped
- 1 large-sized carrot, sliced
- 1 celery stalk, diced
- 2 garlic cloves, minced
- 2 bell peppers, seeded and chopped
- 1 Hungarian wax pepper, seeded and minced
- 1 teaspoon cayenne pepper
- 1 tablespoon Hungarian paprika
- 1 teaspoon coarse salt
- 1/2 teaspoon ground black pepper
- 1/2 teaspoon poultry seasoning
- 6 ounces sour cream
- 1 tablespoon arrowroot powder
- 1 cup water

Directions
1. Press the "Sauté" button to heat up the Instant Pot. Now, melt the lard until hot; sear the chicken thighs for 2 to 3 minutes per side.
2. Add the tomato puree, 1 ½ cups of water, onion, carrot, celery, garlic, peppers, and seasonings.
3. Secure the lid. Choose the "Manual" setting and cook for 20 minutes at High pressure. Once cooking is complete, use a quick pressure release; carefully remove the lid.
4. In the meantime, thoroughly combine sour cream, arrowroot powder and 1 cup of water; whisk to combine well.
5. Add the sour cream mixture to the Instant Pot to thicken the cooking liquid. Cook for a couple of minutes on the residual heat.
6. Ladle into individual bowls and serve immediately.

CHICKEN FILLETS WITH CHEESE AND CREAM

Preparation Time: 25 minutes
Servings 6
Nutrition Values: 450 Calories; 24.1g Fat; 2.5g Total Carbs; 53.6g Protein; 0.2g Sugars

Ingredients
- 1 ¼ cups water
- 10 ounces Ricotta cheese, crumbled
- 6 chicken fillets
- Salt, to taste
- 1/2 teaspoon cayenne pepper
- 6 tablespoons bacon crumbles
- 4 ounces Monterey-Jack cheese
- 1 tablespoon chicken bouillon granules

Directions
1. Add water to the bottom of the Instant Pot. Add Ricotta cheese and chicken fillets; sprinkle with salt and cayenne pepper.
2. Secure the lid. Choose "Manual" mode and High pressure; cook for 18 minutes. Once cooking is complete, use a quick pressure release.
3. Now, shred the chicken with two forks and return it back to the Instant Pot. Stir in bacon crumbles, cheese, and chicken bouillon granules.
4. Place the lid back on the Instant Pot, press the "Sauté" button and cook an additional 4 minutes. Divide among serving plates and serve immediately. Bon appétit!

YUMMY CHICKEN DRUMSTICKS

Preparation Time: 20 minutes
Servings 6
Nutrition Values: 351 Calories; 15.7g Fat; 5g Total Carbs; 43.5g Protein; 2.3g Sugars

Ingredients
- 2 ripe tomatoes, chopped
- 1/2 cup roasted vegetable broth, preferably homemade

- 1 red onion, chopped
- 1 red bell pepper, seeded and chopped
- 1 green bell pepper, seeded and chopped
- 4 cloves garlic
- 1 teaspoon curry powder
- 1/2 teaspoon paprika
- 1/4 teaspoon ground black pepper
- Sea salt, to taste
- A pinch of grated nutmeg
- 1/2 teaspoon ground cumin
- 2 pounds chicken drumsticks, boneless, skinless
- 2 tablespoons butter
- 1/3 cup double cream
- 1 tablespoon flaxseed meal

Directions
1. Add tomatoes, vegetable broth, onion, peppers, garlic, curry powder, paprika, black pepper, salt, grated nutmeg, and ground cumin to the bottom of your Instant Pot.
2. Add chicken drumsticks. Secure the lid. Choose "Manual" mode and High pressure; cook for 12 minutes. Once cooking is complete, use a natural pressure release.
3. Allow it to cool completely and reserve the chicken.
4. In a mixing dish, whisk the remaining ingredients and add this mixture to the Instant Pot; press the "Sauté" button and bring it to a boil.
5. Now, add the chicken back to the cooking liquid. Press the "Cancel" button and serve immediately. Bon appétit!

SPECIAL BEEF SALAD
Preparation Time: 1 hour 35 minutes
Servings 6
Nutrition Values: 346 Calories; 24.8g Fat; 5.7g Total Carbs; 24.2g Protein; 2.1g Sugars
Ingredients
- 1 tablespoon champagne vinegar
- 1/3 cup dry white wine
- 2 tablespoons Shoyu sauce
- 1 cup broth, preferably homemade
- 1 teaspoon finely grated fresh ginger
- 1 tablespoon stone-ground mustard
- 1 teaspoon celery seeds
- 1 ½ pounds beef rump steak
- 1 cup green onions, chopped
- 1 cup cherry tomatoes, halved
- 2 cucumbers, thinly sliced
- 1 bunch fresh coriander, leaves picked
- 1 bunch fresh mint, leaves picked
- 2 tablespoons fresh chives, chopped
- 2 tablespoons fresh lemon juice
- 2 tablespoons extra-virgin olive oil

Directions
1. In a mixing dish, thoroughly combine the vinegar, white wine, Shoyu sauce, broth, fresh ginger, mustard, and celery seeds.
2. Add the beef steak and allow it to marinate for 40 minutes to 1 hour in your refrigerator.
3. Add beef steak, along with its marinade to the Instant Pot. Add enough water to cover the beef.
4. Secure the lid. Choose "Meat/Stew" mode and High pressure; cook for 35 minutes. Once cooking is complete, use a natural pressure release; carefully remove the lid.
5. Allow the beef to cool completely. Now, slice it into strips and transfer to a nice salad bowl.
6. Now, add the vegetables, coriander, mint, and fresh chives; toss to combine. Afterwards, drizzle the salad with lemon juice and olive oil. Toss to combine and serve well-chilled. Bon appétit!

COZY BEEF SOUP
Preparation Time: 20 minutes
Servings 6
Nutrition Values: 239 Calories; 14.2g Fat; 4.5g Total Carbs; 24g Protein; 1.6g Sugars
Ingredients
- 2 tablespoons butter, at room temperature
- 1 ½ pounds beef short ribs
- 6 cups water
- 2 cloves garlic, smashed
- 1 cup scallions, chopped
- 1 carrot, chopped
- 1 celery, chopped
- 3 beef stock cubes
- Kosher salt and ground black pepper, to taste
- 1 cup Swiss chard, torn into pieces

Directions
1. Press the "Sauté" button to heat up the Instant Pot. Then, melt the butter; once hot, cook the ribs for 2 to 4 minutes on each side.
2. Add the water, garlic, scallions, carrot, celery, beef stock cube, salt, and black pepper to the Instant Pot.
3. Choose "Manual" mode and High pressure; cook for 15 minutes. Once cooking is complete, use a natural pressure release; carefully remove the lid.

MEXICAN-STYLE BEEF CHILI

Preparation Time: 15 minutes
Servings 6

Nutrition Values: 238 Calories; 13.6g Fat; 6g Total Carbs; 23.8g Protein; 2.8g Sugars

Ingredients
- 2 tablespoons olive oil
- 1 ½ pounds ground chuck
- 1 green bell pepper, chopped
- 1 red bell pepper, chopped
- 2 red chilies, minced
- 1 red onion
- 2 garlic cloves, smashed
- 1 teaspoon cumin
- 1 teaspoon Mexican oregano
- 1 teaspoon cayenne pepper
- 1 teaspoon smoked paprika
- Salt and freshly ground black pepper, to taste
- 1 ½ cups puréed tomatoes
- 4 cups kale, fresh

Directions
1. Press the "Sauté" button to heat up the Instant Pot. Then, heat the oil; once hot, cook the ground chuck for 2 minutes, crumbling it with a fork or a wide spatula.
2. Add the pepper, onions, and garlic; cook an additional 2 minutes or until fragrant. Stir in the remaining ingredients, minus kale leaves.
3. Choose the "Manual" setting and cook for 6 minutes at High pressure. Once cooking is complete, use a natural pressure release; carefully remove the lid.
4. Add kale, cover with the lid and allow the kale leaves to wilt completely. Bon appétit!

HOT AND SPICY BEEF CURRY

Preparation Time: 30 minutes
Servings 6

Nutrition Values: 446 Calories; 21.5g Fat; 5g Total Carbs; 60g Protein; 2.1g Sugars

Ingredients
- 1 teaspoon coconut oil
- 2 pounds beef braising steak, cut into bite-sized pieces
- 1/2 cup banana shallots, chopped
- 1 ½ tablespoons curry powder
- 1 cinnamon stick
- 2 cloves garlic, crushed
- 1 teaspoon fresh ginger, peeled and grated
- 1 cup full-fat coconut milk
- Sea salt and freshly ground black pepper, to taste
- 1 teaspoon chili powder
- 1/2 teaspoon paprika
- 1/2 teaspoon ground cumin
- 8 ounces natural yogurt
- 2 teaspoons garam masala
- 1 handful fresh coriander, chopped

Directions
1. Press the "Sauté" button to heat up the Instant Pot. Then, warm the coconut oil and cook the beef approximately 3 minutes, stirring occasionally.
2. Add shallots and cook for 2 minutes longer or until they're softened.
3. Add the curry powder, cinnamon, garlic, ginger, milk, salt, black pepper, chili powder, paprika, and cumin; stir to combine well.
4. Secure the lid. Choose "Meat/Stew" mode and High pressure; cook for 20 minutes. Once cooking is complete, use a quick pressure release; carefully remove the lid.
5. Afterwards, add natural yogurt and garam masala; cover and let it stand until heated through. Bon appétit!
1.

1000-DAY MEAL

DAY	BREAKFAST	LUNCH/DINNER	DESSERT
1	Mixed Mushroom Pate	Rice With Chicken And Veggies	Coconut Cake
2	Black Bean & Egg Casserole	Tomato Cream	Yogurt Vanilla Lighter Cheesecake
3	Chicken Liver Breakfast	Carrot Soup	Molten Lava Cake
4	Spice Oatmeal	Simple Chili	Stuffed Peaches
5	Barbeque Tofu	Lentils Soup	Blueberry Jam
6	Instant Pot Cauliflower Soup	Easy Chicken Cacciatore	Vanilla Rice Pudding
7	Beef Bourguignon Recipe	Sweet Paprika Pork Chops	Pressure Cooked Brownies
8	Beef Kale Patties	Simple Pork Roast	Almond Tapioca Pudding
9	Eggs with Mushrooms	Mackerel And Orange Sauce	Lemon and Blackberry Compote
10	Coconut Cherry Pancakes	Fish Curry	Caramel Flan
11	Chicken with Spinach	Shrimp And Tomatoes Mix	Poached Gingery Orange Pears
12	Pork with Mushrooms	Cabbage And Beef Stew	Pear Ricotta Cake
13	Mushroom Chicken with Eggs	Lemon Shrimp	Peach Crumb
14	Keto Vanilla Chia Seeds	Fish Soup	Gingery Applesauce
15	Turkey Soup	Italian Shrimp Mix	Blondies with Peanut Butter
16	Beef Chuck Shoulder Roast Stew	Coconut Chicken Mix	Strawberry Cream
17	Cinnamon Bars	Broccoli Cream	Berry Compote
18	Eggs with Scallions	Salmon, Peas And Parsley Dressing	Creamy Coconut Peach Dessert
19	Mushroom and Eggs Casserole	Shrimp, Tomatoes And Potatoes	Banana and Almond Butter Bars
20	Bacon Brussels Sprouts	Tomato Shrimp	Fruity Sauce with Apples
21	Almond Porridge	Chili Salmon	Brown Fudge Cake
22	Raspberry Mug Cake	Mexican Pork and Okra Salad	Cherry Cheesecake
23	Chicken Veal Stew	Pork and Kale Meatballs	Tapioca Pudding
24	Cinnamon Pancakes	Pork and Baby Spinach	Chocolate Crème Brûlée
25	Beef Stew with Eggplants	Cinnamon Turkey Curry	Nutmeg Apple Crisp
26	Beef Black Pepper Stew	Cod and Tomato Passata	Crème Brûlée
27	Deviled Eggs	Mushroom and Chicken Soup	Almond Cheesecake
28	Pork Tenderloin Stew	Basil Shrimp and Eggplants	Maple-Glazed Flan
29	Lamb Stew	Chicken and Mustard Sauce	Blueberry Cheesecake
30	Beef Chili	Chicken and Avocado Mix	Chocolate Cheesecake
31	Mixed Mushroom Pate	Rice With Chicken And Veggies	Coconut Cake
32	Black Bean & Egg Casserole	Tomato Cream	Yogurt Vanilla Lighter Cheesecake
33	Chicken Liver Breakfast	Carrot Soup	Molten Lava Cake
34	Spice Oatmeal	Simple Chili	Stuffed Peaches
35	Barbeque Tofu	Lentils Soup	Blueberry Jam
36	Instant Pot Cauliflower Soup	Easy Chicken Cacciatore	Vanilla Rice Pudding
37	Beef Bourguignon Recipe	Sweet Paprika Pork Chops	Pressure Cooked Brownies
38	Beef Kale Patties	Simple Pork Roast	Almond Tapioca Pudding
39	Eggs with Mushrooms	Mackerel And Orange Sauce	Lemon and Blackberry Compote

40	Coconut Cherry Pancakes	Fish Curry	Caramel Flan
41	Chicken with Spinach	Shrimp And Tomatoes Mix	Poached Gingery Orange Pears
42	Pork with Mushrooms	Cabbage And Beef Stew	Pear Ricotta Cake
43	Mushroom Chicken with Eggs	Lemon Shrimp	Peach Crumb
44	Keto Vanilla Chia Seeds	Fish Soup	Gingery Applesauce
45	Turkey Soup	Italian Shrimp Mix	Blondies with Peanut Butter
46	Beef Chuck Shoulder Roast Stew	Coconut Chicken Mix	Strawberry Cream
47	Cinnamon Bars	Broccoli Cream	Berry Compote
48	Eggs with Scallions	Salmon, Peas And Parsley Dressing	Creamy Coconut Peach Dessert
49	Mushroom and Eggs Casserole	Shrimp, Tomatoes And Potatoes	Banana and Almond Butter Bars
50	Bacon Brussels Sprouts	Tomato Shrimp	Fruity Sauce with Apples
51	Almond Porridge	Chili Salmon	Brown Fudge Cake
52	Raspberry Mug Cake	Mexican Pork and Okra Salad	Cherry Cheesecake
53	Chicken Veal Stew	Pork and Kale Meatballs	Tapioca Pudding
54	Cinnamon Pancakes	Pork and Baby Spinach	Chocolate Crème Brûlée
55	Beef Stew with Eggplants	Cinnamon Turkey Curry	Nutmeg Apple Crisp
56	Beef Black Pepper Stew	Cod and Tomato Passata	Crème Brûlée
57	Deviled Eggs	Mushroom and Chicken Soup	Almond Cheesecake
58	Pork Tenderloin Stew	Basil Shrimp and Eggplants	Maple-Glazed Flan
59	Lamb Stew	Chicken and Mustard Sauce	Blueberry Cheesecake
60	Beef Chili	Chicken and Avocado Mix	Chocolate Cheesecake
61	Mixed Mushroom Pate	Rice With Chicken And Veggies	Coconut Cake
62	Black Bean & Egg Casserole	Tomato Cream	Yogurt Vanilla Lighter Cheesecake
63	Chicken Liver Breakfast	Carrot Soup	Molten Lava Cake
64	Spice Oatmeal	Simple Chili	Stuffed Peaches
65	Barbeque Tofu	Lentils Soup	Blueberry Jam
66	Instant Pot Cauliflower Soup	Easy Chicken Cacciatore	Vanilla Rice Pudding
67	Beef Bourguignon Recipe	Sweet Paprika Pork Chops	Pressure Cooked Brownies
68	Beef Kale Patties	Simple Pork Roast	Almond Tapioca Pudding
69	Eggs with Mushrooms	Mackerel And Orange Sauce	Lemon and Blackberry Compote
70	Coconut Cherry Pancakes	Fish Curry	Caramel Flan
71	Chicken with Spinach	Shrimp And Tomatoes Mix	Poached Gingery Orange Pears
72	Pork with Mushrooms	Cabbage And Beef Stew	Pear Ricotta Cake
73	Mushroom Chicken with Eggs	Lemon Shrimp	Peach Crumb
74	Keto Vanilla Chia Seeds	Fish Soup	Gingery Applesauce
75	Turkey Soup	Italian Shrimp Mix	Blondies with Peanut Butter
76	Beef Chuck Shoulder Roast Stew	Coconut Chicken Mix	Strawberry Cream
77	Cinnamon Bars	Broccoli Cream	Berry Compote
78	Eggs with Scallions	Salmon, Peas And Parsley Dressing	Creamy Coconut Peach Dessert
79	Mushroom and Eggs Casserole	Shrimp, Tomatoes And Potatoes	Banana and Almond Butter Bars
80	Bacon Brussels Sprouts	Tomato Shrimp	Fruity Sauce with Apples
81	Almond Porridge	Chili Salmon	Brown Fudge Cake
82	Raspberry Mug Cake	Mexican Pork and Okra Salad	Cherry Cheesecake

83	Chicken Veal Stew	Pork and Kale Meatballs	Tapioca Pudding
84	Cinnamon Pancakes	Pork and Baby Spinach	Chocolate Crème Brûlée
85	Beef Stew with Eggplants	Cinnamon Turkey Curry	Nutmeg Apple Crisp
86	Beef Black Pepper Stew	Cod and Tomato Passata	Crème Brûlée
87	Deviled Eggs	Mushroom and Chicken Soup	Almond Cheesecake
88	Pork Tenderloin Stew	Basil Shrimp and Eggplants	Maple-Glazed Flan
89	Lamb Stew	Chicken and Mustard Sauce	Blueberry Cheesecake
90	Beef Chili	Chicken and Avocado Mix	Chocolate Cheesecake
91	Mixed Mushroom Pate	Rice With Chicken And Veggies	Coconut Cake
92	Black Bean & Egg Casserole	Tomato Cream	Yogurt Vanilla Lighter Cheesecake
93	Chicken Liver Breakfast	Carrot Soup	Molten Lava Cake
94	Spice Oatmeal	Simple Chili	Stuffed Peaches
95	Barbeque Tofu	Lentils Soup	Blueberry Jam
96	Instant Pot Cauliflower Soup	Easy Chicken Cacciatore	Vanilla Rice Pudding
97	Beef Bourguignon Recipe	Sweet Paprika Pork Chops	Pressure Cooked Brownies
98	Beef Kale Patties	Simple Pork Roast	Almond Tapioca Pudding
99	Eggs with Mushrooms	Mackerel And Orange Sauce	Lemon and Blackberry Compote
100	Coconut Cherry Pancakes	Fish Curry	Caramel Flan
101	Chicken with Spinach	Shrimp And Tomatoes Mix	Poached Gingery Orange Pears
102	Pork with Mushrooms	Cabbage And Beef Stew	Pear Ricotta Cake
103	Mushroom Chicken with Eggs	Lemon Shrimp	Peach Crumb
104	Keto Vanilla Chia Seeds	Fish Soup	Gingery Applesauce
105	Turkey Soup	Italian Shrimp Mix	Blondies with Peanut Butter
106	Beef Chuck Shoulder Roast Stew	Coconut Chicken Mix	Strawberry Cream
107	Cinnamon Bars	Broccoli Cream	Berry Compote
108	Eggs with Scallions	Salmon, Peas And Parsley Dressing	Creamy Coconut Peach Dessert
109	Mushroom and Eggs Casserole	Shrimp, Tomatoes And Potatoes	Banana and Almond Butter Bars
110	Bacon Brussels Sprouts	Tomato Shrimp	Fruity Sauce with Apples
111	Almond Porridge	Chili Salmon	Brown Fudge Cake
112	Raspberry Mug Cake	Mexican Pork and Okra Salad	Cherry Cheesecake
113	Chicken Veal Stew	Pork and Kale Meatballs	Tapioca Pudding
114	Cinnamon Pancakes	Pork and Baby Spinach	Chocolate Crème Brûlée
115	Beef Stew with Eggplants	Cinnamon Turkey Curry	Nutmeg Apple Crisp
116	Beef Black Pepper Stew	Cod and Tomato Passata	Crème Brûlée
117	Deviled Eggs	Mushroom and Chicken Soup	Almond Cheesecake
118	Pork Tenderloin Stew	Basil Shrimp and Eggplants	Maple-Glazed Flan
119	Lamb Stew	Chicken and Mustard Sauce	Blueberry Cheesecake
120	Beef Chili	Chicken and Avocado Mix	Chocolate Cheesecake
121	Mixed Mushroom Pate	Rice With Chicken And Veggies	Coconut Cake
122	Black Bean & Egg Casserole	Tomato Cream	Yogurt Vanilla Lighter Cheesecake
123	Chicken Liver Breakfast	Carrot Soup	Molten Lava Cake
124	Spice Oatmeal	Simple Chili	Stuffed Peaches
125	Barbeque Tofu	Lentils Soup	Blueberry Jam

126	Instant Pot Cauliflower Soup	Easy Chicken Cacciatore	Vanilla Rice Pudding
127	Beef Bourguignon Recipe	Sweet Paprika Pork Chops	Pressure Cooked Brownies
128	Beef Kale Patties	Simple Pork Roast	Almond Tapioca Pudding
129	Eggs with Mushrooms	Mackerel And Orange Sauce	Lemon and Blackberry Compote
130	Coconut Cherry Pancakes	Fish Curry	Caramel Flan
131	Chicken with Spinach	Shrimp And Tomatoes Mix	Poached Gingery Orange Pears
132	Pork with Mushrooms	Cabbage And Beef Stew	Pear Ricotta Cake
133	Mushroom Chicken with Eggs	Lemon Shrimp	Peach Crumb
134	Keto Vanilla Chia Seeds	Fish Soup	Gingery Applesauce
135	Turkey Soup	Italian Shrimp Mix	Blondies with Peanut Butter
136	Beef Chuck Shoulder Roast Stew	Coconut Chicken Mix	Strawberry Cream
137	Cinnamon Bars	Broccoli Cream	Berry Compote
138	Eggs with Scallions	Salmon, Peas And Parsley Dressing	Creamy Coconut Peach Dessert
139	Mushroom and Eggs Casserole	Shrimp, Tomatoes And Potatoes	Banana and Almond Butter Bars
140	Bacon Brussels Sprouts	Tomato Shrimp	Fruity Sauce with Apples
141	Almond Porridge	Chili Salmon	Brown Fudge Cake
142	Raspberry Mug Cake	Mexican Pork and Okra Salad	Cherry Cheesecake
143	Chicken Veal Stew	Pork and Kale Meatballs	Tapioca Pudding
144	Cinnamon Pancakes	Pork and Baby Spinach	Chocolate Crème Brûlée
145	Beef Stew with Eggplants	Cinnamon Turkey Curry	Nutmeg Apple Crisp
146	Beef Black Pepper Stew	Cod and Tomato Passata	Crème Brûlée
147	Deviled Eggs	Mushroom and Chicken Soup	Almond Cheesecake
148	Pork Tenderloin Stew	Basil Shrimp and Eggplants	Maple-Glazed Flan
149	Lamb Stew	Chicken and Mustard Sauce	Blueberry Cheesecake
150	Beef Chili	Chicken and Avocado Mix	Chocolate Cheesecake
151	Mixed Mushroom Pate	Rice With Chicken And Veggies	Coconut Cake
152	Black Bean & Egg Casserole	Tomato Cream	Yogurt Vanilla Lighter Cheesecake
153	Chicken Liver Breakfast	Carrot Soup	Molten Lava Cake
154	Spice Oatmeal	Simple Chili	Stuffed Peaches
155	Barbeque Tofu	Lentils Soup	Blueberry Jam
156	Instant Pot Cauliflower Soup	Easy Chicken Cacciatore	Vanilla Rice Pudding
157	Beef Bourguignon Recipe	Sweet Paprika Pork Chops	Pressure Cooked Brownies
158	Beef Kale Patties	Simple Pork Roast	Almond Tapioca Pudding
159	Eggs with Mushrooms	Mackerel And Orange Sauce	Lemon and Blackberry Compote
160	Coconut Cherry Pancakes	Fish Curry	Caramel Flan
161	Chicken with Spinach	Shrimp And Tomatoes Mix	Poached Gingery Orange Pears
162	Pork with Mushrooms	Cabbage And Beef Stew	Pear Ricotta Cake
163	Mushroom Chicken with Eggs	Lemon Shrimp	Peach Crumb
164	Keto Vanilla Chia Seeds	Fish Soup	Gingery Applesauce
165	Turkey Soup	Italian Shrimp Mix	Blondies with Peanut Butter
166	Beef Chuck Shoulder Roast Stew	Coconut Chicken Mix	Strawberry Cream
167	Cinnamon Bars	Broccoli Cream	Berry Compote
168	Eggs with Scallions	Salmon, Peas And Parsley Dressing	Creamy Coconut Peach Dessert

#	Breakfast	Lunch/Dinner	Dessert
169	Mushroom and Eggs Casserole	Shrimp, Tomatoes And Potatoes	Banana and Almond Butter Bars
170	Bacon Brussels Sprouts	Tomato Shrimp	Fruity Sauce with Apples
171	Almond Porridge	Chili Salmon	Brown Fudge Cake
172	Raspberry Mug Cake	Mexican Pork and Okra Salad	Cherry Cheesecake
173	Chicken Veal Stew	Pork and Kale Meatballs	Tapioca Pudding
174	Cinnamon Pancakes	Pork and Baby Spinach	Chocolate Crème Brûlée
175	Beef Stew with Eggplants	Cinnamon Turkey Curry	Nutmeg Apple Crisp
176	Beef Black Pepper Stew	Cod and Tomato Passata	Crème Brûlée
177	Deviled Eggs	Mushroom and Chicken Soup	Almond Cheesecake
178	Pork Tenderloin Stew	Basil Shrimp and Eggplants	Maple-Glazed Flan
179	Lamb Stew	Chicken and Mustard Sauce	Blueberry Cheesecake
180	Beef Chili	Chicken and Avocado Mix	Chocolate Cheesecake
181	Mixed Mushroom Pate	Rice With Chicken And Veggies	Coconut Cake
182	Black Bean & Egg Casserole	Tomato Cream	Yogurt Vanilla Lighter Cheesecake
183	Chicken Liver Breakfast	Carrot Soup	Molten Lava Cake
184	Spice Oatmeal	Simple Chili	Stuffed Peaches
185	Barbeque Tofu	Lentils Soup	Blueberry Jam
186	Instant Pot Cauliflower Soup	Easy Chicken Cacciatore	Vanilla Rice Pudding
187	Beef Bourguignon Recipe	Sweet Paprika Pork Chops	Pressure Cooked Brownies
188	Beef Kale Patties	Simple Pork Roast	Almond Tapioca Pudding
189	Eggs with Mushrooms	Mackerel And Orange Sauce	Lemon and Blackberry Compote
190	Coconut Cherry Pancakes	Fish Curry	Caramel Flan
191	Chicken with Spinach	Shrimp And Tomatoes Mix	Poached Gingery Orange Pears
192	Pork with Mushrooms	Cabbage And Beef Stew	Pear Ricotta Cake
193	Mushroom Chicken with Eggs	Lemon Shrimp	Peach Crumb
194	Keto Vanilla Chia Seeds	Fish Soup	Gingery Applesauce
195	Turkey Soup	Italian Shrimp Mix	Blondies with Peanut Butter
196	Beef Chuck Shoulder Roast Stew	Coconut Chicken Mix	Strawberry Cream
197	Cinnamon Bars	Broccoli Cream	Berry Compote
198	Eggs with Scallions	Salmon, Peas And Parsley Dressing	Creamy Coconut Peach Dessert
199	Mushroom and Eggs Casserole	Shrimp, Tomatoes And Potatoes	Banana and Almond Butter Bars
200	Bacon Brussels Sprouts	Tomato Shrimp	Fruity Sauce with Apples
201	Almond Porridge	Chili Salmon	Brown Fudge Cake
202	Raspberry Mug Cake	Mexican Pork and Okra Salad	Cherry Cheesecake
203	Chicken Veal Stew	Pork and Kale Meatballs	Tapioca Pudding
204	Cinnamon Pancakes	Pork and Baby Spinach	Chocolate Crème Brûlée
205	Beef Stew with Eggplants	Cinnamon Turkey Curry	Nutmeg Apple Crisp
206	Beef Black Pepper Stew	Cod and Tomato Passata	Crème Brûlée
207	Deviled Eggs	Mushroom and Chicken Soup	Almond Cheesecake
208	Pork Tenderloin Stew	Basil Shrimp and Eggplants	Maple-Glazed Flan
209	Lamb Stew	Chicken and Mustard Sauce	Blueberry Cheesecake
210	Beef Chili	Chicken and Avocado Mix	Chocolate Cheesecake
211	Mixed Mushroom Pate	Rice With Chicken And Veggies	Coconut Cake

212	Black Bean & Egg Casserole	Tomato Cream	Yogurt Vanilla Lighter Cheesecake
213	Chicken Liver Breakfast	Carrot Soup	Molten Lava Cake
214	Spice Oatmeal	Simple Chili	Stuffed Peaches
215	Barbeque Tofu	Lentils Soup	Blueberry Jam
216	Instant Pot Cauliflower Soup	Easy Chicken Cacciatore	Vanilla Rice Pudding
217	Beef Bourguignon Recipe	Sweet Paprika Pork Chops	Pressure Cooked Brownies
218	Beef Kale Patties	Simple Pork Roast	Almond Tapioca Pudding
219	Eggs with Mushrooms	Mackerel And Orange Sauce	Lemon and Blackberry Compote
220	Coconut Cherry Pancakes	Fish Curry	Caramel Flan
221	Chicken with Spinach	Shrimp And Tomatoes Mix	Poached Gingery Orange Pears
222	Pork with Mushrooms	Cabbage And Beef Stew	Pear Ricotta Cake
223	Mushroom Chicken with Eggs	Lemon Shrimp	Peach Crumb
224	Keto Vanilla Chia Seeds	Fish Soup	Gingery Applesauce
225	Turkey Soup	Italian Shrimp Mix	Blondies with Peanut Butter
226	Beef Chuck Shoulder Roast Stew	Coconut Chicken Mix	Strawberry Cream
227	Cinnamon Bars	Broccoli Cream	Berry Compote
228	Eggs with Scallions	Salmon, Peas And Parsley Dressing	Creamy Coconut Peach Dessert
229	Mushroom and Eggs Casserole	Shrimp, Tomatoes And Potatoes	Banana and Almond Butter Bars
230	Bacon Brussels Sprouts	Tomato Shrimp	Fruity Sauce with Apples
231	Almond Porridge	Chili Salmon	Brown Fudge Cake
232	Raspberry Mug Cake	Mexican Pork and Okra Salad	Cherry Cheesecake
233	Chicken Veal Stew	Pork and Kale Meatballs	Tapioca Pudding
234	Cinnamon Pancakes	Pork and Baby Spinach	Chocolate Crème Brûlée
235	Beef Stew with Eggplants	Cinnamon Turkey Curry	Nutmeg Apple Crisp
236	Beef Black Pepper Stew	Cod and Tomato Passata	Crème Brûlée
237	Deviled Eggs	Mushroom and Chicken Soup	Almond Cheesecake
238	Pork Tenderloin Stew	Basil Shrimp and Eggplants	Maple-Glazed Flan
239	Lamb Stew	Chicken and Mustard Sauce	Blueberry Cheesecake
240	Beef Chili	Chicken and Avocado Mix	Chocolate Cheesecake
241	Mixed Mushroom Pate	Rice With Chicken And Veggies	Coconut Cake
242	Black Bean & Egg Casserole	Tomato Cream	Yogurt Vanilla Lighter Cheesecake
243	Chicken Liver Breakfast	Carrot Soup	Molten Lava Cake
244	Spice Oatmeal	Simple Chili	Stuffed Peaches
245	Barbeque Tofu	Lentils Soup	Blueberry Jam
246	Instant Pot Cauliflower Soup	Easy Chicken Cacciatore	Vanilla Rice Pudding
247	Beef Bourguignon Recipe	Sweet Paprika Pork Chops	Pressure Cooked Brownies
248	Beef Kale Patties	Simple Pork Roast	Almond Tapioca Pudding
249	Eggs with Mushrooms	Mackerel And Orange Sauce	Lemon and Blackberry Compote
250	Coconut Cherry Pancakes	Fish Curry	Caramel Flan
251	Chicken with Spinach	Shrimp And Tomatoes Mix	Poached Gingery Orange Pears
252	Pork with Mushrooms	Cabbage And Beef Stew	Pear Ricotta Cake
253	Mushroom Chicken with Eggs	Lemon Shrimp	Peach Crumb
254	Keto Vanilla Chia Seeds	Fish Soup	Gingery Applesauce

255	Turkey Soup	Italian Shrimp Mix	Blondies with Peanut Butter
256	Beef Chuck Shoulder Roast Stew	Coconut Chicken Mix	Strawberry Cream
257	Cinnamon Bars	Broccoli Cream	Berry Compote
258	Eggs with Scallions	Salmon, Peas And Parsley Dressing	Creamy Coconut Peach Dessert
259	Mushroom and Eggs Casserole	Shrimp, Tomatoes And Potatoes	Banana and Almond Butter Bars
260	Bacon Brussels Sprouts	Tomato Shrimp	Fruity Sauce with Apples
261	Almond Porridge	Chili Salmon	Brown Fudge Cake
262	Raspberry Mug Cake	Mexican Pork and Okra Salad	Cherry Cheesecake
263	Chicken Veal Stew	Pork and Kale Meatballs	Tapioca Pudding
264	Cinnamon Pancakes	Pork and Baby Spinach	Chocolate Crème Brûlée
265	Beef Stew with Eggplants	Cinnamon Turkey Curry	Nutmeg Apple Crisp
266	Beef Black Pepper Stew	Cod and Tomato Passata	Crème Brûlée
267	Deviled Eggs	Mushroom and Chicken Soup	Almond Cheesecake
268	Pork Tenderloin Stew	Basil Shrimp and Eggplants	Maple-Glazed Flan
269	Lamb Stew	Chicken and Mustard Sauce	Blueberry Cheesecake
270	Beef Chili	Chicken and Avocado Mix	Chocolate Cheesecake
271	Mixed Mushroom Pate	Rice With Chicken And Veggies	Coconut Cake
272	Black Bean & Egg Casserole	Tomato Cream	Yogurt Vanilla Lighter Cheesecake
273	Chicken Liver Breakfast	Carrot Soup	Molten Lava Cake
274	Spice Oatmeal	Simple Chili	Stuffed Peaches
275	Barbeque Tofu	Lentils Soup	Blueberry Jam
276	Instant Pot Cauliflower Soup	Easy Chicken Cacciatore	Vanilla Rice Pudding
277	Beef Bourguignon Recipe	Sweet Paprika Pork Chops	Pressure Cooked Brownies
278	Beef Kale Patties	Simple Pork Roast	Almond Tapioca Pudding
279	Eggs with Mushrooms	Mackerel And Orange Sauce	Lemon and Blackberry Compote
280	Coconut Cherry Pancakes	Fish Curry	Caramel Flan
281	Chicken with Spinach	Shrimp And Tomatoes Mix	Poached Gingery Orange Pears
282	Pork with Mushrooms	Cabbage And Beef Stew	Pear Ricotta Cake
283	Mushroom Chicken with Eggs	Lemon Shrimp	Peach Crumb
284	Keto Vanilla Chia Seeds	Fish Soup	Gingery Applesauce
285	Turkey Soup	Italian Shrimp Mix	Blondies with Peanut Butter
286	Beef Chuck Shoulder Roast Stew	Coconut Chicken Mix	Strawberry Cream
287	Cinnamon Bars	Broccoli Cream	Berry Compote
288	Eggs with Scallions	Salmon, Peas And Parsley Dressing	Creamy Coconut Peach Dessert
289	Mushroom and Eggs Casserole	Shrimp, Tomatoes And Potatoes	Banana and Almond Butter Bars
290	Bacon Brussels Sprouts	Tomato Shrimp	Fruity Sauce with Apples
291	Almond Porridge	Chili Salmon	Brown Fudge Cake
292	Raspberry Mug Cake	Mexican Pork and Okra Salad	Cherry Cheesecake
293	Chicken Veal Stew	Pork and Kale Meatballs	Tapioca Pudding
294	Cinnamon Pancakes	Pork and Baby Spinach	Chocolate Crème Brûlée
295	Beef Stew with Eggplants	Cinnamon Turkey Curry	Nutmeg Apple Crisp
296	Beef Black Pepper Stew	Cod and Tomato Passata	Crème Brûlée
297	Deviled Eggs	Mushroom and Chicken Soup	Almond Cheesecake

298	Pork Tenderloin Stew	Basil Shrimp and Eggplants	Maple-Glazed Flan
299	Lamb Stew	Chicken and Mustard Sauce	Blueberry Cheesecake
300	Beef Chili	Chicken and Avocado Mix	Chocolate Cheesecake
301	Mixed Mushroom Pate	Rice With Chicken And Veggies	Coconut Cake
302	Black Bean & Egg Casserole	Tomato Cream	Yogurt Vanilla Lighter Cheesecake
303	Chicken Liver Breakfast	Carrot Soup	Molten Lava Cake
304	Spice Oatmeal	Simple Chili	Stuffed Peaches
305	Barbeque Tofu	Lentils Soup	Blueberry Jam
306	Instant Pot Cauliflower Soup	Easy Chicken Cacciatore	Vanilla Rice Pudding
307	Beef Bourguignon Recipe	Sweet Paprika Pork Chops	Pressure Cooked Brownies
308	Beef Kale Patties	Simple Pork Roast	Almond Tapioca Pudding
309	Eggs with Mushrooms	Mackerel And Orange Sauce	Lemon and Blackberry Compote
310	Coconut Cherry Pancakes	Fish Curry	Caramel Flan
311	Chicken with Spinach	Shrimp And Tomatoes Mix	Poached Gingery Orange Pears
312	Pork with Mushrooms	Cabbage And Beef Stew	Pear Ricotta Cake
313	Mushroom Chicken with Eggs	Lemon Shrimp	Peach Crumb
314	Keto Vanilla Chia Seeds	Fish Soup	Gingery Applesauce
315	Turkey Soup	Italian Shrimp Mix	Blondies with Peanut Butter
316	Beef Chuck Shoulder Roast Stew	Coconut Chicken Mix	Strawberry Cream
317	Cinnamon Bars	Broccoli Cream	Berry Compote
318	Eggs with Scallions	Salmon, Peas And Parsley Dressing	Creamy Coconut Peach Dessert
319	Mushroom and Eggs Casserole	Shrimp, Tomatoes And Potatoes	Banana and Almond Butter Bars
320	Bacon Brussels Sprouts	Tomato Shrimp	Fruity Sauce with Apples
321	Almond Porridge	Chili Salmon	Brown Fudge Cake
322	Raspberry Mug Cake	Mexican Pork and Okra Salad	Cherry Cheesecake
323	Chicken Veal Stew	Pork and Kale Meatballs	Tapioca Pudding
324	Cinnamon Pancakes	Pork and Baby Spinach	Chocolate Crème Brûlée
325	Beef Stew with Eggplants	Cinnamon Turkey Curry	Nutmeg Apple Crisp
326	Beef Black Pepper Stew	Cod and Tomato Passata	Crème Brûlée
327	Deviled Eggs	Mushroom and Chicken Soup	Almond Cheesecake
328	Pork Tenderloin Stew	Basil Shrimp and Eggplants	Maple-Glazed Flan
329	Lamb Stew	Chicken and Mustard Sauce	Blueberry Cheesecake
330	Beef Chili	Chicken and Avocado Mix	Chocolate Cheesecake
331	Mixed Mushroom Pate	Rice With Chicken And Veggies	Coconut Cake
332	Black Bean & Egg Casserole	Tomato Cream	Yogurt Vanilla Lighter Cheesecake
333	Chicken Liver Breakfast	Carrot Soup	Molten Lava Cake
334	Spice Oatmeal	Simple Chili	Stuffed Peaches
335	Barbeque Tofu	Lentils Soup	Blueberry Jam
336	Instant Pot Cauliflower Soup	Easy Chicken Cacciatore	Vanilla Rice Pudding
337	Beef Bourguignon Recipe	Sweet Paprika Pork Chops	Pressure Cooked Brownies
338	Beef Kale Patties	Simple Pork Roast	Almond Tapioca Pudding
339	Eggs with Mushrooms	Mackerel And Orange Sauce	Lemon and Blackberry Compote
340	Coconut Cherry Pancakes	Fish Curry	Caramel Flan

341	Chicken with Spinach	Shrimp And Tomatoes Mix	Poached Gingery Orange Pears
342	Pork with Mushrooms	Cabbage And Beef Stew	Pear Ricotta Cake
343	Mushroom Chicken with Eggs	Lemon Shrimp	Peach Crumb
344	Keto Vanilla Chia Seeds	Fish Soup	Gingery Applesauce
345	Turkey Soup	Italian Shrimp Mix	Blondies with Peanut Butter
346	Beef Chuck Shoulder Roast Stew	Coconut Chicken Mix	Strawberry Cream
347	Cinnamon Bars	Broccoli Cream	Berry Compote
348	Eggs with Scallions	Salmon, Peas And Parsley Dressing	Creamy Coconut Peach Dessert
349	Mushroom and Eggs Casserole	Shrimp, Tomatoes And Potatoes	Banana and Almond Butter Bars
350	Bacon Brussels Sprouts	Tomato Shrimp	Fruity Sauce with Apples
351	Almond Porridge	Chili Salmon	Brown Fudge Cake
352	Raspberry Mug Cake	Mexican Pork and Okra Salad	Cherry Cheesecake
353	Chicken Veal Stew	Pork and Kale Meatballs	Tapioca Pudding
354	Cinnamon Pancakes	Pork and Baby Spinach	Chocolate Crème Brûlée
355	Beef Stew with Eggplants	Cinnamon Turkey Curry	Nutmeg Apple Crisp
356	Beef Black Pepper Stew	Cod and Tomato Passata	Crème Brûlée
357	Deviled Eggs	Mushroom and Chicken Soup	Almond Cheesecake
358	Pork Tenderloin Stew	Basil Shrimp and Eggplants	Maple-Glazed Flan
359	Lamb Stew	Chicken and Mustard Sauce	Blueberry Cheesecake
360	Beef Chili	Chicken and Avocado Mix	Chocolate Cheesecake
361	Mixed Mushroom Pate	Rice With Chicken And Veggies	Coconut Cake
362	Black Bean & Egg Casserole	Tomato Cream	Yogurt Vanilla Lighter Cheesecake
363	Chicken Liver Breakfast	Carrot Soup	Molten Lava Cake
364	Spice Oatmeal	Simple Chili	Stuffed Peaches
365	Barbeque Tofu	Lentils Soup	Blueberry Jam
366	Instant Pot Cauliflower Soup	Easy Chicken Cacciatore	Vanilla Rice Pudding
367	Beef Bourguignon Recipe	Sweet Paprika Pork Chops	Pressure Cooked Brownies
368	Beef Kale Patties	Simple Pork Roast	Almond Tapioca Pudding
369	Eggs with Mushrooms	Mackerel And Orange Sauce	Lemon and Blackberry Compote
370	Coconut Cherry Pancakes	Fish Curry	Caramel Flan
371	Chicken with Spinach	Shrimp And Tomatoes Mix	Poached Gingery Orange Pears
372	Pork with Mushrooms	Cabbage And Beef Stew	Pear Ricotta Cake
373	Mushroom Chicken with Eggs	Lemon Shrimp	Peach Crumb
374	Keto Vanilla Chia Seeds	Fish Soup	Gingery Applesauce
375	Turkey Soup	Italian Shrimp Mix	Blondies with Peanut Butter
376	Beef Chuck Shoulder Roast Stew	Coconut Chicken Mix	Strawberry Cream
377	Cinnamon Bars	Broccoli Cream	Berry Compote
378	Eggs with Scallions	Salmon, Peas And Parsley Dressing	Creamy Coconut Peach Dessert
379	Mushroom and Eggs Casserole	Shrimp, Tomatoes And Potatoes	Banana and Almond Butter Bars
380	Bacon Brussels Sprouts	Tomato Shrimp	Fruity Sauce with Apples
381	Almond Porridge	Chili Salmon	Brown Fudge Cake
382	Raspberry Mug Cake	Mexican Pork and Okra Salad	Cherry Cheesecake
383	Chicken Veal Stew	Pork and Kale Meatballs	Tapioca Pudding

384	Cinnamon Pancakes	Pork and Baby Spinach	Chocolate Crème Brûlée
385	Beef Stew with Eggplants	Cinnamon Turkey Curry	Nutmeg Apple Crisp
386	Beef Black Pepper Stew	Cod and Tomato Passata	Crème Brûlée
387	Deviled Eggs	Mushroom and Chicken Soup	Almond Cheesecake
388	Pork Tenderloin Stew	Basil Shrimp and Eggplants	Maple-Glazed Flan
389	Lamb Stew	Chicken and Mustard Sauce	Blueberry Cheesecake
390	Beef Chili	Chicken and Avocado Mix	Chocolate Cheesecake
391	Mixed Mushroom Pate	Rice With Chicken And Veggies	Coconut Cake
392	Black Bean & Egg Casserole	Tomato Cream	Yogurt Vanilla Lighter Cheesecake
393	Chicken Liver Breakfast	Carrot Soup	Molten Lava Cake
394	Spice Oatmeal	Simple Chili	Stuffed Peaches
395	Barbeque Tofu	Lentils Soup	Blueberry Jam
396	Instant Pot Cauliflower Soup	Easy Chicken Cacciatore	Vanilla Rice Pudding
397	Beef Bourguignon Recipe	Sweet Paprika Pork Chops	Pressure Cooked Brownies
398	Beef Kale Patties	Simple Pork Roast	Almond Tapioca Pudding
399	Eggs with Mushrooms	Mackerel And Orange Sauce	Lemon and Blackberry Compote
400	Coconut Cherry Pancakes	Fish Curry	Caramel Flan
401	Chicken with Spinach	Shrimp And Tomatoes Mix	Poached Gingery Orange Pears
402	Pork with Mushrooms	Cabbage And Beef Stew	Pear Ricotta Cake
403	Mushroom Chicken with Eggs	Lemon Shrimp	Peach Crumb
404	Keto Vanilla Chia Seeds	Fish Soup	Gingery Applesauce
405	Turkey Soup	Italian Shrimp Mix	Blondies with Peanut Butter
406	Beef Chuck Shoulder Roast Stew	Coconut Chicken Mix	Strawberry Cream
407	Cinnamon Bars	Broccoli Cream	Berry Compote
408	Eggs with Scallions	Salmon, Peas And Parsley Dressing	Creamy Coconut Peach Dessert
409	Mushroom and Eggs Casserole	Shrimp, Tomatoes And Potatoes	Banana and Almond Butter Bars
410	Bacon Brussels Sprouts	Tomato Shrimp	Fruity Sauce with Apples
411	Almond Porridge	Chili Salmon	Brown Fudge Cake
412	Raspberry Mug Cake	Mexican Pork and Okra Salad	Cherry Cheesecake
413	Chicken Veal Stew	Pork and Kale Meatballs	Tapioca Pudding
414	Cinnamon Pancakes	Pork and Baby Spinach	Chocolate Crème Brûlée
415	Beef Stew with Eggplants	Cinnamon Turkey Curry	Nutmeg Apple Crisp
416	Beef Black Pepper Stew	Cod and Tomato Passata	Crème Brûlée
417	Deviled Eggs	Mushroom and Chicken Soup	Almond Cheesecake
418	Pork Tenderloin Stew	Basil Shrimp and Eggplants	Maple-Glazed Flan
419	Lamb Stew	Chicken and Mustard Sauce	Blueberry Cheesecake
420	Beef Chili	Chicken and Avocado Mix	Chocolate Cheesecake
421	Mixed Mushroom Pate	Rice With Chicken And Veggies	Coconut Cake
422	Black Bean & Egg Casserole	Tomato Cream	Yogurt Vanilla Lighter Cheesecake
423	Chicken Liver Breakfast	Carrot Soup	Molten Lava Cake
424	Spice Oatmeal	Simple Chili	Stuffed Peaches
425	Barbeque Tofu	Lentils Soup	Blueberry Jam
426	Instant Pot Cauliflower Soup	Easy Chicken Cacciatore	Vanilla Rice Pudding

427	Beef Bourguignon Recipe	Sweet Paprika Pork Chops	Pressure Cooked Brownies
428	Beef Kale Patties	Simple Pork Roast	Almond Tapioca Pudding
429	Eggs with Mushrooms	Mackerel And Orange Sauce	Lemon and Blackberry Compote
430	Coconut Cherry Pancakes	Fish Curry	Caramel Flan
431	Chicken with Spinach	Shrimp And Tomatoes Mix	Poached Gingery Orange Pears
432	Pork with Mushrooms	Cabbage And Beef Stew	Pear Ricotta Cake
433	Mushroom Chicken with Eggs	Lemon Shrimp	Peach Crumb
434	Keto Vanilla Chia Seeds	Fish Soup	Gingery Applesauce
435	Turkey Soup	Italian Shrimp Mix	Blondies with Peanut Butter
436	Beef Chuck Shoulder Roast Stew	Coconut Chicken Mix	Strawberry Cream
437	Cinnamon Bars	Broccoli Cream	Berry Compote
438	Eggs with Scallions	Salmon, Peas And Parsley Dressing	Creamy Coconut Peach Dessert
439	Mushroom and Eggs Casserole	Shrimp, Tomatoes And Potatoes	Banana and Almond Butter Bars
440	Bacon Brussels Sprouts	Tomato Shrimp	Fruity Sauce with Apples
441	Almond Porridge	Chili Salmon	Brown Fudge Cake
442	Raspberry Mug Cake	Mexican Pork and Okra Salad	Cherry Cheesecake
443	Chicken Veal Stew	Pork and Kale Meatballs	Tapioca Pudding
444	Cinnamon Pancakes	Pork and Baby Spinach	Chocolate Crème Brûlée
445	Beef Stew with Eggplants	Cinnamon Turkey Curry	Nutmeg Apple Crisp
446	Beef Black Pepper Stew	Cod and Tomato Passata	Crème Brûlée
447	Deviled Eggs	Mushroom and Chicken Soup	Almond Cheesecake
448	Pork Tenderloin Stew	Basil Shrimp and Eggplants	Maple-Glazed Flan
449	Lamb Stew	Chicken and Mustard Sauce	Blueberry Cheesecake
450	Beef Chili	Chicken and Avocado Mix	Chocolate Cheesecake
451	Mixed Mushroom Pate	Rice With Chicken And Veggies	Coconut Cake
452	Black Bean & Egg Casserole	Tomato Cream	Yogurt Vanilla Lighter Cheesecake
453	Chicken Liver Breakfast	Carrot Soup	Molten Lava Cake
454	Spice Oatmeal	Simple Chili	Stuffed Peaches
455	Barbeque Tofu	Lentils Soup	Blueberry Jam
456	Instant Pot Cauliflower Soup	Easy Chicken Cacciatore	Vanilla Rice Pudding
457	Beef Bourguignon Recipe	Sweet Paprika Pork Chops	Pressure Cooked Brownies
458	Beef Kale Patties	Simple Pork Roast	Almond Tapioca Pudding
459	Eggs with Mushrooms	Mackerel And Orange Sauce	Lemon and Blackberry Compote
460	Coconut Cherry Pancakes	Fish Curry	Caramel Flan
461	Chicken with Spinach	Shrimp And Tomatoes Mix	Poached Gingery Orange Pears
462	Pork with Mushrooms	Cabbage And Beef Stew	Pear Ricotta Cake
463	Mushroom Chicken with Eggs	Lemon Shrimp	Peach Crumb
464	Keto Vanilla Chia Seeds	Fish Soup	Gingery Applesauce
465	Turkey Soup	Italian Shrimp Mix	Blondies with Peanut Butter
466	Beef Chuck Shoulder Roast Stew	Coconut Chicken Mix	Strawberry Cream
467	Cinnamon Bars	Broccoli Cream	Berry Compote
468	Eggs with Scallions	Salmon, Peas And Parsley Dressing	Creamy Coconut Peach Dessert
469	Mushroom and Eggs Casserole	Shrimp, Tomatoes And Potatoes	Banana and Almond Butter Bars

470	Bacon Brussels Sprouts	Tomato Shrimp	Fruity Sauce with Apples
471	Almond Porridge	Chili Salmon	Brown Fudge Cake
472	Raspberry Mug Cake	Mexican Pork and Okra Salad	Cherry Cheesecake
473	Chicken Veal Stew	Pork and Kale Meatballs	Tapioca Pudding
474	Cinnamon Pancakes	Pork and Baby Spinach	Chocolate Crème Brûlée
475	Beef Stew with Eggplants	Cinnamon Turkey Curry	Nutmeg Apple Crisp
476	Beef Black Pepper Stew	Cod and Tomato Passata	Crème Brûlée
477	Deviled Eggs	Mushroom and Chicken Soup	Almond Cheesecake
478	Pork Tenderloin Stew	Basil Shrimp and Eggplants	Maple-Glazed Flan
479	Lamb Stew	Chicken and Mustard Sauce	Blueberry Cheesecake
480	Beef Chili	Chicken and Avocado Mix	Chocolate Cheesecake
481	Mixed Mushroom Pate	Rice With Chicken And Veggies	Coconut Cake
482	Black Bean & Egg Casserole	Tomato Cream	Yogurt Vanilla Lighter Cheesecake
483	Chicken Liver Breakfast	Carrot Soup	Molten Lava Cake
484	Spice Oatmeal	Simple Chili	Stuffed Peaches
485	Barbeque Tofu	Lentils Soup	Blueberry Jam
486	Instant Pot Cauliflower Soup	Easy Chicken Cacciatore	Vanilla Rice Pudding
487	Beef Bourguignon Recipe	Sweet Paprika Pork Chops	Pressure Cooked Brownies
488	Beef Kale Patties	Simple Pork Roast	Almond Tapioca Pudding
489	Eggs with Mushrooms	Mackerel And Orange Sauce	Lemon and Blackberry Compote
490	Coconut Cherry Pancakes	Fish Curry	Caramel Flan
491	Chicken with Spinach	Shrimp And Tomatoes Mix	Poached Gingery Orange Pears
492	Pork with Mushrooms	Cabbage And Beef Stew	Pear Ricotta Cake
493	Mushroom Chicken with Eggs	Lemon Shrimp	Peach Crumb
494	Keto Vanilla Chia Seeds	Fish Soup	Gingery Applesauce
495	Turkey Soup	Italian Shrimp Mix	Blondies with Peanut Butter
496	Beef Chuck Shoulder Roast Stew	Coconut Chicken Mix	Strawberry Cream
497	Cinnamon Bars	Broccoli Cream	Berry Compote
498	Eggs with Scallions	Salmon, Peas And Parsley Dressing	Creamy Coconut Peach Dessert
499	Mushroom and Eggs Casserole	Shrimp, Tomatoes And Potatoes	Banana and Almond Butter Bars
500	Bacon Brussels Sprouts	Tomato Shrimp	Fruity Sauce with Apples
501	Almond Porridge	Chili Salmon	Brown Fudge Cake
502	Raspberry Mug Cake	Mexican Pork and Okra Salad	Cherry Cheesecake
503	Chicken Veal Stew	Pork and Kale Meatballs	Tapioca Pudding
504	Cinnamon Pancakes	Pork and Baby Spinach	Chocolate Crème Brûlée
505	Beef Stew with Eggplants	Cinnamon Turkey Curry	Nutmeg Apple Crisp
506	Beef Black Pepper Stew	Cod and Tomato Passata	Crème Brûlée
507	Deviled Eggs	Mushroom and Chicken Soup	Almond Cheesecake
508	Pork Tenderloin Stew	Basil Shrimp and Eggplants	Maple-Glazed Flan
509	Lamb Stew	Chicken and Mustard Sauce	Blueberry Cheesecake
510	Beef Chili	Chicken and Avocado Mix	Chocolate Cheesecake
511	Mixed Mushroom Pate	Rice With Chicken And Veggies	Coconut Cake
512	Black Bean & Egg Casserole	Tomato Cream	Yogurt Vanilla Lighter Cheesecake

513	Chicken Liver Breakfast	Carrot Soup	Molten Lava Cake
514	Spice Oatmeal	Simple Chili	Stuffed Peaches
515	Barbeque Tofu	Lentils Soup	Blueberry Jam
516	Instant Pot Cauliflower Soup	Easy Chicken Cacciatore	Vanilla Rice Pudding
517	Beef Bourguignon Recipe	Sweet Paprika Pork Chops	Pressure Cooked Brownies
518	Beef Kale Patties	Simple Pork Roast	Almond Tapioca Pudding
519	Eggs with Mushrooms	Mackerel And Orange Sauce	Lemon and Blackberry Compote
520	Coconut Cherry Pancakes	Fish Curry	Caramel Flan
521	Chicken with Spinach	Shrimp And Tomatoes Mix	Poached Gingery Orange Pears
522	Pork with Mushrooms	Cabbage And Beef Stew	Pear Ricotta Cake
523	Mushroom Chicken with Eggs	Lemon Shrimp	Peach Crumb
524	Keto Vanilla Chia Seeds	Fish Soup	Gingery Applesauce
525	Turkey Soup	Italian Shrimp Mix	Blondies with Peanut Butter
526	Beef Chuck Shoulder Roast Stew	Coconut Chicken Mix	Strawberry Cream
527	Cinnamon Bars	Broccoli Cream	Berry Compote
528	Eggs with Scallions	Salmon, Peas And Parsley Dressing	Creamy Coconut Peach Dessert
529	Mushroom and Eggs Casserole	Shrimp, Tomatoes And Potatoes	Banana and Almond Butter Bars
530	Bacon Brussels Sprouts	Tomato Shrimp	Fruity Sauce with Apples
531	Almond Porridge	Chili Salmon	Brown Fudge Cake
532	Raspberry Mug Cake	Mexican Pork and Okra Salad	Cherry Cheesecake
533	Chicken Veal Stew	Pork and Kale Meatballs	Tapioca Pudding
534	Cinnamon Pancakes	Pork and Baby Spinach	Chocolate Crème Brûlée
535	Beef Stew with Eggplants	Cinnamon Turkey Curry	Nutmeg Apple Crisp
536	Beef Black Pepper Stew	Cod and Tomato Passata	Crème Brûlée
537	Deviled Eggs	Mushroom and Chicken Soup	Almond Cheesecake
538	Pork Tenderloin Stew	Basil Shrimp and Eggplants	Maple-Glazed Flan
539	Lamb Stew	Chicken and Mustard Sauce	Blueberry Cheesecake
540	Beef Chili	Chicken and Avocado Mix	Chocolate Cheesecake
541	Mixed Mushroom Pate	Rice With Chicken And Veggies	Coconut Cake
542	Black Bean & Egg Casserole	Tomato Cream	Yogurt Vanilla Lighter Cheesecake
543	Chicken Liver Breakfast	Carrot Soup	Molten Lava Cake
544	Spice Oatmeal	Simple Chili	Stuffed Peaches
545	Barbeque Tofu	Lentils Soup	Blueberry Jam
546	Instant Pot Cauliflower Soup	Easy Chicken Cacciatore	Vanilla Rice Pudding
547	Beef Bourguignon Recipe	Sweet Paprika Pork Chops	Pressure Cooked Brownies
548	Beef Kale Patties	Simple Pork Roast	Almond Tapioca Pudding
549	Eggs with Mushrooms	Mackerel And Orange Sauce	Lemon and Blackberry Compote
550	Coconut Cherry Pancakes	Fish Curry	Caramel Flan
551	Chicken with Spinach	Shrimp And Tomatoes Mix	Poached Gingery Orange Pears
552	Pork with Mushrooms	Cabbage And Beef Stew	Pear Ricotta Cake
553	Mushroom Chicken with Eggs	Lemon Shrimp	Peach Crumb
554	Keto Vanilla Chia Seeds	Fish Soup	Gingery Applesauce
555	Turkey Soup	Italian Shrimp Mix	Blondies with Peanut Butter

556	Beef Chuck Shoulder Roast Stew	Coconut Chicken Mix	Strawberry Cream
557	Cinnamon Bars	Broccoli Cream	Berry Compote
558	Eggs with Scallions	Salmon, Peas And Parsley Dressing	Creamy Coconut Peach Dessert
559	Mushroom and Eggs Casserole	Shrimp, Tomatoes And Potatoes	Banana and Almond Butter Bars
560	Bacon Brussels Sprouts	Tomato Shrimp	Fruity Sauce with Apples
561	Almond Porridge	Chili Salmon	Brown Fudge Cake
562	Raspberry Mug Cake	Mexican Pork and Okra Salad	Cherry Cheesecake
563	Chicken Veal Stew	Pork and Kale Meatballs	Tapioca Pudding
564	Cinnamon Pancakes	Pork and Baby Spinach	Chocolate Crème Brûlée
565	Beef Stew with Eggplants	Cinnamon Turkey Curry	Nutmeg Apple Crisp
566	Beef Black Pepper Stew	Cod and Tomato Passata	Crème Brûlée
567	Deviled Eggs	Mushroom and Chicken Soup	Almond Cheesecake
568	Pork Tenderloin Stew	Basil Shrimp and Eggplants	Maple-Glazed Flan
569	Lamb Stew	Chicken and Mustard Sauce	Blueberry Cheesecake
570	Beef Chili	Chicken and Avocado Mix	Chocolate Cheesecake
571	Mixed Mushroom Pate	Rice With Chicken And Veggies	Coconut Cake
572	Black Bean & Egg Casserole	Tomato Cream	Yogurt Vanilla Lighter Cheesecake
573	Chicken Liver Breakfast	Carrot Soup	Molten Lava Cake
574	Spice Oatmeal	Simple Chili	Stuffed Peaches
575	Barbeque Tofu	Lentils Soup	Blueberry Jam
576	Instant Pot Cauliflower Soup	Easy Chicken Cacciatore	Vanilla Rice Pudding
577	Beef Bourguignon Recipe	Sweet Paprika Pork Chops	Pressure Cooked Brownies
578	Beef Kale Patties	Simple Pork Roast	Almond Tapioca Pudding
579	Eggs with Mushrooms	Mackerel And Orange Sauce	Lemon and Blackberry Compote
580	Coconut Cherry Pancakes	Fish Curry	Caramel Flan
581	Chicken with Spinach	Shrimp And Tomatoes Mix	Poached Gingery Orange Pears
582	Pork with Mushrooms	Cabbage And Beef Stew	Pear Ricotta Cake
583	Mushroom Chicken with Eggs	Lemon Shrimp	Peach Crumb
584	Keto Vanilla Chia Seeds	Fish Soup	Gingery Applesauce
585	Turkey Soup	Italian Shrimp Mix	Blondies with Peanut Butter
586	Beef Chuck Shoulder Roast Stew	Coconut Chicken Mix	Strawberry Cream
587	Cinnamon Bars	Broccoli Cream	Berry Compote
588	Eggs with Scallions	Salmon, Peas And Parsley Dressing	Creamy Coconut Peach Dessert
589	Mushroom and Eggs Casserole	Shrimp, Tomatoes And Potatoes	Banana and Almond Butter Bars
590	Bacon Brussels Sprouts	Tomato Shrimp	Fruity Sauce with Apples
591	Almond Porridge	Chili Salmon	Brown Fudge Cake
592	Raspberry Mug Cake	Mexican Pork and Okra Salad	Cherry Cheesecake
593	Chicken Veal Stew	Pork and Kale Meatballs	Tapioca Pudding
594	Cinnamon Pancakes	Pork and Baby Spinach	Chocolate Crème Brûlée
595	Beef Stew with Eggplants	Cinnamon Turkey Curry	Nutmeg Apple Crisp
596	Beef Black Pepper Stew	Cod and Tomato Passata	Crème Brûlée
597	Deviled Eggs	Mushroom and Chicken Soup	Almond Cheesecake
598	Pork Tenderloin Stew	Basil Shrimp and Eggplants	Maple-Glazed Flan

599	Lamb Stew	Chicken and Mustard Sauce	Blueberry Cheesecake
600	Beef Chili	Chicken and Avocado Mix	Chocolate Cheesecake
601	Mixed Mushroom Pate	Rice With Chicken And Veggies	Coconut Cake
602	Black Bean & Egg Casserole	Tomato Cream	Yogurt Vanilla Lighter Cheesecake
603	Chicken Liver Breakfast	Carrot Soup	Molten Lava Cake
604	Spice Oatmeal	Simple Chili	Stuffed Peaches
605	Barbeque Tofu	Lentils Soup	Blueberry Jam
606	Instant Pot Cauliflower Soup	Easy Chicken Cacciatore	Vanilla Rice Pudding
607	Beef Bourguignon Recipe	Sweet Paprika Pork Chops	Pressure Cooked Brownies
608	Beef Kale Patties	Simple Pork Roast	Almond Tapioca Pudding
609	Eggs with Mushrooms	Mackerel And Orange Sauce	Lemon and Blackberry Compote
610	Coconut Cherry Pancakes	Fish Curry	Caramel Flan
611	Chicken with Spinach	Shrimp And Tomatoes Mix	Poached Gingery Orange Pears
612	Pork with Mushrooms	Cabbage And Beef Stew	Pear Ricotta Cake
613	Mushroom Chicken with Eggs	Lemon Shrimp	Peach Crumb
614	Keto Vanilla Chia Seeds	Fish Soup	Gingery Applesauce
615	Turkey Soup	Italian Shrimp Mix	Blondies with Peanut Butter
616	Beef Chuck Shoulder Roast Stew	Coconut Chicken Mix	Strawberry Cream
617	Cinnamon Bars	Broccoli Cream	Berry Compote
618	Eggs with Scallions	Salmon, Peas And Parsley Dressing	Creamy Coconut Peach Dessert
619	Mushroom and Eggs Casserole	Shrimp, Tomatoes And Potatoes	Banana and Almond Butter Bars
620	Bacon Brussels Sprouts	Tomato Shrimp	Fruity Sauce with Apples
621	Almond Porridge	Chili Salmon	Brown Fudge Cake
622	Raspberry Mug Cake	Mexican Pork and Okra Salad	Cherry Cheesecake
623	Chicken Veal Stew	Pork and Kale Meatballs	Tapioca Pudding
624	Cinnamon Pancakes	Pork and Baby Spinach	Chocolate Crème Brûlée
625	Beef Stew with Eggplants	Cinnamon Turkey Curry	Nutmeg Apple Crisp
626	Beef Black Pepper Stew	Cod and Tomato Passata	Crème Brûlée
627	Deviled Eggs	Mushroom and Chicken Soup	Almond Cheesecake
628	Pork Tenderloin Stew	Basil Shrimp and Eggplants	Maple-Glazed Flan
629	Lamb Stew	Chicken and Mustard Sauce	Blueberry Cheesecake
630	Beef Chili	Chicken and Avocado Mix	Chocolate Cheesecake
631	Mixed Mushroom Pate	Rice With Chicken And Veggies	Coconut Cake
632	Black Bean & Egg Casserole	Tomato Cream	Yogurt Vanilla Lighter Cheesecake
633	Chicken Liver Breakfast	Carrot Soup	Molten Lava Cake
634	Spice Oatmeal	Simple Chili	Stuffed Peaches
635	Barbeque Tofu	Lentils Soup	Blueberry Jam
636	Instant Pot Cauliflower Soup	Easy Chicken Cacciatore	Vanilla Rice Pudding
637	Beef Bourguignon Recipe	Sweet Paprika Pork Chops	Pressure Cooked Brownies
638	Beef Kale Patties	Simple Pork Roast	Almond Tapioca Pudding
639	Eggs with Mushrooms	Mackerel And Orange Sauce	Lemon and Blackberry Compote
640	Coconut Cherry Pancakes	Fish Curry	Caramel Flan
641	Chicken with Spinach	Shrimp And Tomatoes Mix	Poached Gingery Orange Pears

642	Pork with Mushrooms	Cabbage And Beef Stew	Pear Ricotta Cake
643	Mushroom Chicken with Eggs	Lemon Shrimp	Peach Crumb
644	Keto Vanilla Chia Seeds	Fish Soup	Gingery Applesauce
645	Turkey Soup	Italian Shrimp Mix	Blondies with Peanut Butter
646	Beef Chuck Shoulder Roast Stew	Coconut Chicken Mix	Strawberry Cream
647	Cinnamon Bars	Broccoli Cream	Berry Compote
648	Eggs with Scallions	Salmon, Peas And Parsley Dressing	Creamy Coconut Peach Dessert
649	Mushroom and Eggs Casserole	Shrimp, Tomatoes And Potatoes	Banana and Almond Butter Bars
650	Bacon Brussels Sprouts	Tomato Shrimp	Fruity Sauce with Apples
651	Almond Porridge	Chili Salmon	Brown Fudge Cake
652	Raspberry Mug Cake	Mexican Pork and Okra Salad	Cherry Cheesecake
653	Chicken Veal Stew	Pork and Kale Meatballs	Tapioca Pudding
654	Cinnamon Pancakes	Pork and Baby Spinach	Chocolate Crème Brûlée
655	Beef Stew with Eggplants	Cinnamon Turkey Curry	Nutmeg Apple Crisp
656	Beef Black Pepper Stew	Cod and Tomato Passata	Crème Brûlée
657	Deviled Eggs	Mushroom and Chicken Soup	Almond Cheesecake
658	Pork Tenderloin Stew	Basil Shrimp and Eggplants	Maple-Glazed Flan
659	Lamb Stew	Chicken and Mustard Sauce	Blueberry Cheesecake
660	Beef Chili	Chicken and Avocado Mix	Chocolate Cheesecake
661	Mixed Mushroom Pate	Rice With Chicken And Veggies	Coconut Cake
662	Black Bean & Egg Casserole	Tomato Cream	Yogurt Vanilla Lighter Cheesecake
663	Chicken Liver Breakfast	Carrot Soup	Molten Lava Cake
664	Spice Oatmeal	Simple Chili	Stuffed Peaches
665	Barbeque Tofu	Lentils Soup	Blueberry Jam
666	Instant Pot Cauliflower Soup	Easy Chicken Cacciatore	Vanilla Rice Pudding
667	Beef Bourguignon Recipe	Sweet Paprika Pork Chops	Pressure Cooked Brownies
668	Beef Kale Patties	Simple Pork Roast	Almond Tapioca Pudding
669	Eggs with Mushrooms	Mackerel And Orange Sauce	Lemon and Blackberry Compote
670	Coconut Cherry Pancakes	Fish Curry	Caramel Flan
671	Chicken with Spinach	Shrimp And Tomatoes Mix	Poached Gingery Orange Pears
672	Pork with Mushrooms	Cabbage And Beef Stew	Pear Ricotta Cake
673	Mushroom Chicken with Eggs	Lemon Shrimp	Peach Crumb
674	Keto Vanilla Chia Seeds	Fish Soup	Gingery Applesauce
675	Turkey Soup	Italian Shrimp Mix	Blondies with Peanut Butter
676	Beef Chuck Shoulder Roast Stew	Coconut Chicken Mix	Strawberry Cream
677	Cinnamon Bars	Broccoli Cream	Berry Compote
678	Eggs with Scallions	Salmon, Peas And Parsley Dressing	Creamy Coconut Peach Dessert
679	Mushroom and Eggs Casserole	Shrimp, Tomatoes And Potatoes	Banana and Almond Butter Bars
680	Bacon Brussels Sprouts	Tomato Shrimp	Fruity Sauce with Apples
681	Almond Porridge	Chili Salmon	Brown Fudge Cake
682	Raspberry Mug Cake	Mexican Pork and Okra Salad	Cherry Cheesecake
683	Chicken Veal Stew	Pork and Kale Meatballs	Tapioca Pudding
684	Cinnamon Pancakes	Pork and Baby Spinach	Chocolate Crème Brûlée

685	Beef Stew with Eggplants	Cinnamon Turkey Curry	Nutmeg Apple Crisp
686	Beef Black Pepper Stew	Cod and Tomato Passata	Crème Brûlée
687	Deviled Eggs	Mushroom and Chicken Soup	Almond Cheesecake
688	Pork Tenderloin Stew	Basil Shrimp and Eggplants	Maple-Glazed Flan
689	Lamb Stew	Chicken and Mustard Sauce	Blueberry Cheesecake
690	Beef Chili	Chicken and Avocado Mix	Chocolate Cheesecake
691	Mixed Mushroom Pate	Rice With Chicken And Veggies	Coconut Cake
692	Black Bean & Egg Casserole	Tomato Cream	Yogurt Vanilla Lighter Cheesecake
693	Chicken Liver Breakfast	Carrot Soup	Molten Lava Cake
694	Spice Oatmeal	Simple Chili	Stuffed Peaches
695	Barbeque Tofu	Lentils Soup	Blueberry Jam
696	Instant Pot Cauliflower Soup	Easy Chicken Cacciatore	Vanilla Rice Pudding
697	Beef Bourguignon Recipe	Sweet Paprika Pork Chops	Pressure Cooked Brownies
698	Beef Kale Patties	Simple Pork Roast	Almond Tapioca Pudding
699	Eggs with Mushrooms	Mackerel And Orange Sauce	Lemon and Blackberry Compote
700	Coconut Cherry Pancakes	Fish Curry	Caramel Flan
701	Chicken with Spinach	Shrimp And Tomatoes Mix	Poached Gingery Orange Pears
702	Pork with Mushrooms	Cabbage And Beef Stew	Pear Ricotta Cake
703	Mushroom Chicken with Eggs	Lemon Shrimp	Peach Crumb
704	Keto Vanilla Chia Seeds	Fish Soup	Gingery Applesauce
705	Turkey Soup	Italian Shrimp Mix	Blondies with Peanut Butter
706	Beef Chuck Shoulder Roast Stew	Coconut Chicken Mix	Strawberry Cream
707	Cinnamon Bars	Broccoli Cream	Berry Compote
708	Eggs with Scallions	Salmon, Peas And Parsley Dressing	Creamy Coconut Peach Dessert
709	Mushroom and Eggs Casserole	Shrimp, Tomatoes And Potatoes	Banana and Almond Butter Bars
710	Bacon Brussels Sprouts	Tomato Shrimp	Fruity Sauce with Apples
711	Almond Porridge	Chili Salmon	Brown Fudge Cake
712	Raspberry Mug Cake	Mexican Pork and Okra Salad	Cherry Cheesecake
713	Chicken Veal Stew	Pork and Kale Meatballs	Tapioca Pudding
714	Cinnamon Pancakes	Pork and Baby Spinach	Chocolate Crème Brûlée
715	Beef Stew with Eggplants	Cinnamon Turkey Curry	Nutmeg Apple Crisp
716	Beef Black Pepper Stew	Cod and Tomato Passata	Crème Brûlée
717	Deviled Eggs	Mushroom and Chicken Soup	Almond Cheesecake
718	Pork Tenderloin Stew	Basil Shrimp and Eggplants	Maple-Glazed Flan
719	Lamb Stew	Chicken and Mustard Sauce	Blueberry Cheesecake
720	Beef Chili	Chicken and Avocado Mix	Chocolate Cheesecake
721	Mixed Mushroom Pate	Rice With Chicken And Veggies	Coconut Cake
722	Black Bean & Egg Casserole	Tomato Cream	Yogurt Vanilla Lighter Cheesecake
723	Chicken Liver Breakfast	Carrot Soup	Molten Lava Cake
724	Spice Oatmeal	Simple Chili	Stuffed Peaches
725	Barbeque Tofu	Lentils Soup	Blueberry Jam
726	Instant Pot Cauliflower Soup	Easy Chicken Cacciatore	Vanilla Rice Pudding
727	Beef Bourguignon Recipe	Sweet Paprika Pork Chops	Pressure Cooked Brownies

728	Beef Kale Patties	Simple Pork Roast	Almond Tapioca Pudding
729	Eggs with Mushrooms	Mackerel And Orange Sauce	Lemon and Blackberry Compote
730	Coconut Cherry Pancakes	Fish Curry	Caramel Flan
731	Chicken with Spinach	Shrimp And Tomatoes Mix	Poached Gingery Orange Pears
732	Pork with Mushrooms	Cabbage And Beef Stew	Pear Ricotta Cake
733	Mushroom Chicken with Eggs	Lemon Shrimp	Peach Crumb
734	Keto Vanilla Chia Seeds	Fish Soup	Gingery Applesauce
735	Turkey Soup	Italian Shrimp Mix	Blondies with Peanut Butter
736	Beef Chuck Shoulder Roast Stew	Coconut Chicken Mix	Strawberry Cream
737	Cinnamon Bars	Broccoli Cream	Berry Compote
738	Eggs with Scallions	Salmon, Peas And Parsley Dressing	Creamy Coconut Peach Dessert
739	Mushroom and Eggs Casserole	Shrimp, Tomatoes And Potatoes	Banana and Almond Butter Bars
740	Bacon Brussels Sprouts	Tomato Shrimp	Fruity Sauce with Apples
741	Almond Porridge	Chili Salmon	Brown Fudge Cake
742	Raspberry Mug Cake	Mexican Pork and Okra Salad	Cherry Cheesecake
743	Chicken Veal Stew	Pork and Kale Meatballs	Tapioca Pudding
744	Cinnamon Pancakes	Pork and Baby Spinach	Chocolate Crème Brûlée
745	Beef Stew with Eggplants	Cinnamon Turkey Curry	Nutmeg Apple Crisp
746	Beef Black Pepper Stew	Cod and Tomato Passata	Crème Brûlée
747	Deviled Eggs	Mushroom and Chicken Soup	Almond Cheesecake
748	Pork Tenderloin Stew	Basil Shrimp and Eggplants	Maple-Glazed Flan
749	Lamb Stew	Chicken and Mustard Sauce	Blueberry Cheesecake
750	Beef Chili	Chicken and Avocado Mix	Chocolate Cheesecake
751	Mixed Mushroom Pate	Rice With Chicken And Veggies	Coconut Cake
752	Black Bean & Egg Casserole	Tomato Cream	Yogurt Vanilla Lighter Cheesecake
753	Chicken Liver Breakfast	Carrot Soup	Molten Lava Cake
754	Spice Oatmeal	Simple Chili	Stuffed Peaches
755	Barbeque Tofu	Lentils Soup	Blueberry Jam
756	Instant Pot Cauliflower Soup	Easy Chicken Cacciatore	Vanilla Rice Pudding
757	Beef Bourguignon Recipe	Sweet Paprika Pork Chops	Pressure Cooked Brownies
758	Beef Kale Patties	Simple Pork Roast	Almond Tapioca Pudding
759	Eggs with Mushrooms	Mackerel And Orange Sauce	Lemon and Blackberry Compote
760	Coconut Cherry Pancakes	Fish Curry	Caramel Flan
761	Chicken with Spinach	Shrimp And Tomatoes Mix	Poached Gingery Orange Pears
762	Pork with Mushrooms	Cabbage And Beef Stew	Pear Ricotta Cake
763	Mushroom Chicken with Eggs	Lemon Shrimp	Peach Crumb
764	Keto Vanilla Chia Seeds	Fish Soup	Gingery Applesauce
765	Turkey Soup	Italian Shrimp Mix	Blondies with Peanut Butter
766	Beef Chuck Shoulder Roast Stew	Coconut Chicken Mix	Strawberry Cream
767	Cinnamon Bars	Broccoli Cream	Berry Compote
768	Eggs with Scallions	Salmon, Peas And Parsley Dressing	Creamy Coconut Peach Dessert
769	Mushroom and Eggs Casserole	Shrimp, Tomatoes And Potatoes	Banana and Almond Butter Bars
770	Bacon Brussels Sprouts	Tomato Shrimp	Fruity Sauce with Apples

771	Almond Porridge	Chili Salmon	Brown Fudge Cake
772	Raspberry Mug Cake	Mexican Pork and Okra Salad	Cherry Cheesecake
773	Chicken Veal Stew	Pork and Kale Meatballs	Tapioca Pudding
774	Cinnamon Pancakes	Pork and Baby Spinach	Chocolate Crème Brûlée
775	Beef Stew with Eggplants	Cinnamon Turkey Curry	Nutmeg Apple Crisp
776	Beef Black Pepper Stew	Cod and Tomato Passata	Crème Brûlée
777	Deviled Eggs	Mushroom and Chicken Soup	Almond Cheesecake
778	Pork Tenderloin Stew	Basil Shrimp and Eggplants	Maple-Glazed Flan
779	Lamb Stew	Chicken and Mustard Sauce	Blueberry Cheesecake
780	Beef Chili	Chicken and Avocado Mix	Chocolate Cheesecake
781	Mixed Mushroom Pate	Rice With Chicken And Veggies	Coconut Cake
782	Black Bean & Egg Casserole	Tomato Cream	Yogurt Vanilla Lighter Cheesecake
783	Chicken Liver Breakfast	Carrot Soup	Molten Lava Cake
784	Spice Oatmeal	Simple Chili	Stuffed Peaches
785	Barbeque Tofu	Lentils Soup	Blueberry Jam
786	Instant Pot Cauliflower Soup	Easy Chicken Cacciatore	Vanilla Rice Pudding
787	Beef Bourguignon Recipe	Sweet Paprika Pork Chops	Pressure Cooked Brownies
788	Beef Kale Patties	Simple Pork Roast	Almond Tapioca Pudding
789	Eggs with Mushrooms	Mackerel And Orange Sauce	Lemon and Blackberry Compote
790	Coconut Cherry Pancakes	Fish Curry	Caramel Flan
791	Chicken with Spinach	Shrimp And Tomatoes Mix	Poached Gingery Orange Pears
792	Pork with Mushrooms	Cabbage And Beef Stew	Pear Ricotta Cake
793	Mushroom Chicken with Eggs	Lemon Shrimp	Peach Crumb
794	Keto Vanilla Chia Seeds	Fish Soup	Gingery Applesauce
795	Turkey Soup	Italian Shrimp Mix	Blondies with Peanut Butter
796	Beef Chuck Shoulder Roast Stew	Coconut Chicken Mix	Strawberry Cream
797	Cinnamon Bars	Broccoli Cream	Berry Compote
798	Eggs with Scallions	Salmon, Peas And Parsley Dressing	Creamy Coconut Peach Dessert
799	Mushroom and Eggs Casserole	Shrimp, Tomatoes And Potatoes	Banana and Almond Butter Bars
800	Bacon Brussels Sprouts	Tomato Shrimp	Fruity Sauce with Apples
801	Almond Porridge	Chili Salmon	Brown Fudge Cake
802	Raspberry Mug Cake	Mexican Pork and Okra Salad	Cherry Cheesecake
803	Chicken Veal Stew	Pork and Kale Meatballs	Tapioca Pudding
804	Cinnamon Pancakes	Pork and Baby Spinach	Chocolate Crème Brûlée
805	Beef Stew with Eggplants	Cinnamon Turkey Curry	Nutmeg Apple Crisp
806	Beef Black Pepper Stew	Cod and Tomato Passata	Crème Brûlée
807	Deviled Eggs	Mushroom and Chicken Soup	Almond Cheesecake
808	Pork Tenderloin Stew	Basil Shrimp and Eggplants	Maple-Glazed Flan
809	Lamb Stew	Chicken and Mustard Sauce	Blueberry Cheesecake
810	Beef Chili	Chicken and Avocado Mix	Chocolate Cheesecake
811	Mixed Mushroom Pate	Rice With Chicken And Veggies	Coconut Cake
812	Black Bean & Egg Casserole	Tomato Cream	Yogurt Vanilla Lighter Cheesecake
813	Chicken Liver Breakfast	Carrot Soup	Molten Lava Cake

814	Spice Oatmeal	Simple Chili	Stuffed Peaches
815	Barbeque Tofu	Lentils Soup	Blueberry Jam
816	Instant Pot Cauliflower Soup	Easy Chicken Cacciatore	Vanilla Rice Pudding
817	Beef Bourguignon Recipe	Sweet Paprika Pork Chops	Pressure Cooked Brownies
818	Beef Kale Patties	Simple Pork Roast	Almond Tapioca Pudding
819	Eggs with Mushrooms	Mackerel And Orange Sauce	Lemon and Blackberry Compote
820	Coconut Cherry Pancakes	Fish Curry	Caramel Flan
821	Chicken with Spinach	Shrimp And Tomatoes Mix	Poached Gingery Orange Pears
822	Pork with Mushrooms	Cabbage And Beef Stew	Pear Ricotta Cake
823	Mushroom Chicken with Eggs	Lemon Shrimp	Peach Crumb
824	Keto Vanilla Chia Seeds	Fish Soup	Gingery Applesauce
825	Turkey Soup	Italian Shrimp Mix	Blondies with Peanut Butter
826	Beef Chuck Shoulder Roast Stew	Coconut Chicken Mix	Strawberry Cream
827	Cinnamon Bars	Broccoli Cream	Berry Compote
828	Eggs with Scallions	Salmon, Peas And Parsley Dressing	Creamy Coconut Peach Dessert
829	Mushroom and Eggs Casserole	Shrimp, Tomatoes And Potatoes	Banana and Almond Butter Bars
830	Bacon Brussels Sprouts	Tomato Shrimp	Fruity Sauce with Apples
831	Almond Porridge	Chili Salmon	Brown Fudge Cake
832	Raspberry Mug Cake	Mexican Pork and Okra Salad	Cherry Cheesecake
833	Chicken Veal Stew	Pork and Kale Meatballs	Tapioca Pudding
834	Cinnamon Pancakes	Pork and Baby Spinach	Chocolate Crème Brûlée
835	Beef Stew with Eggplants	Cinnamon Turkey Curry	Nutmeg Apple Crisp
836	Beef Black Pepper Stew	Cod and Tomato Passata	Crème Brûlée
837	Deviled Eggs	Mushroom and Chicken Soup	Almond Cheesecake
838	Pork Tenderloin Stew	Basil Shrimp and Eggplants	Maple-Glazed Flan
839	Lamb Stew	Chicken and Mustard Sauce	Blueberry Cheesecake
840	Beef Chili	Chicken and Avocado Mix	Chocolate Cheesecake
841	Mixed Mushroom Pate	Rice With Chicken And Veggies	Coconut Cake
842	Black Bean & Egg Casserole	Tomato Cream	Yogurt Vanilla Lighter Cheesecake
843	Chicken Liver Breakfast	Carrot Soup	Molten Lava Cake
844	Spice Oatmeal	Simple Chili	Stuffed Peaches
845	Barbeque Tofu	Lentils Soup	Blueberry Jam
846	Instant Pot Cauliflower Soup	Easy Chicken Cacciatore	Vanilla Rice Pudding
847	Beef Bourguignon Recipe	Sweet Paprika Pork Chops	Pressure Cooked Brownies
848	Beef Kale Patties	Simple Pork Roast	Almond Tapioca Pudding
849	Eggs with Mushrooms	Mackerel And Orange Sauce	Lemon and Blackberry Compote
850	Coconut Cherry Pancakes	Fish Curry	Caramel Flan
851	Chicken with Spinach	Shrimp And Tomatoes Mix	Poached Gingery Orange Pears
852	Pork with Mushrooms	Cabbage And Beef Stew	Pear Ricotta Cake
853	Mushroom Chicken with Eggs	Lemon Shrimp	Peach Crumb
854	Keto Vanilla Chia Seeds	Fish Soup	Gingery Applesauce
855	Turkey Soup	Italian Shrimp Mix	Blondies with Peanut Butter
856	Beef Chuck Shoulder Roast Stew	Coconut Chicken Mix	Strawberry Cream

857	Cinnamon Bars	Broccoli Cream	Berry Compote
858	Eggs with Scallions	Salmon, Peas And Parsley Dressing	Creamy Coconut Peach Dessert
859	Mushroom and Eggs Casserole	Shrimp, Tomatoes And Potatoes	Banana and Almond Butter Bars
860	Bacon Brussels Sprouts	Tomato Shrimp	Fruity Sauce with Apples
861	Almond Porridge	Chili Salmon	Brown Fudge Cake
862	Raspberry Mug Cake	Mexican Pork and Okra Salad	Cherry Cheesecake
863	Chicken Veal Stew	Pork and Kale Meatballs	Tapioca Pudding
864	Cinnamon Pancakes	Pork and Baby Spinach	Chocolate Crème Brûlée
865	Beef Stew with Eggplants	Cinnamon Turkey Curry	Nutmeg Apple Crisp
866	Beef Black Pepper Stew	Cod and Tomato Passata	Crème Brûlée
867	Deviled Eggs	Mushroom and Chicken Soup	Almond Cheesecake
868	Pork Tenderloin Stew	Basil Shrimp and Eggplants	Maple-Glazed Flan
869	Lamb Stew	Chicken and Mustard Sauce	Blueberry Cheesecake
870	Beef Chili	Chicken and Avocado Mix	Chocolate Cheesecake
871	Mixed Mushroom Pate	Rice With Chicken And Veggies	Coconut Cake
872	Black Bean & Egg Casserole	Tomato Cream	Yogurt Vanilla Lighter Cheesecake
873	Chicken Liver Breakfast	Carrot Soup	Molten Lava Cake
874	Spice Oatmeal	Simple Chili	Stuffed Peaches
875	Barbeque Tofu	Lentils Soup	Blueberry Jam
876	Instant Pot Cauliflower Soup	Easy Chicken Cacciatore	Vanilla Rice Pudding
877	Beef Bourguignon Recipe	Sweet Paprika Pork Chops	Pressure Cooked Brownies
878	Beef Kale Patties	Simple Pork Roast	Almond Tapioca Pudding
879	Eggs with Mushrooms	Mackerel And Orange Sauce	Lemon and Blackberry Compote
880	Coconut Cherry Pancakes	Fish Curry	Caramel Flan
881	Chicken with Spinach	Shrimp And Tomatoes Mix	Poached Gingery Orange Pears
882	Pork with Mushrooms	Cabbage And Beef Stew	Pear Ricotta Cake
883	Mushroom Chicken with Eggs	Lemon Shrimp	Peach Crumb
884	Keto Vanilla Chia Seeds	Fish Soup	Gingery Applesauce
885	Turkey Soup	Italian Shrimp Mix	Blondies with Peanut Butter
886	Beef Chuck Shoulder Roast Stew	Coconut Chicken Mix	Strawberry Cream
887	Cinnamon Bars	Broccoli Cream	Berry Compote
888	Eggs with Scallions	Salmon, Peas And Parsley Dressing	Creamy Coconut Peach Dessert
889	Mushroom and Eggs Casserole	Shrimp, Tomatoes And Potatoes	Banana and Almond Butter Bars
890	Bacon Brussels Sprouts	Tomato Shrimp	Fruity Sauce with Apples
891	Almond Porridge	Chili Salmon	Brown Fudge Cake
892	Raspberry Mug Cake	Mexican Pork and Okra Salad	Cherry Cheesecake
893	Chicken Veal Stew	Pork and Kale Meatballs	Tapioca Pudding
894	Cinnamon Pancakes	Pork and Baby Spinach	Chocolate Crème Brûlée
895	Beef Stew with Eggplants	Cinnamon Turkey Curry	Nutmeg Apple Crisp
896	Beef Black Pepper Stew	Cod and Tomato Passata	Crème Brûlée
897	Deviled Eggs	Mushroom and Chicken Soup	Almond Cheesecake
898	Pork Tenderloin Stew	Basil Shrimp and Eggplants	Maple-Glazed Flan
899	Lamb Stew	Chicken and Mustard Sauce	Blueberry Cheesecake

900	Beef Chili	Chicken and Avocado Mix	Chocolate Cheesecake
901	Mixed Mushroom Pate	Rice With Chicken And Veggies	Coconut Cake
902	Black Bean & Egg Casserole	Tomato Cream	Yogurt Vanilla Lighter Cheesecake
903	Chicken Liver Breakfast	Carrot Soup	Molten Lava Cake
904	Spice Oatmeal	Simple Chili	Stuffed Peaches
905	Barbeque Tofu	Lentils Soup	Blueberry Jam
906	Instant Pot Cauliflower Soup	Easy Chicken Cacciatore	Vanilla Rice Pudding
907	Beef Bourguignon Recipe	Sweet Paprika Pork Chops	Pressure Cooked Brownies
908	Beef Kale Patties	Simple Pork Roast	Almond Tapioca Pudding
909	Eggs with Mushrooms	Mackerel And Orange Sauce	Lemon and Blackberry Compote
910	Coconut Cherry Pancakes	Fish Curry	Caramel Flan
911	Chicken with Spinach	Shrimp And Tomatoes Mix	Poached Gingery Orange Pears
912	Pork with Mushrooms	Cabbage And Beef Stew	Pear Ricotta Cake
913	Mushroom Chicken with Eggs	Lemon Shrimp	Peach Crumb
914	Keto Vanilla Chia Seeds	Fish Soup	Gingery Applesauce
915	Turkey Soup	Italian Shrimp Mix	Blondies with Peanut Butter
916	Beef Chuck Shoulder Roast Stew	Coconut Chicken Mix	Strawberry Cream
917	Cinnamon Bars	Broccoli Cream	Berry Compote
918	Eggs with Scallions	Salmon, Peas And Parsley Dressing	Creamy Coconut Peach Dessert
919	Mushroom and Eggs Casserole	Shrimp, Tomatoes And Potatoes	Banana and Almond Butter Bars
920	Bacon Brussels Sprouts	Tomato Shrimp	Fruity Sauce with Apples
921	Almond Porridge	Chili Salmon	Brown Fudge Cake
922	Raspberry Mug Cake	Mexican Pork and Okra Salad	Cherry Cheesecake
923	Chicken Veal Stew	Pork and Kale Meatballs	Tapioca Pudding
924	Cinnamon Pancakes	Pork and Baby Spinach	Chocolate Crème Brûlée
925	Beef Stew with Eggplants	Cinnamon Turkey Curry	Nutmeg Apple Crisp
926	Beef Black Pepper Stew	Cod and Tomato Passata	Crème Brûlée
927	Deviled Eggs	Mushroom and Chicken Soup	Almond Cheesecake
928	Pork Tenderloin Stew	Basil Shrimp and Eggplants	Maple-Glazed Flan
929	Lamb Stew	Chicken and Mustard Sauce	Blueberry Cheesecake
930	Beef Chili	Chicken and Avocado Mix	Chocolate Cheesecake
931	Mixed Mushroom Pate	Rice With Chicken And Veggies	Coconut Cake
932	Black Bean & Egg Casserole	Tomato Cream	Yogurt Vanilla Lighter Cheesecake
933	Chicken Liver Breakfast	Carrot Soup	Molten Lava Cake
934	Spice Oatmeal	Simple Chili	Stuffed Peaches
935	Barbeque Tofu	Lentils Soup	Blueberry Jam
936	Instant Pot Cauliflower Soup	Easy Chicken Cacciatore	Vanilla Rice Pudding
937	Beef Bourguignon Recipe	Sweet Paprika Pork Chops	Pressure Cooked Brownies
938	Beef Kale Patties	Simple Pork Roast	Almond Tapioca Pudding
939	Eggs with Mushrooms	Mackerel And Orange Sauce	Lemon and Blackberry Compote
940	Coconut Cherry Pancakes	Fish Curry	Caramel Flan
941	Chicken with Spinach	Shrimp And Tomatoes Mix	Poached Gingery Orange Pears
942	Pork with Mushrooms	Cabbage And Beef Stew	Pear Ricotta Cake

943	Mushroom Chicken with Eggs	Lemon Shrimp	Peach Crumb
944	Keto Vanilla Chia Seeds	Fish Soup	Gingery Applesauce
945	Turkey Soup	Italian Shrimp Mix	Blondies with Peanut Butter
946	Beef Chuck Shoulder Roast Stew	Coconut Chicken Mix	Strawberry Cream
947	Cinnamon Bars	Broccoli Cream	Berry Compote
948	Eggs with Scallions	Salmon, Peas And Parsley Dressing	Creamy Coconut Peach Dessert
949	Mushroom and Eggs Casserole	Shrimp, Tomatoes And Potatoes	Banana and Almond Butter Bars
950	Bacon Brussels Sprouts	Tomato Shrimp	Fruity Sauce with Apples
951	Almond Porridge	Chili Salmon	Brown Fudge Cake
952	Raspberry Mug Cake	Mexican Pork and Okra Salad	Cherry Cheesecake
953	Chicken Veal Stew	Pork and Kale Meatballs	Tapioca Pudding
954	Cinnamon Pancakes	Pork and Baby Spinach	Chocolate Crème Brûlée
955	Beef Stew with Eggplants	Cinnamon Turkey Curry	Nutmeg Apple Crisp
956	Beef Black Pepper Stew	Cod and Tomato Passata	Crème Brûlée
957	Deviled Eggs	Mushroom and Chicken Soup	Almond Cheesecake
958	Pork Tenderloin Stew	Basil Shrimp and Eggplants	Maple-Glazed Flan
959	Lamb Stew	Chicken and Mustard Sauce	Blueberry Cheesecake
960	Beef Chili	Chicken and Avocado Mix	Chocolate Cheesecake
961	Mixed Mushroom Pate	Rice With Chicken And Veggies	Coconut Cake
962	Black Bean & Egg Casserole	Tomato Cream	Yogurt Vanilla Lighter Cheesecake
963	Chicken Liver Breakfast	Carrot Soup	Molten Lava Cake
964	Spice Oatmeal	Simple Chili	Stuffed Peaches
965	Barbeque Tofu	Lentils Soup	Blueberry Jam
966	Instant Pot Cauliflower Soup	Easy Chicken Cacciatore	Vanilla Rice Pudding
967	Beef Bourguignon Recipe	Sweet Paprika Pork Chops	Pressure Cooked Brownies
968	Beef Kale Patties	Simple Pork Roast	Almond Tapioca Pudding
969	Eggs with Mushrooms	Mackerel And Orange Sauce	Lemon and Blackberry Compote
970	Coconut Cherry Pancakes	Fish Curry	Caramel Flan
971	Chicken with Spinach	Shrimp And Tomatoes Mix	Poached Gingery Orange Pears
972	Pork with Mushrooms	Cabbage And Beef Stew	Pear Ricotta Cake
973	Mushroom Chicken with Eggs	Lemon Shrimp	Peach Crumb
974	Keto Vanilla Chia Seeds	Fish Soup	Gingery Applesauce
975	Turkey Soup	Italian Shrimp Mix	Blondies with Peanut Butter
976	Beef Chuck Shoulder Roast Stew	Coconut Chicken Mix	Strawberry Cream
977	Cinnamon Bars	Broccoli Cream	Berry Compote
978	Eggs with Scallions	Salmon, Peas And Parsley Dressing	Creamy Coconut Peach Dessert
979	Mushroom and Eggs Casserole	Shrimp, Tomatoes And Potatoes	Banana and Almond Butter Bars
980	Bacon Brussels Sprouts	Tomato Shrimp	Fruity Sauce with Apples
981	Almond Porridge	Chili Salmon	Brown Fudge Cake
982	Raspberry Mug Cake	Mexican Pork and Okra Salad	Cherry Cheesecake
983	Chicken Veal Stew	Pork and Kale Meatballs	Tapioca Pudding
984	Cinnamon Pancakes	Pork and Baby Spinach	Chocolate Crème Brûlée
985	Beef Stew with Eggplants	Cinnamon Turkey Curry	Nutmeg Apple Crisp

986	Beef Black Pepper Stew	Cod and Tomato Passata	Crème Brûlée
987	Deviled Eggs	Mushroom and Chicken Soup	Almond Cheesecake
988	Pork Tenderloin Stew	Basil Shrimp and Eggplants	Maple-Glazed Flan
989	Lamb Stew	Chicken and Mustard Sauce	Blueberry Cheesecake
990	Beef Chili	Chicken and Avocado Mix	Chocolate Cheesecake
991	Mixed Mushroom Pate	Rice With Chicken And Veggies	Coconut Cake
992	Black Bean & Egg Casserole	Tomato Cream	Yogurt Vanilla Lighter Cheesecake
993	Chicken Liver Breakfast	Carrot Soup	Molten Lava Cake
994	Spice Oatmeal	Simple Chili	Stuffed Peaches
995	Barbeque Tofu	Lentils Soup	Blueberry Jam
996	Instant Pot Cauliflower Soup	Easy Chicken Cacciatore	Vanilla Rice Pudding
997	Beef Bourguignon Recipe	Sweet Paprika Pork Chops	Pressure Cooked Brownies
998	Beef Kale Patties	Simple Pork Roast	Almond Tapioca Pudding
999	Eggs with Mushrooms	Mackerel And Orange Sauce	Lemon and Blackberry Compote
1000	Coconut Cherry Pancakes	Fish Curry	Caramel Flan

CONCLUSION

Thanks for purchasing this book. I hope the recipes covered in this guide will help you make the most of your instant pot, save you time while still enjoying your meals.

You can take it as a nifty life hack, but to be completely honest with you, it works really well! This hack uses the steam function, which is the most aggressive setting in the Instant Pots of this generation. It dials the Instant Pot straight up to full heat and pressure, and is preset to work for only 5-10 minutes. It is usually used to steam vegetables to clean them from harmful germs and bacteria, but there is a hidden feature in it, or so you may say.

You can reheat your leftovers and frozen meals, and here's exactly how. Just pour 1 cup of water in the Instant Pot, let the moisture build up, and then put it the leftovers in the Instant Pot just like that! There are a few tricks to this. If you are defrosting a pre-packaged meal, remove the plastic rack before you bring it into the pressure, as the food can get spoilt by the plastic, and if you are using any frozen leftovers, put the block in a casserole dish on the rack before putting it in the Instant Pot. Smaller quantities can take less than 3 minutes, while larger portions and whole pre-packaged meals can take 7 to 10 minutes.

All the Instant Pot models currently being sold are capable of switching from one mode to the next simultaneously, and if you think about it carefully, that is a great deal of stress lifted from your shoulders. Remember the time when you had to run around the kitchen handling the sautéing, simmering, cooking and boiling all together, well, with the Instant Pot, it is all a piece of cake!

You can set a timer for when you want the Instant Pot to change modes, or do it manually yourself. For example, you can first sauté onions in the pot, then instantly switch to the pressure cooker and add the beef to continue the recipe without a sweat. It is a lifesaver, as you can increase your productivity in the time you saved, plus you'll need to wash fewer dishes, so it's a win-win on everything!

Start making nutritious and absolutely delicious meals for you, your family, and your friends.

Happy cooking!!

Made in the
USA
Middletown, DE